D0757554

BREAST IMAGING

Each volume of *The Core Curriculum Series* examines one key area in radiology and focuses on the essential information readers need for rotations and later, written board examination. Readers will appreciate the easy-to-follow format, the abundant high-quality illustrations, and the full complement of learning tools—including chapter outlines, bulleted lists, tables, summary boxes, and points for review. Please contact the publisher for additional information on existing and upcoming titles.

Other titles in *The Core Curriculum Series* . . .

Brant: *Ultrasound*
Castillo: *Neuroradiology*
Chew: *Musculoskeletal Imaging*
Kazerooni: *Cardiopulmonary Imaging*

The Core Curriculum

BREAST IMAGING

GILDA CARDENOSA, MS, MD

Medical Director
The Breast Center of Greensboro
Greensboro Radiology Associates and the Moses Cone Health System
Greensboro, North Carolina

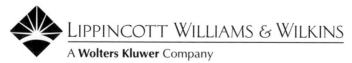
LIPPINCOTT WILLIAMS & WILKINS
A **Wolters Kluwer** Company
Philadelphia • Baltimore • New York • London
Buenos Aires • Hong Kong • Sydney • Tokyo

Acquisitions Editor: Lisa McAllister
Developmental Editor: Scott Scheidt
Production Editor: Rakesh Rampertab
Manufacturing Manager: Benjamin Rivera
Cover Designer: Karen Quigley
Compositor: Lippincott Williams & Wilkins Desktop Division
Printer: Maple Press

© 2004 by LIPPINCOTT WILLIAMS & WILKINS
530 Walnut Street
Philadelphia, PA 19106 USA
LWW.com

Library of Congress Cataloging-in-Publication Data

0-7817-4685-X

Care has been taken to confirm the accuracy of the information presented and to describe generally accepted practices. However, the authors, editors, and publisher are not responsible for errors or omissions or for any consequences from application of the information in this book and make no warranty, expressed or implied, with respect to the currency, completeness, or accuracy of the contents of the publication. Application of this information in a particular situation remains the professional responsibility of the practitioner.

The authors, editors, and publisher have exerted every effort to ensure that drug selection and dosage set forth in this text are in accordance with current recommendations and practice at the time of publication. However, in view of ongoing research, changes in government regulations, and the constant flow of information relating to drug therapy and drug reactions, the reader is urged to check the package insert for each drug for any change in indications and dosage and for added warnings and precautions. This is particularly important when the recommended agent is a new or infrequently employed drug.

Some drugs and medical devices presented in this publication have Food and Drug Administration (FDA) clearance for limited use in restricted research settings. It is the responsibility of the health care provider to ascertain the FDA status of each drug or device planned for use in their clinical practice.

10 9 8 7 6 5 4 3 2 1

In memory of
Dr. Juan M. Taveras
(1919–2002)
Radiologist-in-Chief
Massachusetts General Hospital
(1971–1988)

and

To all of the radiology staff members at the Massachusetts
General Hospital during my residency (1985–1989)

You gave me one of the greatest gifts possible:
the opportunity to learn and to think critically and independently

You have my heartfelt thanks

CONTENTS

PREFACE

This book is intended for two audiences: residents in training who desire an introduction and overview of breast imaging and radiologists in practice who want some practical, workable, common sense tips and guidelines. This is a book that presents a basic, common sense, practical approach to breast imaging—it is *not* a comprehensive scientific review. This is a book with detailed descriptions of an approach to breast imaging that is time tested and promotes better patient care. It is *not* an exhaustive discussion of the topics selected for presentation or all available approaches to breast imaging. Several outstanding books already provide that level of detail and information. I have elected to include as many images as possible in this book to *illustrate* the basic points presented in the text. Inherent in the organization of the book is a certain amount of purposeful repetition. Some entities with corresponding images are seen in multiple chapters. I can only hope that some interest remains in our specialty for this type of book and that we see value in teaching the basics through experience.

Writing a book is rewarding in itself, but it is a long, hard and solitary road with no guarantee as to what your efforts will yield. For medical books, particularly those in a subspecialized area, writing a book is not about retirement security, it is about sharing knowledge. For many, as it has been for me, it is a labor of love. It is the recognition that the best way I can give back to my patients, and honor their courage in battling breast cancer, is to share my experiences, anecdotal as they may be viewed by some. It is an attempt to teach others, who are taking care of patients, what I have learned and continue to learn from my patients. Our approach works and is supported by medical audit data. Much of it is based on common sense and a commitment to providing the best possible patient care experience. Recently, a colleague approached me to tell me that my previous book (*Breast Imaging Companion*) had sparked her interest in Breast Imaging and that she had gone on to do a Breast Imaging fellowship. It was a comment made in passing, but to me it was the greatest reward and honor possible. I am grateful to her for sharing this with me. While spending long hours at work on this book, it was a wonderfully energizing encounter that helped to keep me focused. After all, one of my main goals is to spark interest in Breast Imaging among residents as they contemplate fields to pursue. This is an incredibly rewarding subspecialty that, when undertaken with compassion and commitment, provides a needed and invaluable service. It is a subspecialty through which we save women's lives and improve their quality of life. This is what medicine is all about.

ACKNOWLEDGMENTS

I stand in awe of the *clerical staff* (Amy Davis, Cara Sams, Melody Shelton, Diana Shepherd, Tanya Kempson, Kimberly Cobb, Beth Kurtz, Maxine Hatley, Sue McBride, and Erica Carmichael) and *technical staff* (Marie Allred, Diane Ball, Cindy Church, Pamela J. deFriess, Cheryl A. Hurst, Heather James, Karyn B. Jetty, Vickie Kindl, Christie B. McAdams, Jill Pruitt, Jane E. Salvatti, Elaine U. Ayers, Michelle Bullins, Diane S. Garrett, April H. Pait, Wendy Summers and Roxie Williams) at the Breast Center of Greensboro, North Carolina. I congratulate and thank them for going the extra mile each and every day. They are kind, compassionate, dedicated and loyal. Whatever is requested gets accomplished with enthusiasm and the utmost professionalism. They all know that the answer to any request from our patients and referring physicians is, "Yes, we can do it today," and then they make it happen effortlessly. Margie Glenn, the Breast Center site manager has been helpful in the development, organization, and ongoing success of the center. Her hard work is appreciated.

How can I ever thank my colleagues at the Breast Center? During a time when there is a national shortage of breast imagers, I feel extremely fortunate to work with Drs. Elizabeth Eagle, Elizabeth Brown, Caron Dover, and Dina Arceo; all incredibly talented women, with an unquestionable commitment to the center and our patients, and a keen *common sense* approach to patient care. It is a privilege to work with them. Not a day goes by that we don't learn something new about how to improve on the care we deliver to our patients. I have also had the pleasure of working with Dr. Ericka Coats, our fellow. She is part of the future to whom we pass the clinical breast imaging torch. I am sure that she will use it to light the way through new paths and with her dedication, the field and patient care will be that much better.

Greensboro Radiology Associates, P.A. and Moses Cone Health System have provided me with a wonderful home: the Breast Center of Greensboro, North Carolina, a beautiful, welcoming place for our patients and their families, filled with state-of-the-art equipment and staffed with energetic people. A number of years ago, Greensboro Radiology Associates very wisely recognized that a dedicated, clinically oriented breast center, staffed by radiologists with special training and an interest in breast imaging, could provide the women of Greensboro with an optimal, outcome-based practice complete with compassionate and prompt care. That is what we have created.

The success and uniqueness of our program also reflects significant commitments on the part of Greensboro Pathology Associates, P.A. and Central Carolina Surgery, P.A. Greensboro Pathology Associates have come through with their commitment to provide turn around times of less than 24 hours for all of our patients undergoing imaging guided breast biopsies. Every morning there is a discussion between radiologist and pathologist to ensure adequacy of sampling, congruency of findings and appropriate next steps. They have now recruited a colleague with specialty training in breast pathology. Central Carolina Surgery has agreed to see patients within 24 hours of a breast cancer diagnosis; for many of our patients this is the day after the core biopsy has been done. Every Friday morning, radiology, pathology, surgery, radiation oncology and medical oncology come together to discuss all patients diagnosed with breast cancer in the course of the week. The impact this group effort and commitment has had on the care we deliver is significant and tangible.

At Lippincott Williams & Wilkins I am grateful to Joyce-Rachel John for believing that I could put together another basic breast imaging book and letting me develop it with as many images as possible, to Scott Scheidt for facilitating the editorial process and being patient, and to Rakesh Rampertab for his hard work getting the book through production.

On a personal note, I must include many thanks to previous collaborators I have had the privilege to work with—Drs. G. W. Eklund, Christine A. Quinn, William A. Chilcote, and Philip F. Murphy, all of whom I miss dearly but continue to share experiences with. I would be remiss in not personally thanking Amy Davis. Mrs. Davis is one of those special people one encounters and never forgets. Her selflessness, and commitment to helping others, coupled with common sense, loyalty and quintessential southern hospitality is truly special; this project would not have been completed without her help and support. K. M. Connelly has once again stood by with unwavering support of my efforts; although not a breast imager, she has patiently read through much of what is in these pages with superb editorial suggestions. Lastly, although I wish I had said this many times more than I did when it could be comprehended, a special thanks to my mother who continues to teach me much about life, perseverance, and tenacity and to my father for whom I have a new-found respect as I watch him spend hours by my mother's side wrestling to find a patience he did not know he had. Thank you both for your love and support.

BREAST CANCER, AN OVERVIEW

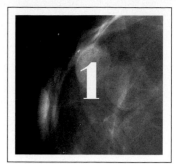

Breast cancer is a common, life-threatening disease. If skin cancers are excluded, breast cancer is the most frequently diagnosed malignancy and a leading cause of cancer mortality among women, second only to lung cancer (1). Women have a 12.5% (1 in 8) lifetime risk for developing breast cancer by 85 years of age (2,3). Although breast cancer incidence rates increased about 4% per year in the 1980s, they have leveled off at about 110 cases per 100,000 women (2,3).

The National Cancer Institute's Surveillance, Epidemiology, and End Results (SEER) program reported decreases in the breast cancer mortality rate for 1989 to 1992 across all age groups. An 8.1% decrease in the mortality rate was reported for 40- to 49-year-old women compared with a 9.3% decrease for 50- to 59-year-old women, a 4.8% decrease for 60- to 69-year-old women, and 3.1% decrease for 70- to 79-year-old women (4). It is estimated that 41,200 breast cancer–related deaths will occur in 2003 (40,800 in women, 400 in men) compared with 43,884 deaths in 1995 when the number of deaths was the highest (1). These decreases in mortality are at least partially attributable to the benefits gained by early detection through screening mammography.

> Women have a 12.5% (1 in 8) lifetime risk for developing breast cancer by 85 years of age.

> It is estimated that 211,300 women and 1,300 men will be diagnosed with invasive ductal carcinoma and that 41,200 (40,800 women and 400 men) breast cancer–related deaths will occur in 2003.

RISK FACTORS

Many factors are reportedly associated with an increased risk for breast cancer, but only a few are considered significant. Included among these are gender, age, a personal or family history of breast cancer, prior breast biopsy with certain histologic diagnoses, mutations in the BRCA1 and BRCA2 genes, and several other relatively rare breast cancer susceptibility genes. Other factors that have been implicated include early menarche, late menopause, late first-term pregnancy, nulliparity, and postmenopausal obesity. For these risk factors, prolonged exposure of breast tissue to estrogen is thought to play a role. A history of high-dose radiation therapy to the chest is another risk factor for breast cancer (1,2).

Women are more likely to develop breast cancer. It is estimated that 211,300 women will be diagnosed with invasive ductal carcinoma in 2003 compared with 1,300 men. The incidence of breast cancer increases with advancing patient age. The risk increases rapidly in premenopausal women and more slowly in postmenopausal women. Women with a

> Significant risk factors for breast cancer include gender, age, personal history of breast cancer, first-degree family member with breast cancer, prior breast biopsy with a risk marker lesion, and mutations in breast cancer susceptibility genes.

A diagnosis of atypical ductal hyperplasia or lobular neoplasia (lobular carcinoma *in situ*) on a prior breast biopsy is associated with a significant risk for the subsequent development of breast cancer.

personal history of breast cancer are at a higher risk for developing another breast cancer compared with women who have never had breast cancer. Women with one or multiple first-degree relatives with breast cancer (mother, father, sisters, brothers, daughters, and sons) are at increased risk, particularly if the breast cancers developed premenopausally are bilateral, or are multiple. Women who have had a breast biopsy, particularly if atypical ductal hyperplasia (ADH) or lobular neoplasia (lobular carcinoma *in situ*, LCIS) was diagnosed, are also at increased risk. With ADH, the lesion itself may represent a precursor, in contrast to lobular neoplasia, which is considered to be more of a marker lesion. Two genes (*BRCA1* and *BRCA2*) have been isolated in some women with breast cancer. It is estimated that 5% to 10% of all breast cancers in the United States are hereditary, related to mutations in the *BRCA1* or *BRCA2* genes. Women with mutations in the *BRCA1* gene are also at increased risk for developing ovarian cancer. The risk for developing breast cancer in women who carry mutations in this gene is 85% by 70 years of age (63% by 70 years of age for ovarian cancer). Women who carry mutations in the *BRCA2* gene are at increased risk for developing breast cancer but not ovarian cancer. Hereditary male breast cancer is associated with mutations in the *BRCA2* gene but not the *BRCA1* gene. Some genetic diseases (e.g., Li-Fraumeni syndrome, Cowden's disease, and ataxia-telangiectasia) are associated with breast cancer susceptibility genes and with an increased risk for breast cancer (2,3,5).

About 5% to 10% of all breast cancers are estimated to be related to mutations in the *BRCA1* or *BRCA2* genes.

Women with mutations in the *BRCA1* gene are at increased risk for developing breast and ovarian cancer.

Hereditary male breast cancer is associated with mutations in *BRCA2*.

Early menarche and the establishment of regular menses are risk factors in breast cancer development. It is estimated that the risk for breast cancer decreases by 10% to 15% with each year or two that menarche is delayed (2,3). Late menopause is another factor associated with increased breast cancer risk. The risk for breast cancer can be decreased by 50% with bilateral oophorectomy before 40 years of age, and it is estimated that women undergoing natural menopause before 45 years of age have half the risk for developing breast cancer than women who undergo menopause after 55 years of age (5). Breast cancer risk is reduced by 50% if the first term pregnancy occurs before 20 years of age compared with after 35 years of age (2,3,5). Women who do not have any pregnancies (nulliparous) and those who are obese after menopause are at increased risk compared with women who have had children and those who are not obese after menopause. Patients who undergo high-dose radiation therapy to the chest for lymphoma or an enlarged thymus are at increased risk for breast cancer (2,3,5). Breast cancer in these patients develops about 10 to 15 years after the radiation therapy and tends to be aggressive.

Patients with a history of high-dose radiation to the chest wall have an increased risk for developing breast cancer 10 to 15 years after the radiation.

Other factors reportedly associated with increased breast cancer risk are controversial. These include oral contraceptive use, alcohol intake, exogenous estrogen use (after 10 years of use), and dietary fat intake (saturated fats). Lactation, exercise, and monounsaturated fat intake may have protective benefits. Although implicated in some studies as a risk factor, cigarette smoking does not appear to be associated with an increased risk for breast cancer (2,3,5).

SCREENING MAMMOGRAPHY AND SCREENING RECOMMENDATIONS

The use and benefits of screening mammography in diagnosing breast cancer have been controversial. The goal of screening mammography is to identify breast cancer as early as possible before it becomes apparent clinically as a lump or with skin changes or distant metastasis. But, how do we know that mammography can show early breast cancers consistently? And if it can, how do we know that finding these early breast cancers is of any benefit to the patient? The ability of mammography to demonstrate small breast cancers consistently and the benefits of detecting these breast cancers through mammography were established by several randomized controlled trials.

Specifically, seven randomized controlled trials of screening mammography have all proved a benefit. Fewer women die from breast cancer among the population invited to undergo screening mammography compared with the control group of women not invited to undergo screening mammography. The reported benefits range from a 20% to 40% reduction in breast cancer mortality among the women invited to screening mammography (6–8). Screening mammography does show breast cancers consistently, and the diagnosis and treatment of the women with breast cancers identified through mammography saves lives.

The issue of screening women who are 40 to 49 years of age has been particularly controversial. However, a statistically significant benefit has been reported from several of the randomized controlled trials, including the Gothenberg and Malmo trials, which reported 44% and 36% reductions in breast cancer mortality, respectively, in this population of women. Also, a statistically significant benefit (26%) of screening 40- to 49-year-old women was reported from a metaanalysis (a statistical test that combines data reported from multiple trials) that used data from the seven population-based screening trials (9). In determining appropriate screening intervals, it is important to consider tumor sojourn times. *Tumor sojourn time*, defined as the time taken for cancers to go from preclinical to clinical mammographic detectability, is 1.7 years in premenopausal women and 3.3 years in postmenopausal women (10). Screening women in their 40s, therefore, is optimally done at annual intervals.

Mammography is not a perfect test. In some women with breast cancer, the cancer is not visible on the mammogram, even under the best of circumstances. The false-negative rates for mammography range from 7% to 15% (11). This is why it is important that women recognize the need for breast self-examination and annual breast examinations by a health care provider. Although there are false-negative mammograms, screening mammography is an effective method for finding early, potentially curable breast cancers and saving lives. It is the best and, currently, the only, reliable defense women have against breast cancer.

Using the cumulative data from all of the randomized controlled screening trials, the American Cancer Society (ACS), in March 1997, issued new screening guidelines recommending annual screening mammography for all women starting at 40 years of age. The baseline study (35 to 40 years of age) is no longer part of the screening guidelines. The ACS also recommends monthly breast self-examination starting at 20 years of age and an annual physical examination by a health care provider every 3 years for women 20 to 33 years of age and annually starting at 40 years of age. Breast cancer is now more commonly diagnosed after screening mammography compared with previously, when most breast cancers were diagnosed by the patient during breast self-examination (12).

Although there have been no rigorous trials to evaluate the use and benefit of screening mammography in high-risk women, many radiologists recommend starting screening mammography at 30 years of age in women in a high-risk category, including those with a family history of breast cancer (first-degree relative), particularly if the family member developed premenopausal, bilateral, or multiple breast cancers. In a woman whose mother developed breast cancer before 40 years of age, consider starting mammographic screening 10 years before the age of detection in the mother. For example, if the mother developed breast cancer at 36 years of age, consider starting mammographic screening in the daughter at 26 years of age.

Mammography provides the ability to diagnose stage 1 and 2 breast cancers as well as, in many patients, noninvasive, intraductal (stage 0) breast cancers. The diagnosis of early, potentially curable breast cancer increases the treatment options for patients and probably renders available treatments more effective. Regardless of the histologic grade (aggressiveness) of a tumor or the status of the axillary lymph nodes, women with breast cancers that are smaller than 1 cm in size have a 12-year survival rate of 95% (13). The goal of screening mammography, therefore, becomes the identification of cancers that are smaller than 1 cm in size. Inclusion of all breast tissue in the images through optimal mammographic positioning; high-contrast, high-resolution, well-exposed images; and the interpretive skills of the radiologist become pivotal in our ability to identify cancers consistently that are less than 1 cm in size.

Several randomized controlled trials have been done to establish the ability of mammography to demonstrate small breast cancers leading to significant reductions in breast cancer mortality rates.

Reported false-negative rates for mammography range from 7% to 15%. False-negative rates vary depending on breast tissue density and lesion type (higher false-negative rates are reported with invasive lobular carcinoma).

Mammography is recommended annually starting at 40 years of age for women at average risk for breast cancer.

At this time, there are insufficient data to establish screening guidelines for women with an increased risk for breast cancer. Options to consider in these women include starting annual screening mammography at 30 years of age, employing shorter screening intervals (e.g., every 6 months), or adding ultrasound or magnetic resonance imaging to the screening examination.

MAMMOGRAPHY QUALITY STANDARDS ACT

In 1992, following several reports of a wide range of problems with mammography in the United States, Congress passed the Mammography Quality Standards Act (MQSA) to establish quality standards for mammography. The legislation, authorized for 5 years, was signed on December 12, 1993 and reauthorized on October 8, 1998, extending it into 2002. MQSA regulates *mammographic modalities*, defined as technologies for radiography of the breast. Stereotactic biopsies, needle localizations, and ductography are procedures currently exempt from the definition of mammographic modality and not regulated under MQSA; ultrasound, magnetic resonance imaging, and nuclear medicine studies are nonradiographic procedures and not regulated under MQSA.

Effective October 1, 1994, all mammography facilities (except those of the Department of Veterans Affairs) must have:

- Accreditation by an approved accrediting body every 3 years
- Certification by the Secretary of Health and Human Services every 3 years
- Annual, on-site inspection by U.S. Food and Drug Administration (FDA) trained and certified federal or state inspectors on behalf of the Department of Health and Human Services

The Federal Register publication of October 28, 1997 (14) provides the final MQSA regulations, which are in effect as of April 28, 1999. Every aspect of a mammographic facility is regulated by this law, and familiarity with the details is advised, particularly for those designated as the lead interpreting physician (refer to the Federal Register publication for all the nuances of the law, which are beyond the scope of this book).

AMERICAN COLLEGE OF RADIOLOGY MAMMOGRAPHY ACCREDITATION PROGRAM

The American College of Radiology (ACR) took a leadership role in the late 1980s in addressing some of the deficiencies with mammographic image quality. The Mammography Accreditation Program developed by the ACR is now the oldest and largest accreditation program in the United States. This program accredits units (FDA-certifies facilities) every 3 years. For accreditation facilities submit the following:

- Completed form providing information on equipment, personnel qualifications, and test image data
- Phantom image for image quality and dose evaluations, using an approved phantom and thermoluminescent dosimeter
- Two normal mammograms (fatty and dense breasts)
- Processor quality control for a 30-day period
- Fee

The facilities are also required to provide an annual update to the ACR. This annual update includes quality-control documentation, the medical physicist's annual survey for each unit, and updated application data (e.g., changes in personnel). The ACR is also required under MQSA to perform on-site surveys of at least 5% of the facilities it accredits; 50% are selected randomly, and others are selected based on problems identified through FDA inspections, serious consumer complaints, or history of noncompliance. A medical physicist, a radiologist, and an ACR staff person make up the survey team. Additionally, random clinical image reviews are required of at least 3% of accredited facilities; facilities are selected randomly.

The ACR has also subsequently developed accreditation programs for stereotactic breast biopsy, diagnostic breast ultrasound, and ultrasound-guided breast biopsy. The reader is encouraged strongly to become familiar with these programs by contacting the ACR or visiting their website.

TREATMENT OPTIONS

Most women diagnosed with breast cancer undergo mastectomy or lumpectomy. In woman who have invasive cancer and in some women who have extensive ductal carcinoma *in situ* (DCIS), assessment of the axilla is undertaken regardless of the surgical procedure elected for the breast.

The goal of lumpectomy is to remove the entire tumor so that there is little, if any, cancer left in the breast. The margins of the specimen are evaluated histologically. If the margins are positive, the patient is usually taken back to the operating room for reexcision of the tumor bed. The goal of reexcision is to achieve negative margins. If the margins are grossly positive after reexcision, the patient may not be a good candidate for conservative therapy, and mastectomy may be more appropriate.

Traditionally, axillary dissections involved the excision of multiple lymph nodes from the axilla. Complications associated with axillary dissections include lymphedema, arm and shoulder numbness, paresthesias involving the arm and shoulder, loss of range of motion at the shoulder, and the formation of fluid pockets (seromas, hematomas) in the axilla. Sentinel lymph node biopsies have now been adopted by many surgeons to minimize the surgery required in the axilla; these minimize dissection and associated complications and have made a significant contribution to patient care and overall quality of life for patients.

The concept of the sentinel lymph node biopsy is fairly simple and first developed in the evaluation of patients with melanoma. If the lymphatic drainage from the breast to the axilla proceeds in an orderly, stepwise manner, one or two lymph nodes in the axilla should receive the lymphatic drainage from the breast first and consistently. If these lymph nodes can be identified reliably and if they reflect the overall status of the axillary lymph nodes accurately, axillary dissections can be minimized to the removal of the sentinel lymph nodes. To identify the sentinel lymph nodes, a vital blue dye, technetium-labeled sulfur colloid particles, or both are injected around the tumor or subcutaneously around the areola. Visual inspection of the axilla by the surgeon for collection of the vital blue dye, or radioactivity detected with a handheld gamma probe, is used to identify the one, two, or sometimes three sentinel lymph nodes (15–18). We inject technetium-labeled sulfur colloid particles around the areola 2 hours before surgery, and the vital blue dye is injected into the tumor by the surgeon intraoperatively. Use of both methods increases the likelihood of identifying the sentinel lymph node in up to 90% of patients, with an overall accuracy of 98.2% and a false-negative rate of 5.8% (19).

At the time the lymph node is excised, a touch prep is done to determine whether there is gross involvement of the lymph node. If the touch prep is positive, the surgeon completes an axillary dissection. If the touch prep is negative, no further lymph nodes are sampled at this time. The touch preps are usually reliable; however, in women with invasive lobular carcinoma, a higher false-negative rate is found. If metastatic disease is identified on the hematoxylin and eosin–stained slides of the lymph node, the patient is scheduled for a completion axillary dissection. Although controversial, we do not routinely do completion axillary dissections in patients with micrometastatic disease identified on the permanent hematoxylin and eosin sections.

Although many questions remain unanswered with respect to sentinel node biopsies in women with breast cancer, data are accumulating rapidly in support of the procedure. It appears that the sentinel lymph node can be identified in most patients and that it reliably reflects the status of the remainder of the axillary lymph nodes (e.g., if there is no breast cancer in the sentinel node, it is unlikely that other lymph nodes are involved). Difficulties in identifying the sentinel lymph node are most commonly encountered in patients in whom the sentinel lymph node is totally replaced with tumor. Discussion remains as to the best method of injecting patients (although this may turn out not to play a significant role). Because the excised lymph node is now scrutinized more carefully histologically (often with reverse transcriptase polymerase chain reaction testing), the significance of isolated tumor cells or micrometastatic disease (defined as metastasis greater than 0.2 mm but not greater than 2.0 mm) in the management of patients is not yet clear. Also, the potential role for lymphoscintigraphy in evaluating the status of internal mammary lymph nodes needs additional research.

Radiation therapy is usually recommended after lumpectomy. In a small number of patients, radiation therapy to the chest wall or axilla is also recommended after mastectomy to reduce the likelihood of chest wall or axillary recurrence. Radiation after lumpectomy is given 5 days a week for 6 weeks. Local control of breast cancer is the purpose of the radiation therapy.

Chemotherapy is commonly recommended in women with metastatic disease to the axillary lymph nodes or with distant metastases. Premenopausal women with negative axillary lymph nodes also appear to benefit from chemotherapy. However, the benefit of chemotherapy in postmenopausal women with node-negative, estrogen and progesterone receptor–positive disease is minimal. These patients may be best managed with tamoxifen. Chemotherapy is usually a combination of drugs given over an 18- to 24-week period.

In most women, surgery for local control and the axillary lymph node biopsy are done before radiation or chemotherapy. In some women with advanced breast cancer at the time of diagnosis or with inflammatory carcinoma, chemotherapy is used first to shrink the tumor (neoadjuvant). Depending on the response of the tumor, this is followed by mastectomy or lumpectomy. Radiation therapy and additional chemotherapy after the surgery may also be used in these patients.

Chemoprevention of breast cancer is controversial and receiving much attention. It may be that drugs such as tamoxifen and raloxifene (selective estrogen receptor modulators) can reduce the risk for developing breast cancer. Tamoxifen is approved for use as a breast cancer preventive agent in premenopausal and postmenopausal women with a significantly increased risk for breast cancer. A study is underway to further evaluate the role of tamoxifen in breast cancer prevention. The Study of Tamoxifen and Raloxifen (STAR) trial is also evaluating the potential role for raloxifene (5).

BREAST CANCER STAGING

Breast cancer is staged based on the size of the tumor (T), the presence or absence regional lymph node (N) involvement, and the presence or absence of cancer cells at sites distant (M) to the breast. This system is referred to as the *TNM system* (20). Numbers are assigned to each of these letters to define the characteristics of the cancer found in an individual patient.

Clinical staging (cTNM) is staging based on information obtained from the clinical evaluation of patients, including a complete physical examination, imaging, biopsy, and surgical exploration before any treatment is given (Boxes 1.1 and 1.2). Pathologic staging (pTNM) is based on information from the clinical evaluation and the complete removal and evaluation of the primary tumor and regional lymph nodes (Box 1.3) after surgery but before treatment (20). After each one of these three components (TNM) is classified (see Box 1.4 for classification of "M"), the patient is assigned into one of several stages (Table 1.1). Recommendations for treatment and the overall prognosis of a patient vary depending on the stage of the breast cancer at the time of diagnosis.

Axillary and internal mammary lymph nodes on the side (ipsilateral) of the primary tumor are the regional lymph nodes in patients with breast cancer. Sentinel lymph node biopsies or axillary dissections are almost always done in women with invasive breast cancer to stage the cancer pathologically. Sentinel lymph node biopsy or axillary dissection is not always done in women with some forms of DCIS. Internal mammary lymph nodes are not usually sampled because they are difficult to access without extensive surgery.

Changes to the TNM classification system for breast cancer have been incorporated in the sixth edition (20) of the American Joint Commission on Cancer staging manual (the reader is encouraged to consult and review this manual for details beyond the scope of this book). Recent changes include the following:

Box 1.1: Primary Tumor (T) Classification

TX	Primary tumor cannot be assessed
T0	No evidence of primary tumor
Tis	Carcinoma *in situ* (DCIS, LCIS, and Paget's disease with no tumor)
T1	Tumor ≤2 cm
T1a	Tumor >0.1 cm but ≤0.5 cm
T1b	Tumor >0.5 cm but ≤1.0 cm
T1c	Tumor >1.0 cm but ≤2.0 cm
T2	Tumor >2 cm but ≤5 cm
T3	Tumor >5 cm
T4	Tumor of any size extending to chest wall or skin
T4a	Tumor extending to chest wall but not including pectoralis muscle
T4b	Edema, ulceration of the skin, or satellite skin nodules confined to same breast
T4c	Both T4a and T4b
T4d	Inflammatory carcinoma

DCIS, ductal carcinoma *in situ*; LCIS, lobular carcinoma *in situ*.
Adapted from the American Joint Commission on Cancer. *Cancer staging manual*, 6th ed. New York: Springer 2002, with permission.

Box 1.2: Regional Lymph Node (N) Classification

Clinical

NX	Regional lymph nodes (LNs) cannot be assessed (previously removed)
N0	No metastasis to the regional LNs
N1	Metastasis to movable ipsilateral axillary LNs
N2	Metastasis to ipsilateral axillary LNs fixed or matted or in clinically apparent ipsilateral internal mammary nodes in the absence of clinically evident axillary LN metastasis
N2a	Metastasis to ipsilateral axillary lymph nodes fixed to one another or to other structures
N2b	Metastasis only in clinically apparent ipsilateral internal mammary nodes and in the absence of clinically evident axillary lymph node metastasis
N3	Metastasis in ipsilateral infraclavicular LNs with or without axillary LN involvement or metastasis to ipsilateral supraclavicular LNs with or without axillary LN involvement or internal mammary LN involvement
N3a	Metastasis in ipsilateral infraclavicular LNs
N3b	Metastasis in ipsilateral internal mammary LNs and axillary LNs
N3c	Metastasis in ipsilateral supraclavicular LNs

Adapted from the American Joint Commission on Cancer. *Cancer staging manual*, 6th ed. New York: Springer 2002, with permission.

Box 1.3: Pathologic Lymph Node (N) Classification

pNX	Regional LN cannot be assessed
pN0	No regional LN metastasis histologically, no study for (ITC)
pN0 (i–)	No regional LN metastasis histologically, negative immunohistochemical (IHC) or molecular studies
pN0 (i+)	No regional LN metastasis histologically, positive IHC no cluster >0.2 mm
pN0 (mol–)	No regional LN metastasis histologically, negative molecular findings
pN0 (mol+)	No regional LN metastasis histologically, positive molecular findings
pN1	Metastasis in 1 to 3 LNs and/or internal mammary LNs with microscopic disease detected by sentinel LN dissection but not clinically apparent
pN1mi	Micrometastasis (>0.2 mm, none >2.0 mm)
pN1a	Metastasis in 1 to 3 axillary LNs
pN1b	Metastasis in internal mammary LN with microscopic disease detected by sentinel LN biopsy but not clinically apparent
pN1c	Metastasis in 1 to 3 axillary LNs and internal mammary LNs with microscopic disease detected by sentinel LN biopsy but not clinically apparent
pN2	Metastasis in 4 to 9 axillary LNs or in clinically apparent internal mammary LNs in the absence of axillary LN metastasis
pN2a	Metastasis in 4 to 9 axillary LNs (at least one tumor deposit >2.0 mm)
pN2b	Metastasis in clinically apparent internal mammary LNs in the absence of axillary LNs
pN3	Metastasis in 10 or more axillary LNs or in infraclavicular LNs or in clinically apparent ipsilateral internal mammary LNs in the presence of 1 or more positive axillary LNs, or in more than 3 axillary LNs with clinically negative microscopic metastasis in internal mammary LNs, or in ipsilateral supraclavicular LNs
pN3a	Metastasis in 10 or more axillary LNs (at least one tumor deposit >2.0 mm) or metastasis to infraclavicular LNs
pN3b	Metastasis in clinically apparent ipsilateral internal mammary LNs or in more than 3 axillary LNs and in internal mammary LNs with microscopic disease detected by sentinel LN biopsy but not clinically apparent
pN3c	Metastasis in ipsilateral supraclavicular LNs

ITC, isolated tumor cells.
Adapted from the American Joint Commission on Cancer. *Cancer staging manual*, 6th ed. New York: Springer 2002, with permission.

Box 1.4: Distant Metastasis

MX	Distant metastasis cannot be assessed
M0	No distant metastasis
M1	Distant metastasis

Adapted from the American Joint Commission on Cancer. *Cancer staging manual*, 6th ed. New York: Springer 2002, with permission.

Table 1.1: Breast Cancer Staging

Stage 0	Tis	N0	M0
Stage I	T1	N0	M0
Stage IIA	T0	N1	M0
	T1	N1	M0
	T2	N0	M0
Stage IIB	T2	N1	M0
	T3	N0	M0
Stage IIIA	T0	N2	M0
	T1	N2	M0
	T2	N2	M0
	T3	N1	M0
	T3	N2	M0
Stage IIIB	T4	N0	M0
	T4	N1	M0
	T4	N2	M0
Stage IIIC	any T	N3	M0
Stage IV	any T	any N	M1

T, primary tumor; N, lymph node; M, distant metastasis.
Adapted from the American Joint Commission on Cancer. *Cancer staging manual*, 6th ed. New York: Springer 2002, with permission.

- Distinction on the basis of size and histologic evidence of malignant activity between isolated tumor cells and micrometastatic disease
- Identifiers to indicate use of sentinel lymph node and immunohistochemical or molecular techniques
- Lymph node status classifications based on number of axillary nodes involved as determined by hematoxylin and eosin or immunohistochemical staining
- Addition of N3, metastasis to infraclavicular nodes, and change from M1, supraclavicular lymph node involvement, to N3
- Reclassification of metastasis to intramammary lymph nodes based on method of detection and the presence or absence of axillary nodal involvement

The prognosis for women with breast cancer is determined by the staging of the breast cancer using the TNM system and the histopathologic grading of tumors. In addition, several tests are performed on the cancer cells that provide information and guide the use of certain treatment options. Some of the more commonly used tests include estrogen and progesterone receptor studies, p53 expression and erbB-2 (HER-2/neu) overexpression. Tumors having estrogen receptors (e.g., estrogen receptor positive) may respond to treatment with tamoxifen and usually have a better prognosis. Tumors that are estrogen and progesterone receptor negative have higher and quicker recurrence and mortality rates than tumors that have estrogen and progesterone receptors (2,3,5). Tumor ploidy and S phase are also routinely obtained. Normally, the p53 protein monitors cells and keeps abnormal cells from dividing. When the p53 protein is abnormal, cells become unstable. Expression of p53 in breast cancers is associated with a poor prognosis. Likewise, overexpression of erbB-2 (HER-2/neu) is associated with a poor prognosis (2,3,5).

SUGGESTIONS FOR DISCUSSION OF PATIENT FILMS IN BREAST IMAGING

As an introduction to the remainder of the textbook, consider the following suggestions for "case" presentations. After completing the textbook, you may want to refer back to these suggestions.

1. When presented with films on a patient for discussion, consider demographic information, relevant clinical issues, and pertinent imaging findings in formulating a logical and reasonable list of diagnostic considerations. This, in conjunction with an understanding of the manifestations of breast diseases, facilitates narrowing the considerations to one or two most likely etiologies. With a logical approach, and recognizing that "common things are common," justifiable management decisions can be routinely made (and if not, one is usually dealing with an obscure entity that in practice would not be a primary consideration anyway).

2. A well-developed, complete, and logical patient ("case") discussion is an art to be mastered. Although getting the "right" answer is often the focus, this is not what counts. The ability to make observations and integrate relevant information in the formulation of appropriate diagnostic considerations and the approach taken in sorting through the differential are what, in the long run, serve patients and referring physicians.

3. Armed with common sense, the best approach in mastering the art of patient discussions is involvement. Review as many films as possible and discuss patients whenever there is an opportunity. Unfortunately, the tendency is to take the path of least resistance and make learning a passive experience. Conferences are given priority over active involvement in patient care, and didactic conferences are requested over patient discussion conferences. There appears to be a widely held belief that becoming a good radiologist can be accomplished by passive participation or nonparticipation at conferences and in the daily activities of a section. Reading has taken a secondary role. Get involved with patient care directly, review as many films as possible, and depend on yourself for teaching by reading critically.

4. Develop a systematic approach to reviewing mammographic images.

5. Evaluate technique:
   - Is the tissue well exposed?
   - Are the images high-contrast images?
   - Is there blurring? (Look specifically for blurring; otherwise, subtle blurring will not be perceived. Remember, too, that blurring does not necessarily involve the image diffusely—blurring can also be focal.)
   - Are there any artifacts that could interfere with interpretation?
   - Are the films labeled appropriately?

6. Evaluate positioning on the mediolateral oblique (MLO) views:
   - Is pectoral muscle seen to the level of the nipple?
   - Is the anterior margin of the pectoral muscle convex?
   - Is the breast lifted up and pulled out?
   - Is the inframammary fold open, and is there a small amount of upper abdomen on the image?
   - Is there tissue to the edge of the film inferiorly (between the pectoral muscle and inframammary fold)?
   - Is there a possibility that tissue, or a lesion, has been excluded from the image?

7. Evaluate positioning on the craniocaudal (CC) views:
   - Is pectoral muscle imaged?
   - If pectoral muscle is not imaged, is cleavage seen?
   - Is there lateral tissue extending to the edge of the film? Should an exaggerated CC view be done?
   - Is there a possibility that tissue, or a lesion, has been excluded from the image?

8. With right and left MLO views back to back, evaluate the following:
   - Upper third of the breasts
   - Middle third of the breasts
   - Lower third of the breasts
   - Usually fatty stripe between pectoral muscle and glandular tissue
   - Uppermost cone of tissue
   - Fat–glandular interfaces

- Retroareolar area
- Inframammary fold area

9. With right and left CC views back to back, evaluate the following:
   - Outer third of the breasts
   - Middle third of the breasts
   - Medial third (usually fatty) of the breasts
   - Retroglandular fat and fat–glandular interfaces
   - Subareolar area

10. If there is a possible abnormality, undertake additional evaluation before making recommendations or drawing significant conclusions (do whatever it takes to resolve the clinical or mammographic issue):
    - Previous films for comparisons
    - Spot compression views
    - Microfocus spot magnification views
    - Tangential views
    - Rolled or change-of-angle views
    - Cleavage views
    - 90-Degree lateral views (mediolateral or lateromedial)
    - Correlative physical examination
    - Breast ultrasound
    - Ductography
    - Cyst aspiration (and possibly pneumocystography)
    - Fine-needle aspiration
    - Imaging-guided needle biopsy

11. Before undertaking additional evaluation or recommending an interventional procedure, procure and review prior studies.

12. If there is something obvious clinically, or on the films, look away and review remaining tissue before returning to consider obvious findings (otherwise, you may miss additional, more subtle lesions).

13. If there is nothing obvious, start talking and systematically go through the images. Send your eyes out and specifically look for microcalcifications, masses, architectural distortion, diffuse changes, and adenopathy. While going through the images, the abnormality usually becomes apparent.

14. Learn your blind spots—areas where you have missed things in the past.

15. When discussing patients, structure the discussion and progress through the four Ds:
    - *Detection*: review films systematically, request or inquire about prior studies
    - *Description*: describe the abnormality, providing relevant positive and negative findings
    - *Differential diagnosis*: based on the description of the findings, construct a logical differential in order of likelihood. Start with possible benign lesions and progress into possible malignant lesions. Try not to go back and forth between benign and malignant lesions, and do not start by saying, "I don't think this is . . . ." Do not discuss what the lesions is *not* likely to be; rather discuss what are reasonable benign and malignant considerations.
    - *Diagnosis*: end the discussion by suggesting what you think is the most likely diagnosis based on the integration of patient demographics, relevant history, described features of the lesion, and your differential considerations.

16. In formulating a differential diagnosis, consider the following:
    - Gender—do not assume all patients are female
    - Age (e.g., fibroadenomas are unlikely to develop in a 70-year-old woman; mucinous carcinomas are more common in older women)
    - Type of study: screening or diagnostic (i.e., asymptomatic or symptomatic patient; whether there are any radiopaque markers or metallic markers on the films and their significance)
    - Prior studies

- Medications (estrogen replacement therapy, tamoxifen, chemotherapy)
- Relevant history—medical and surgical

17. If you don't know something, be willing to admit it—don't try to talk yourself out of situations.

18. Think critically and be succinct with descriptions—verbosity accomplishes little, obscures the message, and often reflects sloppy, imprecise thinking.

19. Be precise with terminology:
   - "There is a large mass." (How is *large* defined? One person's definition of large may be someone's definition of small. Give specific measurements of the lesion.)
   - "There appears to be a mass." (What does *appears* mean? Is there a mass or not? Make up your mind, and do not be afraid to "call a spade a spade.")
   - "There is fatty replacement." (How do you know that anything has been replaced? You need to have prior films available to state that something has been replaced.)
   - Know the ACR's BIRAD lexicon and learn how to use it. How is mass defined? How is density defined? What information should you provide relative to masses? Relative to calcifications?

20. Do not just memorize a list of possible lesions—know the different disease processes, and learn how to sort through them based on patient demographics, presentation, and imaging findings.

21. Know the limitations of the studies under review and how to overcome them. On screening studies, be careful with characterization. Obtain additional mammographic images, ultrasound, ductography, or needle biopsies for characterization.

22. Know what biopsy results need to be discussed with the pathologist directly and under what circumstances the patient should undergo repeat biopsy.

REFERENCES

1. Jemal A, Murray T, Samuels A, et al. Cancer statistics, 2003.   *CA Cancer J Clin* 2003;53:5–26.
2. Bland KI, Copeland EM, eds. *The breast*, 2nd ed. Philadelphia: WB Saunders, 1998.
3. Roses DF. *Breast cancer*. New York: Churchill Livingstone, 1999.
4. Breast cancer death drops: mammography screening listed as factor. *ACR Bull* 1995;51:2:1.
5. Harris JR, Lippman ME, Morrow M, et al. *Diseases of the breast*, 2nd ed. Philadelphia: Lippincott Williams & Wilkins, 2000.
6. Elwood JM, Cox B, Richardson AK. The effectiveness of breast cancer screening by mammography in younger women. *Online J Curr Clin Trials* (serial on line) 1993;2(Doc NR 32).
7. Kerlikowske K, Grady D, Rubin SM, et al. Efficacy of screening mammography: a meta-analysis. *JAMA* 1995;273:149–154.
8. Feig S. Determination of mammographic screening intervals with surrogate measures for women aged 40–49 years. *Radiology* 1994;193:311–314.
9. *Report of the Consensus Development Conference Panel on Breast Cancer Screening for Women Aged 40–49, January 21–23, 1997*. Bethesda, MD: National Institute of Health, 1997.
10. Tabar L, Fagerberg G, Day NE, et al. Breast cancer treatment and natural history: new insights from result of screening. *Lancet* 1992;1:412–414.
11. Linver MN, Osuch JR, Brenner RJ, et al. The mammography audit: a primer for the Mammography Quality Standards Act (MQSA). *AJR Am J Roentgenol* 1995;165:19–25.
12. Smith RA, Mettlin CJ, Johnston Davis K, Eyre H. American Cancer Society Guidelines for the early detection of cancer. *CA Cancer J Clin* 2000;50:34–49.
13. Tabar L, Fagerberg G, Duffy SW, et al. Update of the Swedish two-county program of mammographic screening for breast cancer. *Radiol Clin North Am* 1992;30:187–210.
14. *Quality mammography standards, final rule*. Federal Register October 28, 1997; 62:55852–55993. Department of Health and Human Services. Food and Drug Administration. 21 CFR parts 16 and 900.
15. Krag D, Weaver D, Ashikaga T, et al. The sentinel node is breast cancer. *N Engl J Med* 1998;339: 941–946.
16. McIntosh SA, Purushotham AD. Lymphatic mapping and sentinel node biopsy in breast cancer. *Br J Surg* 1998;85:1347–1356.

17. Liberman L, Cody HS, Hill ADK, et al. Sentinel lymph node biopsy after percutaneous diagnosis of nonpalpable breast cancer. *Radiology* 1999;211:835–844.

18. DeAngelis GA, Gizienski T, Moore MM. Axillary sentinel node biopsy in breast cancer staging. *Appl Radiol* 1999;(June):8–11.

19. Donegan WL, Spratt JS. *Cancer of the breast*, 5th ed. Philadelphia: WB Saunders, 2002.

20. American Joint Commission on Cancer. *Cancer staging manual*, 6th ed. New York: Springer, 2002.

SCREENING MAMMOGRAPHY

QUALITY-CONTROL TESTS

Quality-control tests done daily, weekly, monthly, quarterly, and semiannually by the technologists, as required under the Mammography Quality Standards Act (MQSA) (1) and the American College of Radiology (ACR) *Mammography Quality Control Manual* (2), are listed in Table 2.1. The reader is advised to consult this manual for details on how each test is done and interpreted. Any failures in daily processor quality control, weekly phantom images, semiannual darkroom fog, screen-film contact, and compression require corrective action before clinical imaging can be done (1,2). Failures in repeat analysis and fixer retention require corrective actions within 30 days of the test date.

Quality-control tests that should be done at least once annually by a physicist are listed in Box 2.1. Corrective action needs to be taken within 30 days of the test date for failures in collimation assessment, system resolution, kilovolt (peak) [kV(p)] accuracy and reproducibility, automatic exposure control, system performance assessment, and uniformity of screen speed. Average glandular dose to an average (4.2-cm compressed) breast must not exceed 3 mGy (0.3 rad) per view for screen-film image receptors. The condition of the focal spot is evaluated by determining the system resolution and should be 13 line pairs per millimeter with the bars parallel to the anode–cathode axis and 11 line pairs per millimeter with the bars perpendicular to the anode–cathode axis. The kV(p) should be ±5% of indicated kV(p) (1,2).

Corrective action must be taken before any clinical imaging is done if daily processor quality control, weekly phantom images, and the semiannual darkroom fog or compression tests fail.

Table 2.1: Quality-Control Tests (Technologist)

Daily	Weekly	Monthly	Quarterly	Semiannual
Darkroom cleanliness	Screen cleanliness	Visual checklist	Repeat analysis	Darkroom fog
Processor quality control	Viewboxes		Analysis of fixer retention	Screen-film contact
	Viewing conditions			Compression
	Phantom images			

Box 2.1: *Quality-Control Tests (Physicist)*

Mammography unit assembly
Collimation assessment
Evaluation of system resolution
kV(p) accuracy and reproducibility
Beam quality assessment (half-value layer measurement)
Assessment of automatic exposure control system performance
Uniformity of screen speed
Breast entrance exposure dose, average glandular dose, AEC reproducibility
Image quality evaluation
Artifact evaluation
Viewbox luminance and room illuminance

---

kV(p), Kilovolt (peak); AEC, Automatic Exposure Control.

PHANTOM IMAGES

At a minimum, the four largest fibers, three largest speck groups, and three largest masses should be seen on images of the phantom.

A basic understanding of phantom images is important because these serve to check that the x-ray imaging system and film processors are operating optimally with respect to film density, contrast (density differences), uniformity, and overall image quality. As part of the quality assessment and quality-control program, phantom images are done weekly. Phantom images are also done after equipment is serviced, when film or screen type is changed, or as needed when troubleshooting problems with the imaging chain. Although beyond the scope of this book, the reader is encouraged to review and understand how phantom images are obtained, evaluated, and scored (2). The phantom (Radiation Measurement, Inc. RMI 156 or Nuclear Associates 18-220) simulates a 4.2-cm thick compressed breast composed of 50% glandular tissue and 50% fatty tissue. It contains six fibers (range, 1.56 to 0.4 mm), five specks (range, 1.56 to 0.4 mm in diameter) and five masses (range, 2.00 to 0.25 mm in diameter). An acrylic disk (4-mm thick, 1 cm in diameter) is placed, or permanently attached to the phantom.

Operating levels for background optical density should be at least 1.40 ± 0.20 and should never be less than 1.2.

At a minimum, the four largest fibers, three largest speck groups, and three largest masses should be seen. The image is also reviewed for artifacts, and these are factored into the scoring (Figure 2.1). Operating levels for background optical density should be at least 1.40 ± 0.20; background film optical density should never be less than 1.2, and the density difference due to the 4.0-mm acrylic disk should be at least 0.40 ± 0.05.

FILM LABELING

Mammography films are legal documents and must be labeled appropriately as required under MQSA (1). A permanent identification label *must* include the items listed in Box 2.2.

It is strongly recommended that a flash card with patient and location information be used. This is permanent and reproduces on copy films. The information should fit squarely in the designated space, be legible and not cut off. It is also recommended that technical factors used in obtaining the exposure be available as part of the permanent record. Fortunately, most new units flash some of the technical information onto the identification label. Troubleshooting suboptimal films, reproducibility, and comparison of technique from one year to the next are facilitated when the technical factors listed in Box 2.3 are known.

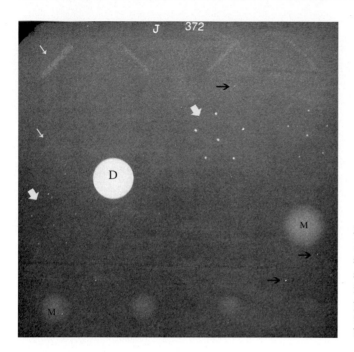

Figure 2.1 *Phantom image.* Radiation Measurement, Inc. (RMI 156) phantom image demonstrating fibers (*thin white arrows*), specks (*thick white arrow*), and masses (M). Acrylic disc (D) attached to phantom is used in calculating density difference. Artifacts (*black arrows*) are noted and factored into the scoring of the phantom images. As part of the quality assessment and quality control program, phantom images are done weekly; the images should be retained for the past full year.

Box 2.2: Required Information on Films

Patient name
Unique patient identifying number
Date of study
Radiopaque laterality and projection markers placed closest to axilla
Facility name
Facility location (minimum: city, state, and zip code)
Technologist identification
Cassette/screen identification number
Mammography unit identification number (if more than one unit/facility)

Box 2.3: Technical Factors Helpful in Troubleshooting Films

Target–filter combination
Milliampere-second (mAs)
Kilovolt (peak): kV(p)
Exposure time
Compression force
Compressed breast thickness
Photo cell positioning
Degree of obliquity on MLOs

MLO, mediolateral oblique views.

IMAGING ALGORITHM

As part of the screening study, anterior compression and exaggerated craniocaudal views are obtained in a small number of women to compress anterior tissue and image lateral tissue, respectively.

By definition, screening mammography is done in asymptomatic women. We recommend annual screening mammography starting at 40 years of age. In women with a strong family history of breast cancer, we start screening annually at 30 years of age. Craniocaudal (CC) and mediolateral oblique (MLO) views of each breast are obtained for screening (3). At the discretion of the technologist, anterior compression and exaggerated craniocaudal (XCCL) views are obtained in a small number of women. A metallic BB is used to mark any prominent skin lesions that may be mistaken for a breast lesion. We require that the technologist document on the patient's history form, the location and reason for using skin markers. Likewise, the presence of surgical scars is documented on a diagram of the breast provided for the technologist on the history form. We do not routinely use radiopaque markers on biopsy scars or the nipples.

In women with implants, we obtain four views of each breast: CC and MLO views with the implants in the field of view and CC and MLO views with displacement of the implants (1,2,4). If there is significant encapsulation, implant-displaced views may not be obtainable. If these views cannot be done, it is documented in the mammography report and by the technologist in the patient's history form. We do not obtain written consent for a mammogram from women who have implants.

IMAGING THE SMALL FEMALE BREAST OR MALE BREAST

In women with small breasts, or in male patients, it can be hard for the technologist to maintain the breast in place as compression is applied without scraping the skin over the knuckles. Compression paddles that are half the width of the standard compression paddle are available to overcome these limitations. These paddles are also helpful for achieving the implant-displaced views in women with implants.

IMAGING THE LARGE FEMALE BREAST

Image receptors, compression paddles, and cassettes come in two different sizes (18 × 24 cm and 24 × 30 cm). Selection should be based on the woman's breast size. The large image receptor should not be used for women with small breasts. Likewise, a small image receptor should not be used on a woman with large breasts (Figure 2.2). In women with large breasts, a 24 × 30 cm image receptor is used, and more than two views of each breast may be needed to image all breast tissue adequately.

MEDIOLATERAL OBLIQUE VIEWS

Maximal tissue inclusion on mediolateral oblique views requires selection of a patient-specific angle of obliquity, relaxation of the pectoral muscle, and medial mobilization of the breast and underlying pectoral muscle.

Factors to consider in obtaining optimal tissue positioning on MLO views are listed in Box 2.4.

The angle of obliquity for MLO varies for different patients and is determined by the orientation of the pectoral muscle fibers. Tall women have a more vertically oriented pectoral muscle than short women. Our goal is to image as much breast tissue as possible and, because the breasts are skin appendages, pulling parallel to underlying relaxed muscle fibers maximizes the amount of tissue that is pulled away from the body (4).

Relaxation of the pectoral muscle requires that the patient inwardly rotate her humeral head and hold her arm down (behind or on the bucky). The patient should not lift her arm to hold onto the unit. The pectoralis major muscle inserts on the upper third of the humerus such that the muscle tenses when the arm is elevated and the humeral

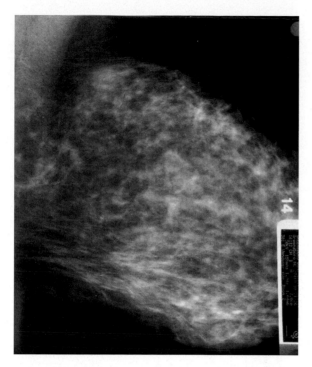

Figure 2.2 *Inappropriate image receptor.* Image receptor size needs to be matched to breast size. The anterior portion of this patient's breast has been cut off from the image, and the cassette number and identification label partially obscure anterior tissue. This patient should have been imaged on a 24 × 30 cm cassette.

head is externally rotated. Relaxing the pectoral muscle reduces the amount of resistance encountered during positioning so that a greater amount of tissue and muscle is routinely included on the images.

Breast tissue in the lateral and inferior quadrants of the breast is mobile (Figure 2.3A). Tissue in the upper, and particularly the inner quadrants, has little inherent mobility. Unfortunately, most of our equipment is designed so that, for MLO views, the compression paddle travels from the upper inner quadrant to the lower outer quadrant (Figure 2.3B). As the compression paddle is put in motion, it attempts to mobilize tissue in the

---

Box 2.4: Factors to Consider in Positioning for Mediolateral Oblique Views

Technologist works from behind and medial side of patient
Angle of obliquity
    Specific for every patient
    Determined by technologist
    Based on obliquity of pectoral muscle
Relaxation of pectoral muscle
    Inward rotation of humeral head
    Ipsilateral arm down
Medial mobilization of breast tissue and pectoral muscle
    Need to maintain medial mobilization
    Minimizes skin stretching upper inner quadrant
Patient needs to stay in unit
Breast out and up
    Open inframammary fold
    Include a small amount of abdomen

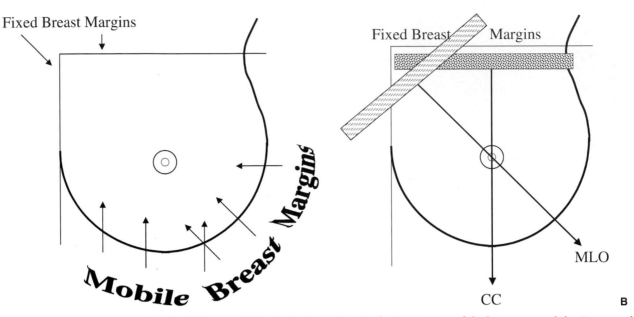

Figure 2.3 *Breast mobility. A. The lateral and inferior portions of the breast are mobile. Upper and medial tissue is fixed in position. During positioning, tissue should be mobilized to minimize the amount of fixed tissue passed over by the compression paddle. B. For the mediolateral oblique (MLO) view, the compression paddle moves from the upper inner quadrant toward the lower outer quadrant. With little inherent mobility, upper inner quadrant tissue is excluded from the field of view as the compression paddle is mobilized for the MLO views. Associated skin stretching results from the paddle scraping over this tissue. For the craniocaudal view (CC), the compression paddle moves from the upper quadrants toward the lower quadrants. As the paddle moves downward, superior tissue can roll out from the under the paddle, and skin stretching leads to patient discomfort.*

upper inner quadrants with little inherent mobility. This results in the exclusion of variable amounts of tissue and potential lesions from the field of view and is associated with skin stretching that can be quite uncomfortable. The tissue rolls out as compression is applied. If we use natural breast mobility effectively, we can minimize the amount of excluded tissue and associated skin stretching (4). Therein lies the importance of medial mobilization of breast tissue and underlying muscle during positioning for MLO views. Every 1 mm of medial tissue mobilization represents 1 mm less of compression paddle traveling over fixed tissue.

The tip of the film holder is positioned at the apex of the axilla so that the film holder is snug against the body along the mid-axillary line. There should be no air gap between the pectoral muscle and upper portion of the breast and the film holder; otherwise, the pectoral muscle appears overexposed (Figure 2.4). Also, there should be no space between the film holder and the breast posteriorly; otherwise, posterior tissue is excluded. The technologist should not be able to advance her index finger into the apex of the axilla.

In assessing the adequacy of positioning on MLO views, consider the factors listed in Box 2.5. The length and shape of the pectoral muscle is evaluated in assessing the quality of positioning on MLO views (5). Pectoral muscle should be wide at the axilla, have an anterior convex margin, and extend to the level of the nipple (Figure 2.5). Lack of muscle relaxation, selection of an inappropriate angle of obliquity, failure to medially mobilize or maintain medial mobilization of breast tissue, or allowing the patient to lean back slightly can result in a concave pectoral muscle edge, a triangular pectoral muscle, or a muscle that is parallel to the edge of the film (Figure 2.6). The inframammary fold (IMF)

The appearance of the pectoral muscle is helpful in assessing adequacy of positioning on MLO views. The muscle should widen at the axilla, extend to the level of the nipple, and have a convex anterior margin.

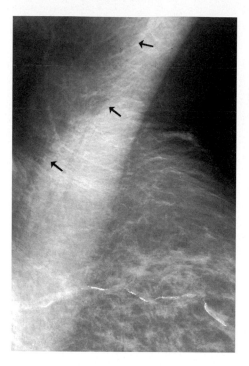

Figure 2.4 *Uneven exposure, air gap.* The upper portion of the breast and pectoral muscle need to be directly on the film holder. This area of uneven exposure (*arrows*) is an indication that the tissue was not directly up against the film holder. An air gap is present. When areas like this are seen, evaluate the tissue carefully for blur because compression is not optimal in this area. Artificial calcification is incidentally noted.

Box 2.5: *Assessing Positioning on Mediolateral Oblique Views*

Wide muscle (thick) at the axilla
Pectoral muscle to level of nipple
Convex anterior margin of pectoral muscle
Open inframammary fold
Small amount of upper abdomen
Breast pulled out and up (no sagging)

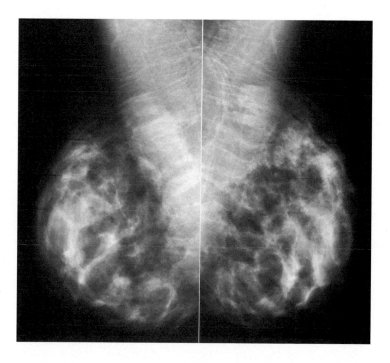

Figure 2.5 *Mediolateral oblique view.* The pectoral muscles are thick in the axillary region, the anterior borders are convex and extend to the level of the nipple. The tissue is pulled up and out and is well compressed. With a bright light, the inframammary fold is noted and is open.

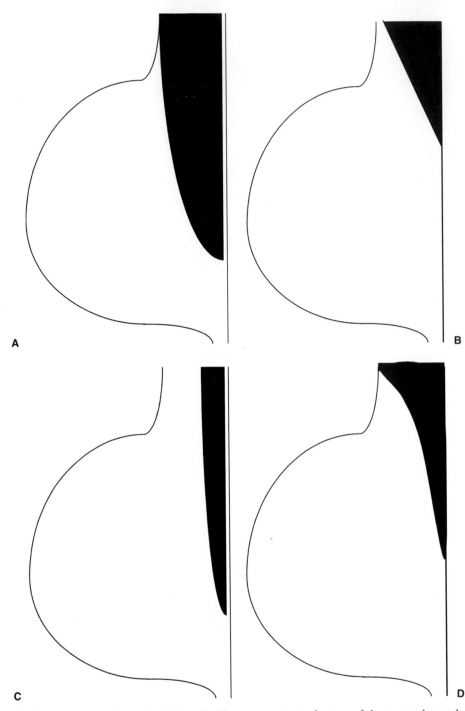

Figure 2.6 *The pectoral muscle and mediolateral oblique views. A.* Evaluation of the pectoral muscle is helpful in assessing positioning on mediolateral oblique views. Ideally, the pectoral muscle is thick at the axilla, has a convex anterior border, and extends to the level of the nipple. To accomplish this, the patient needs to be cooperative, and the technologist needs to match the angle of obliquity to the patient's body habitus. Additionally, the pectoral muscle needs to be relaxed, mobilized medially, and maintained medially as compression is applied. When these principles are not followed, the muscle may be triangular in shape (*B*), be parallel to the edge of the film (*C*), or have a concave anterior margin (*D*).

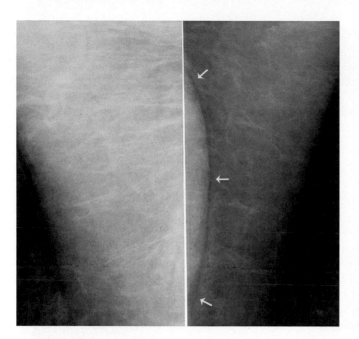

Figure 2.7 *Skin fold.* This skin fold develops laterally as the breast is being mobilized medially. Because the skin fold develops up against the film holder, the technologist does not see it during positioning. The lucency is air outlining the edge of the skin fold (*arrows*). Tissue surrounding skin folds needs to be evaluated carefully for blur. If the skin fold is adequately penetrated and there is no associated blur, it is not absolutely necessary to repeat this image.

should be open, and a small amount of abdomen is included on the image. The technologist should exercise care not to include too much abdomen or to allow a skin fold to develop up against the bucky laterally because this may limit compression (Figure 2.7). A small triangular density, superimposed on the pectoralis major muscle in a small number of women, is the pectoralis minor muscle (Figure 2.8).

In some women, positioning may be limited secondary to a physical disability such as kyphosis, paraplegia, frozen shoulder, Parkinson's disease, or absence of the pectoral muscle (Poland's syndrome) (6) (Figure 2.9). We work closely with these women to obtain the best images possible. We document on the patient's history form the patient's limitations and our efforts to obtain adequate images.

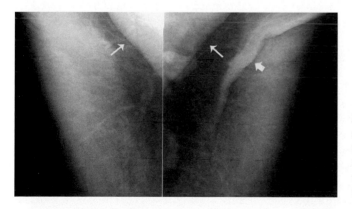

Figure 2.8 *Pectoralis minor muscle.* A triangular density seen superimposed on the pectoral major muscle is the pectoralis minor muscle (*thin arrows*). In this patient, the pectoralis minor muscle is seen bilaterally. A skin fold is noted on the left (*thick arrow*). Also note the air gap with uneven exposure particularly prominent on the left.

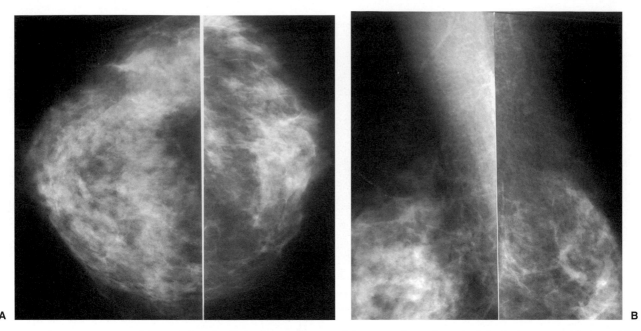

Figure 2.9 *Poland's syndrome. Absence of the pectoral muscle on the left. A.* Craniocaudal views. The left breast is smaller than the right. *B.* Mediolateral oblique views. No pectoral muscle is imaged on the left. As in this patient, the breast on the affected side is usually smaller than the contralateral breast. Other ipsilateral chest wall abnormalities may be seen in patients with Poland's syndrome.

CRANIOCAUDAL VIEWS

In assessing adequacy of positioning on craniocaudal views, pectoral muscle should be seen in 30% to 40% of patients (4) (Figure 2.10A). If pectoral muscle is not seen, look for cleavage (Figure 2.10B). If pectoral muscle or cleavage is seen, you are assured that medial tissue has not be excluded from the image; if neither is seen, consider measuring the posterior nipple line (PNL; discussed later). Laterally, retroglandular fat should be seen; if tissue is seen to the edge of the film, an exaggerated craniocaudal view may be indicated.

Factors to consider in obtaining optimal tissue positioning on CC views are listed in Box 2.6.

In positioning for the CC view, the technologist should work from the medial side of the breast being imaged. As with MLO views, natural breast mobility is used to maximize the amount of tissue included on the images and to minimize skin stretching and tissue exclusion superiorly. The breast is taken at the neutral IMF position, lifted to the natural extent of mobility of the IMF, and pulled out away from the body (4). The bucky should not be placed higher than the elevated IMF position; otherwise, posterior tissue is excluded. As the breast is lifted, the technologist needs to be careful that a skin fold does not develop between the inferior aspect of the breast and the IMF. When present, this skin fold can simulate the pectoral muscle. A sharp lucency (air) outlines the edge of the skin fold but is not seen associated with the pectoral muscle (Figure 2.11). The position of the contralateral breast also needs to be considered. If the contralateral breast is left pendulous, it can be an impediment to the bucky going back against the chest wall. By placing the contralateral breast on the edge of the film holder, the bucky can be properly positioned against the chest wall. The technologist should ascertain that there is no space (air gap) between the chest wall and bucky (film holder); the technologist should not be able to place an index finger through the cleavage area.

The inclusion of medial tissue on CC views needs to be emphasized; however, as much as 2 cm of lateral tissue can be pulled into the image without giving up medial tis-

Maximal tissue inclusion on craniocaudal views requires upward and outward pull of breast tissue as well as active tugging of lateral tissue without giving up any medial tissue.

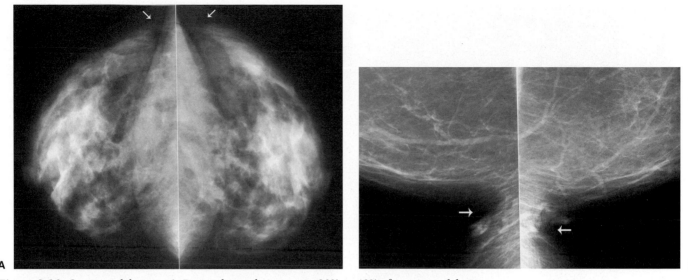

Figure 2.10 *Craniocaudal views. A.* Pectoral muscle is seen in 30% to 40% of craniocaudal views. When pectoral muscle is seen, we are ensured that posterior tissue has been maximally included in the image. Retroglandular fat should be seen laterally (*arrows*). *B.* If pectoral muscle is not seen, look for cleavage (*arrows*). When cleavage is seen on craniocaudal views, we are ensured that medial tissue has not been excluded. It also indicates that the contralateral breast has been positioned appropriately so that the film holder can go back to the chest wall. If neither pectoral muscle nor cleavage is seen, measure the posterior nipple line to ensure that no significant amounts of tissue have been excluded from the craniocaudal view.

sue (Figure 2.12). The lateral aspect of the breast is mobile and has to be pulled actively into the image by the technologist as compression is applied. A skin fold may develop laterally as the technologist pulls lateral tissue in. This skin fold can be rolled out from underneath the paddle without losing tissue.

In some women, the pectoral muscle is atrophied, and only the sternal insertion is seen medially on the CC view. The rounded or triangular appearance of the muscle in these women can simulate a mass (Figure 2.13). Alternatively, a round density seen on the CC view medially can represent the sternalis muscle. In some patients, the sternalis muscle can be seen in conjunction with the pectoral muscle (Figure 2.14). The sternalis muscle is an uncommon normal variant in chest wall musculature; it is a remnant of a muscle that would extend from the infraclavicular region to the caudal aspect of the sternum. It is commonly a unilateral finding. When the MLO is reviewed in these patients, no abnormality is seen.

Measuring the posterior nipple line is helpful in evaluating positioning on craniocaudal views in which no pectoral muscle or cleavage is seen.

Box 2.6: Factors to Consider in Positioning for Craniocaudal Views

Technologist works from medial side of patient
Identify neutral inframammary fold position
   Lift breast up to extent of natural mobility of inframammary fold
Pull breast tissue out
Lateral tug: active pull of lateral tissue into field of view
Contralateral breast up on bucky (not left pendulous)
Bucky back to chest wall

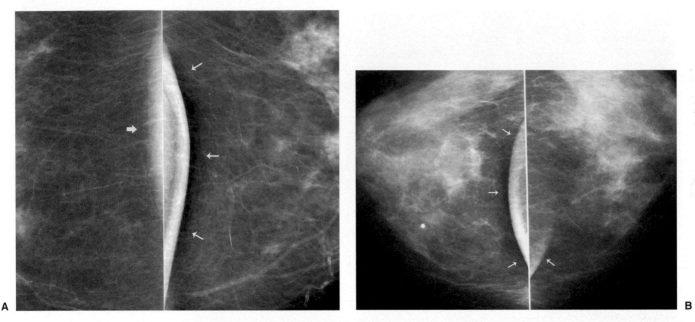

Figure 2.11 *Skin fold. A.* As the breast is mobilized upward, a skin fold can develop inferiorly. This skin fold can simulate the pectoral muscle. If evaluated carefully, however, a lucency (air) outlines the skin fold (*thin arrows*); this is not seen with the pectoral muscle (*thick arrow*). Because the skin fold develops up against the film holder, the technologist does not see it during positioning. *B.* Bilateral skin fold inferiorly (*arrows*). On the right, the skin fold simulates the pectoral muscle; however, because air outlines the edge, a lucency is seen (not seen with pectoral muscle). Skin fold on the left is smaller.

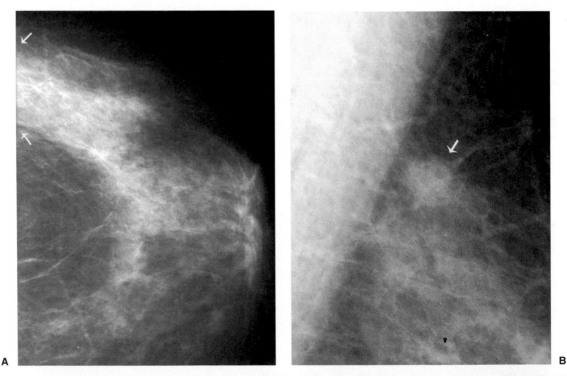

Figure 2.12 *Lateral tug for craniocaudal views. Invasive ductal carcinomas.* Craniocaudal (CC) (*A*) and mediolateral oblique (MLO) (*B*) views. Tissue is seen extending to the edge of the film laterally on the CC view (*arrows*). A density is seen on the MLO view (*arrow*).

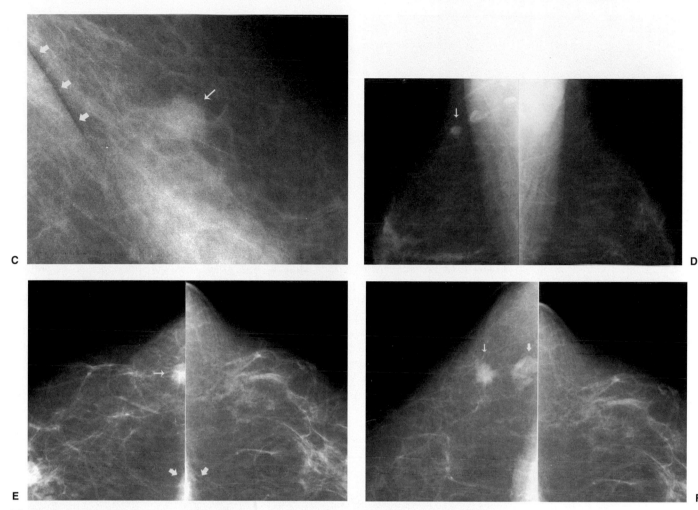

Figure 2.12 **(continued)** *C.* CC view with lateral tug. Having the technologist actively tug on the lateral aspect of the breast brings the mass (*thin arrow*) into the image, and no medial tissue is given up. A skin fold (*thick arrows*) often develops laterally as the technologist tugs the lateral tissue into the field of view. *D.* Different patient. MLO views demonstrate a mass in the right breast (*arrow*). *E.* CC views. Mass is partially seen (*thin arrow*) laterally on the right. Pectoral muscle is seen (*thick arrows*). *F.* Repeat CC view with lateral tug. Mass (*thin arrow*) and additional posterior tissue, including a lymph node (*thick arrow*), are now included on the image. During positioning for CC views, the technologist should actively tug on the lateral aspect of the breast. This will routinely increase the amount of lateral tissue that is imaged.

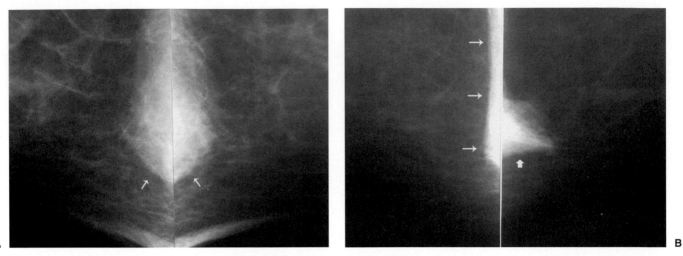

Figure 2.13 *Pectoral muscle insertion, medially.* A. A round, masslike appearance of the pectoral muscle (*arrows*). B. In some patients, the pectoral insertion may have a triangular shape (*thick arrow*). A more characteristic appearance of the pectoral muscle is shown on the right (*thin arrows*).

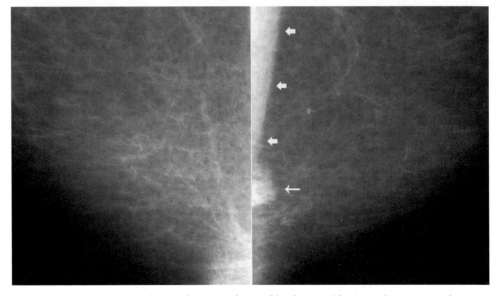

Figure 2.14 *Sternalis muscle.* Rarely, a round, masslike density (*thin arrow*) is seen on the craniocaudal view either in isolation or overlying the pectoral muscle (*thick arrows*), as in this patient. No abnormality is seen on the mediolateral oblique view (not shown).

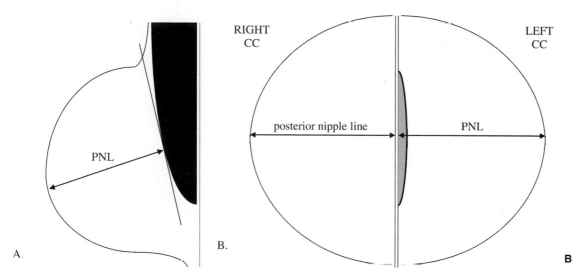

Figure 2.15 *Posterior nipple line.* A. The posterior nipple line (PNL) is used to assess inclusion of posterior tissue on craniocaudal views when pectoral muscle or cleavage is not seen. It is most useful when measured on an optimally positioned mediolateral oblique view. The distance from the nipple to the anterior edge of the pectoral muscle is measured. This is the PNL. B. On the craniocaudal view, the distance from the nipple to the edge of the film is measured. These two measurements should be within 1 cm of each other.

Posterior Nipple Line

The PNL is used to determine whether a significant amount of posterior tissue is excluded when no pectoral muscle or cleavage is seen on the CC view. This is most accurate when measured on a well-positioned MLO view (Figure 2.15A). The distance from the nipple to the anterior edge of the muscle is first measured on the MLO view, then the distance from the nipple to the edge of the film is then measured on the CC view (Figure 2.15B). These two measurements should be within 1 cm of each other. If the PNL measures 10 cm and 8 cm on MLO and CC views, respectively, posterior tissue is excluded on the CC view, and it should be repeated (4,5).

Exaggerated Craniocaudal Views

There are two indications for XCCL views. In the screening setting, when tissue extends to the edge of the film on the CC view after the lateral tug is done and tissue is seen projecting over the upper aspect of the pectoral muscle on the MLO view, an XCCL view is done to image lateral breast tissue in the CC projection (Figure 2.16). In the problem-solving setting, the XCCL projection can be combined with spot compression to evaluate potential lesions in the lateral aspect of the breast (Figure 2.17).

Factors to consider in positioning for XCCL views are listed in Box 2.7.

In positioning for an XCCL view, the woman is asked to rotate slightly so that the film holder is placed at the mid-axillary line. The tube may need to be angled slightly so that the compression paddle clears the humeral head (4). The tube should not, however, be angled more than 5 degrees, and the patient should not be leaned back; otherwise, a shallow oblique rather than a CC view is obtained. If the pectoral muscle seen on the XCCL is prominent, convex, and bulging (like what is seen on MLO views), it is likely that the tube was angled more than 5 degrees or the patient was leaned back during positioning. Factors to consider in assessing adequacy of positioning on XCCL views include seeing the following:

- Retroglandular fat laterally
- Small amount of pectoral muscle laterally

Consider obtaining an XCCL view when tissue extends to the edge of the film on the CC view and tissue projects on the pectoral muscle on the MLO view.

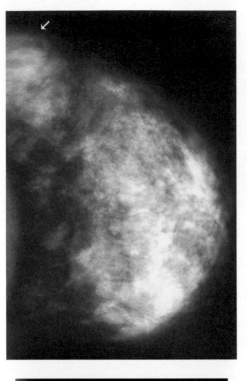

A

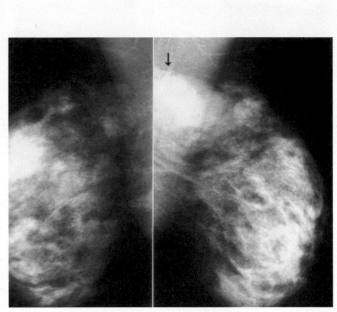

B

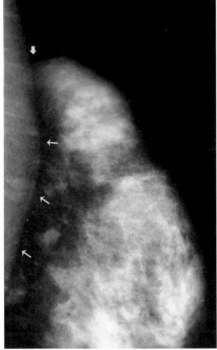

C

Figure 2.16 *Exaggerated craniocaudal view.* Craniocaudal (CC) (*A*) and mediolateral oblique (MLO) (*B*) views are shown. Glandular tissue is seen to the edge of the film on the CC view (*arrow*). On the MLO view, dense tissue is noted superimposed on the left pectoral muscle. Although the lateral tug may add some additional lateral tissue on the CC view, it is unlikely to include this large island of accessory tissue. An exaggerated craniocaudal (XCCL) view is indicated in this patient on the left. *C.* Left XCCL view. On this view, the accessory tissue can be evaluated in the CC projection. Retroglandular fat is now seen (*thick arrow*). A small amount of pectoral muscle (*thin arrows*) is included on all well-positioned XCCL views.

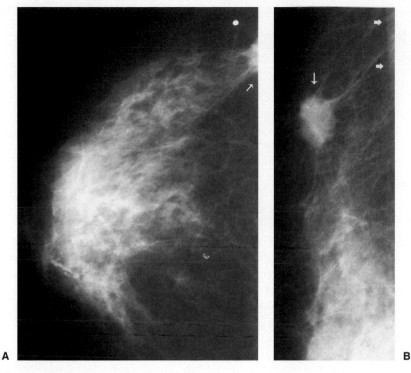

A   B

Figure 2.17 *Exaggerated craniocaudal view. Invasive ductal carcinoma.* Craniocaudal (CC) (*A*) and exaggerated craniocaudal (XCCL) (*B*) views are shown. A mass (*arrow*) is partially seen laterally on the CC view (*arrow*). The mass (*thin arrow*) is seen in its entirety on an XCCL view. Retroglandular fat is now seen. On a well-positioned XCCL view, a small amount of pectoral muscle is seen (*thick arrows*).

Box 2.7: Factors to Consider in Positioning for Exaggerated Craniocaudal Views

Rotate patient slightly
   Film holder placed at midaxillary line
Angle x-ray tube (to clear humeral)
   Not more than 5 degrees
   Do not lean patient back

> ### Box 2.8: Assessing Adequacy of Compression
>
> Blurring (motion) (Fig. 2.18)
> Uneven exposure (Fig. 2.19)
> Inadequate exposure (Fig 2.20)
> Poor separation of parenchymal densities (Fig. 2.21)

COMPRESSION AND ANTERIOR COMPRESSION VIEWS

Specifically evaluate images for adequacy of compression. Look for blurring, uneven or inadequate exposure, and poor separation of parenchymal densities.

Maximal tissue compression is ideal for optimal image quality (4,5). As breast tissue is thinned, optimal exposure with lower radiation doses is facilitated, and scatter radiation, a deterrent to optimal contrast, is reduced. Immobilization of the breast minimizes geometric unsharpness, and as tissue is thinned, superimposition is decreased so that lesions can become more apparent. Detrimental effects on image quality related to inadequate compression are listed in Box 2.8. These effects can be focal or involve the entire image (Figures 2.18 to 2.21).

In evaluating images for blurring, it is important to prepare your brain to see it; otherwise, it may go undetected. For detection of blurring, consider the following (Figure 2.22):

- Trabecular pattern: is it sharp? (Figure 2.18A)
- Pectoral muscle edge: is it sharp? (Figure 2.18A)

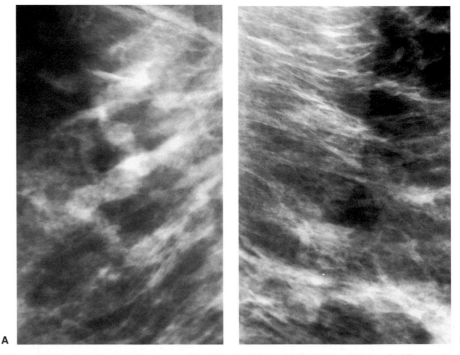

A   B

Figure 2.18 *Geometric unsharpness (blur).* Right (*A*) and left (*B*) mediolateral oblique views. Compare the trabecular pattern and pectoral muscle edges on these two images. There is blurring of the trabecula and pectoral muscle edge on the right. Apparent loss of contrast on the right is noted on images with significant blurring. Our brains perceive blur as an apparent loss of contrast. Adequate compression is critical in minimizing the likelihood of motion.

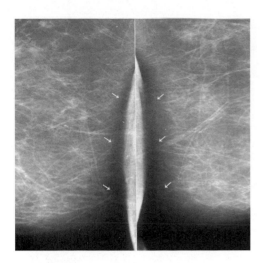

Figure 2.19 *Uneven exposure.* Areas of uneven exposure (*arrows*), in this case secondary to skin folds, can be seen when compression is compromised.

- If there are vessels or calcifications, are they sharp? (Figure 2.23)
- Evaluate subareolar areas
- Evaluate tissue just above the IMF on MLO views

Recognizing factors that can limit compression is important in preventing suboptimal studies and troubleshooting blurry images. Potential limiting factors to adequate compression include the following:

- Patient issues
- Breast thickness
- Prominent pectoral muscles
- Inclusion of other body parts (upper arm, chin, abdomen)
- Skin folds

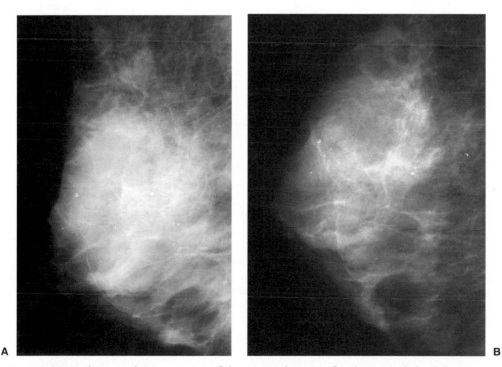

A   B

Figure 2.20 *Underexposed image.* A. One of the potential causes of underexposed glandular tissue is suboptimal compression. B. Repeat image with improved compression. Marked improvement in the exposure of the glandular tissue is noted.

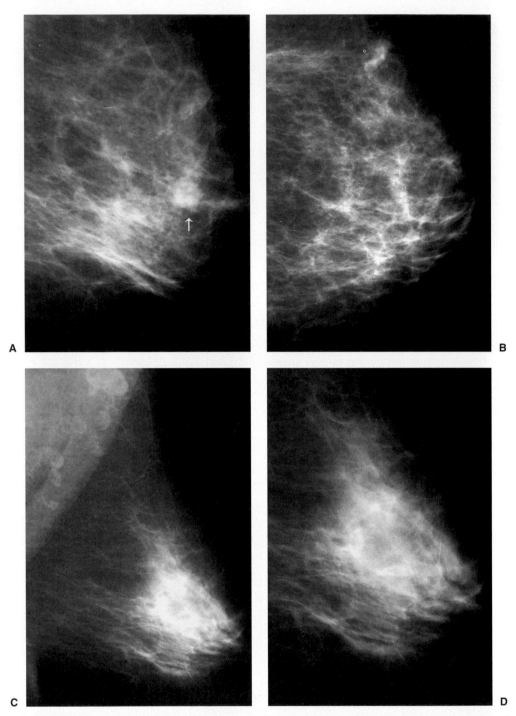

Figure 2.21 *Poor separation of parenchyma. A.* Mediolateral oblique (MLO) view. Poor separation of parenchymal tissue is noted anteriorly, and there is the suggestion of a lesion (*arrow*). Also note relative underexposure of tissue and poor contrast. *B.* Anterior compression view obtained by the technologist at the time of the screening study. Parenchyma is now adequately compressed. No abnormality is present. Tissue is better exposed, and contrast is improved. Patient recall was averted. *C.* Different patient, MLO view. Thick, prominent pectoral muscle, limiting compression of anterior tissue, and poor separation of parenchyma are seen. *D.* Photographic cone down, anterior portion of MLO view. Poor separation of parenchymal densities, underexposure, and poor contrast reflect inadequate compression of tissue anteriorly.

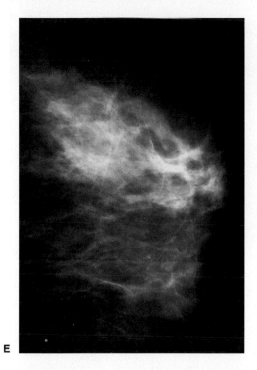

E

Figure 2.21 (continued) *E.* Anterior compression view obtained by the technologist at the time of the screening study. Tissue is now well compressed. Exposure and contrast are improved. Suboptimal compression can lead to missing lesions or calling patients back for technically inadequate studies.

- Technique used for exposure
- Aging compression paddle

The technologist needs to work closely with the patient. Although the importance of compression is explained and the amount of time the breast is compressed is approximated, the patient is made to feel in charge of how much compression is applied; when she finds it uncomfortable, compression can be stopped (4). If the patient's breast discomfort is cyclical, scheduling the exam when her breast tissue is less sensitive may be helpful. Alternatively, the patient can try taking an analgesic half an hour to an hour before the mammogram to decrease any associated discomfort.

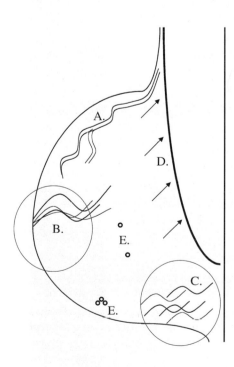

Figure 2.22 *Detection of motion.* It is important to evaluate images for blurring. Do not settle for images with blur because lesions are easily "tomogramed" off the image. Specifically evaluate vascular structures (*A*), the subareolar and inframammary fold areas (*B*, *C*), the pectoral muscle edge (*D*), and calcifications (*E*) (if any are present). Are these structures sharp? Is there an apparent loss of contrast?

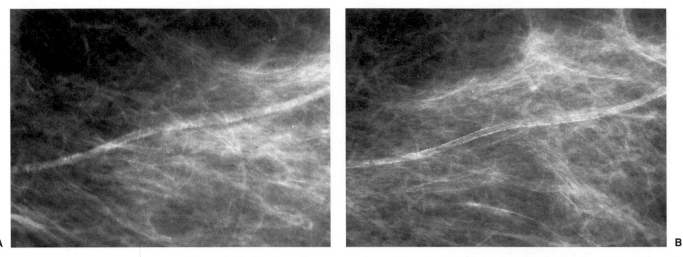

Figure 2.23 *Motion, effect on vascular calcification.* A. This image shows blurring of vessel, associated calcifications that are difficult to recognize, and apparent loss of contrast. B. Repeat image with no motion demonstrates sharp vessel with associated calcification. In evaluating images for blur, specifically look at vessels and any calcifications. Do they look sharp?

The breast is a conical structure with the base as the thickest part. Consequently, as compression is applied, the base of the breast is the factor that limits compression. If the base of the breast is thick, anterior tissue may be inadequately compressed (Figure 2.24). Likewise, in women with prominent pectoral muscles, the thick muscle may limit compression. In these women, obtaining an anterior compression view may be indicated so that evaluation of anterior tissue is optimized. For anterior compression views, the compression paddle is moved forward off the base of the breast, or the pectoral muscle, so that

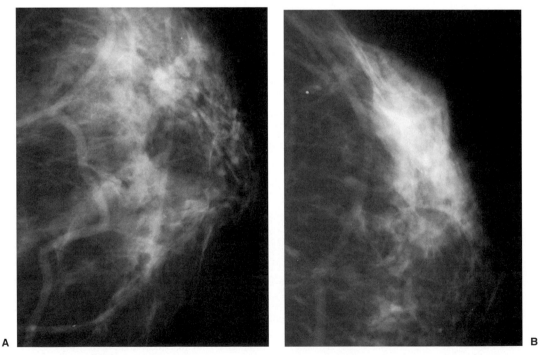

Figure 2.24 *Poor compression. Anterior compression view. Invasive ductal carcinoma.* Craniocaudal (CC) (A) and mediolateral oblique (MLO) (B) views (5.6 cm of compression). The base of the breast is thick. Poor separation of parenchymal densities anteriorly.

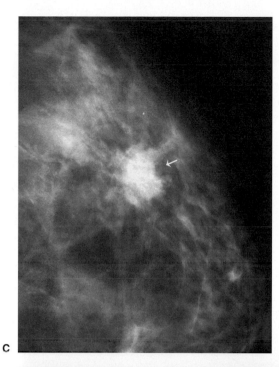

C

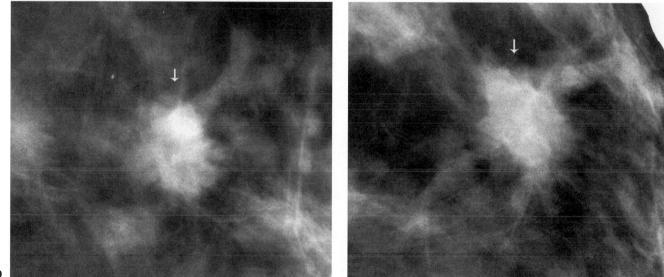

D   E

Figure 2.24 (continued) C. Anterior compression (4.4 cm of compression) in the craniocaudal projection obtained by the technologist as part of the screening study. A possible lesion (*arrow*) is detected on this image. The CC (*D*) and MLO (*E*) spot compression views (3.4 cm of compression) confirm the presence of a spiculated mass, which would not have been seen on the suboptimally compressed routine views. Technologists should be encouraged to obtain anterior compression views if, during positioning, they determine that the anterior aspect of the breast is inadequately compressed.

maximal compression of anterior tissue is obtained. In some patients, anterior compression views can be done using a spot compression paddle.

Interposition of other body parts (e.g., chin, upper arm) between the compression paddle and the bucky can compromise compression. Uneven exposures, or blurring, can be seen in these images limited to the upper portion of the breast on the MLO views. If the chin or arm is visible on the image, focus your attention on the upper part of the breast to ensure that image quality has not been compromised. If the breast is sagging (Figure 2.25), too much abdomen (Figure 2.26) is included on the image, or a skin fold is seen posterolaterally on the MLO view, compression may be compromised, particularly in the area of the IMF. Uneven exposure (Figure 2.26) and blurring, limited to tissue just above the IMF, can sometimes be seen in these patients. Large skin folds can also lead to inadequate compression and often result in uneven exposures.

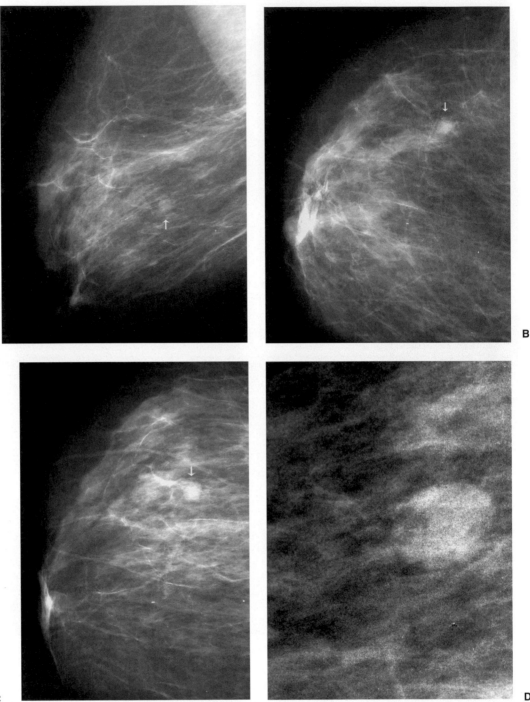

Figure 2.25 *Poor compression, sagging breast. Invasive ductal carcinoma with ductal carcinoma* in situ *of the micropapillary and cribriform type, low nuclear grade. A.* Mediolateral oblique (MLO) view (7.5 cm of compression; 32 kV; 122 mAs) in a 72-year-old patient with large breasts, prominent pectoral muscle, and sagging of anterior portion of breast shows poor separation of parenchyma densities. The nodule (*arrow*) is not readily appreciated on this view. *B.* Craniocaudal (CC) view showing a mass (*arrow*) not seen on prior studies (not shown). *C.* Anterior compression (5 cm of compression; 27 kV; 75 mAs), MLO projection obtained by the technologist as part of the screening study. Anterior tissue is now well compressed. Mass can now be seen (*arrow*). MLO (*D*) and CC (*E*) spot compression views show a mass with indistinct margins. *F.* Solid round mass (*arrow*) seen sonographically corresponding to the mass seen mammographically. A new solid mass in a 72-year-old patient warrants biopsy. Ultrasound guided biopsy was done.

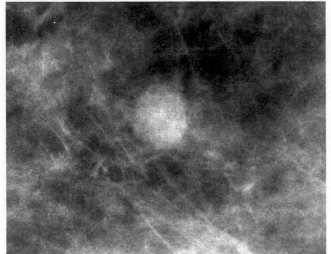
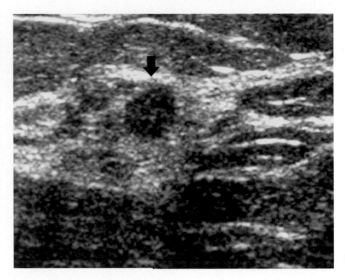

E   F

Figure 2.25 (continued)

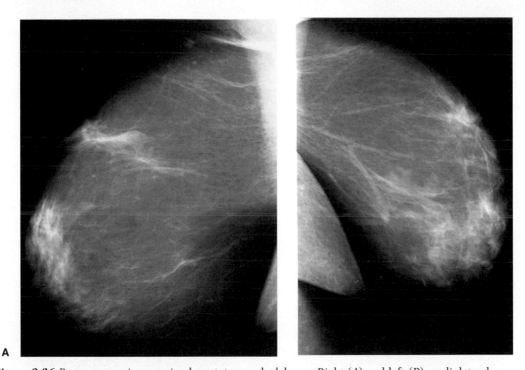

A   B

Figure 2.26 *Poor compression; sagging breast, too much abdomen.* Right (*A*) and left (*B*) mediolateral oblique views demonstrate sagging of breast anteriorly and too much abdomen included on the images. Notice uneven exposure in the area of the inframammary fold, consistent with suboptimal compression. Anterior compression views are indicated.

IMAGING WOMEN WITH IMPLANTS

In women with implants, four views of each breast are done: CC and MLO views with the implants in the field of view and CC and MLO views with the implants displaced out of the field of view. A minimal amount of compression is used for the images with the implants in the field of view—just enough to immobilize the breast (7). On these images,

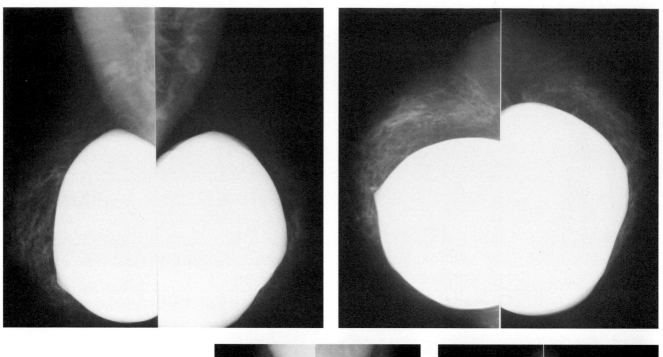

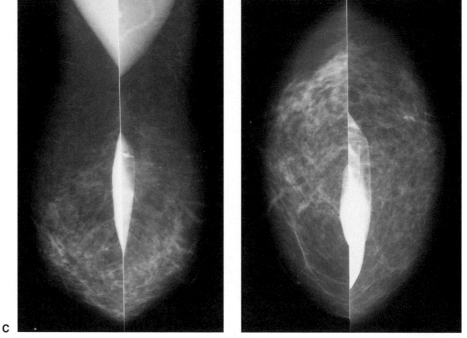

Figure 2.27 *Implants, subglandular location.* Mediolateral oblique (*A*) and craniocaudal (*B*) views with the implant in the field of view. Mediolateral oblique (*C*) and craniocaudal (*D*) views following implant displacement.

the implants are the limiting factor to compression. Consequently, increasing compression of the implant only serves to increase tissue superimposition and underexposure. The implants impinge and push out on the tissue, trapping it against the skin.

For the implant-displaced views, anterior and lateral tissue is pulled out away from the implant while the implant is pushed back toward the chest wall. Compression is applied over tissue with the implants out of the field of view (7). Depending on the location of the implants (e.g., subglandular or subpectoral) and the amount of encapsulation, variable amounts of tissue are imaged on displaced views (Figure 2.27). As a general rule,

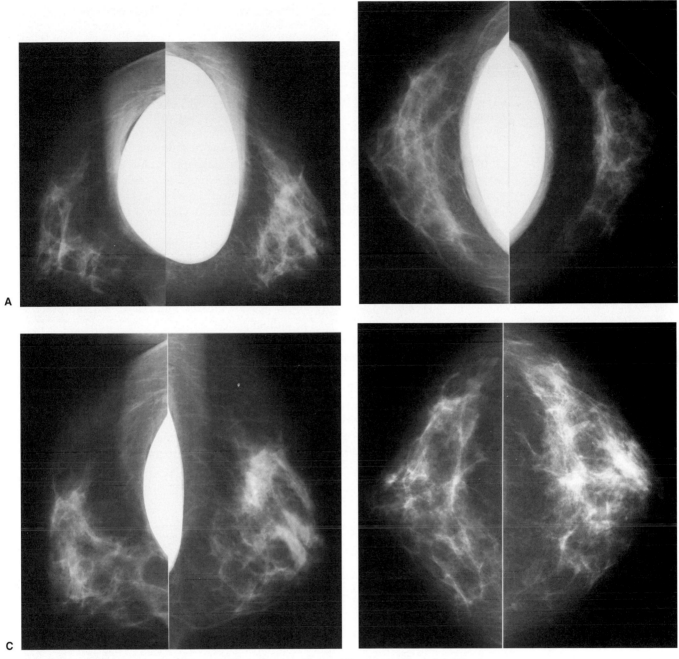

Figure 2.28 *Implants, subpectoral location.* Mediolateral oblique (*A*) and craniocaudal (*B*) views with implants in the field of view. Pectoral muscle can be seen as a density around the implants. Mediolateral oblique (*C*) and craniocaudal (*D*) views with implant displacement views.

more tissue is imaged when the implants are subpectoral in location (Figure 2.28). With subglandular implants and significant encapsulation, tissue visualization may be limited significantly.

CONTRAST AND EXPOSURE

High-contrast images are critical in the quest to identify small breast cancers (5). Depending on the energy of the x-rays used for an exposure, different tissue types absorb different amounts of radiation. The amount of radiation absorbed by 1 cm of tissue at different kiloelectron volts is quantified by using linear attenuation coefficients. Lower-photon x-rays are used in mammography because the linear attenuation coefficients of fat, glandular tissue, and breast cancers are more distinct than the linear attenuation coefficients of these tissues at higher-proton energies.

The final contrast seen on an image is a function of subject and film contrast. Subject contrast is independent of film contrast. It reflects radiation absorption differences of the tissues being imaged and varies depending on the quality of the radiation beam and the amount of scatter radiation (Figure 2.29). Radiation absorption differences depend on the amount of tissue compression, tissue thickness, and atomic number. The quality of the radiation used is dependent on the target material, kilovoltage, and filtration. Scatter radiation is minimized by the use of grids, maximal compression, selected kilovoltage, and collimation. Film contrast is dependent on subject contrast, scatter radiation, film and screen type used, correct film orientation in the cassette (Figure 2.30), processing, photographic density, and fog.

Ideally, the peak kilovoltage selected is as low as possible to obtain an adequate exposure (Figure 2.31). In some patients, a high peak kilovoltage is needed to penetrate the tissue adequately; however, this is obtained at the expense of contrast. Lower kilovoltage peaks, however, are associated with higher radiation doses; as the peak kilovoltage is lowered, the penetrating power of the x-ray beam decreases, and scatter radiation increases. Beam intensity is controlled by the milliamperage output. As milliamperage output is increased, exposure times decrease, and the optical density of the film increases (e.g., darker film). When the density setting is changed, milliamperage remains constant, but exposure time is changed. Each step in density setting changes the milliamperage by 12% to 15%. Film optical density in areas of glandular tissue should be 1.4 to 1.6 and should never be less than 0.7.

Glandular tissue needs to be adequately exposed. When phototiming images, the photocell needs to be positioned correctly under the glandular tissue (Figure 2.32). Maximizing compression and selecting a kilovoltage peak high enough to penetrate through the

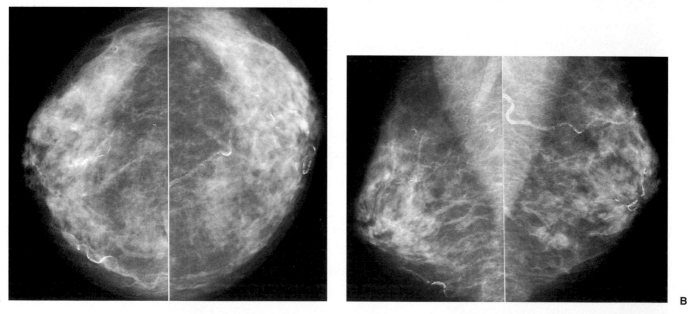

Figure 2.29 *Poor contrast.* Craniocaudal *(A)* and mediolateral oblique *(B)* views show poor contrast. The fatty tissue appears gray, and there is visualization of the skin line and subcutaneous fat. This is a "pancake" breast. There is not much that can be done to improve the contrast in this type of a situation. This reflects "poor" subject contrast. The kilovoltage (23 kV) is as low as possible, with a low milliamperage (32 mAs) and marked thinning of the breast (1.5 cm of compression). Incidentally noted is vascular calcification.

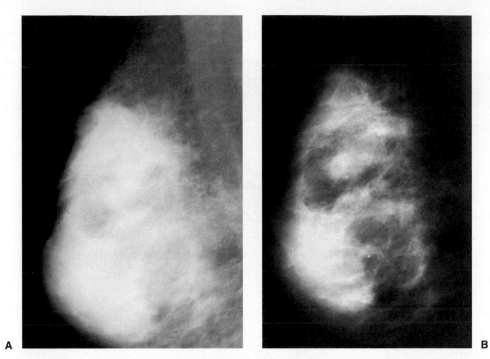

A   B

Figure 2.30 *Poor contrast; film upside down in cassette.* A. Low-contrast, low-resolution image. Gray image (note appearance of fatty tissue) with inadequate exposure. B. Repeat high-contrast image. Mammography film is single emulsion film and must be placed in the cassette correctly with the emulsion side of the film in direct contact with the screen. Ideally, it is recommended that 15 minutes be allowed between loading film into the cassettes and taking images. This allows the film to settle into full contact with the screen.

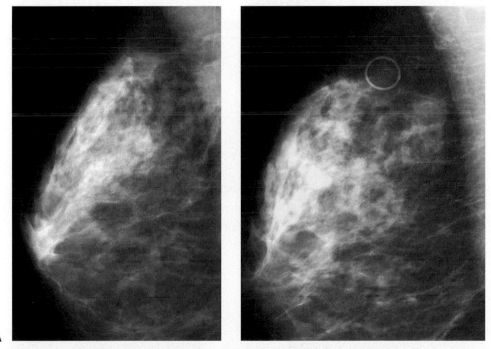

A   B

Figure 2.31 *Suboptimal contrast. Effect of kilovoltage.* A. Mediolateral oblique (MLO) view demonstrating suboptimal contrast with gray fatty tissue (27 kV; 27 mAs). Given the low milliamperage, exposure time is not an issue. The kilovoltage can be lowered to improve contrast. B. Repeat MLO view showing improved contrast. Compare the differences in the appearance of the fatty tissue (25 kV; 200 mAs). The selection of kilovoltage is a balancing act. It needs to be high enough to penetrate the glandular tissue; however, as it is increased, contrast decreases. The kilovoltage should be as low as possible to obtain an adequate exposure with no blurring (i.e., as it is lowered, exposure times increase). Round radio-opaque matter is on a skin lesion.

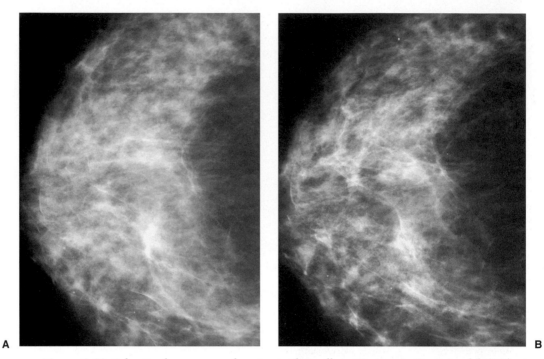

A   **B**

Figure 2.32 *Suboptimal exposure and contrast. Photocell positioning. A.* Craniocaudal (CC) view demonstrates underexposure and poor contrast. The photocell was placed closest to the chest wall. *B.* In this repeat CC view, with repositioning of the photocell, glandular tissue is now well exposed, and contrast is optimal.

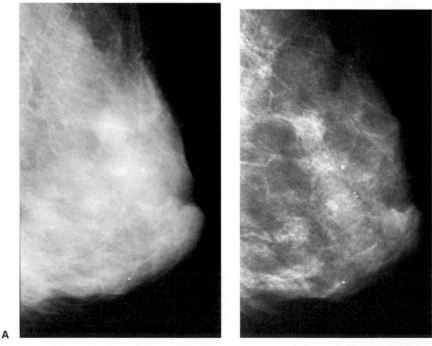

A   **B**

Figure 2.33 *Inadequate exposure. A.* Left mediolateral oblique view. Glandular tissue is inadequately penetrated. *B.* Repeat image demonstrating improved exposure of glandular tissue. Multiple clusters of calcifications are now apparent. In a well-exposed image, the trabecular pattern and vasculature should be seen through the glandular tissue. Do not settle for underexposed images and hide behind disclaimers. Some cases of purportedly extremely dense, heterogeneous tissue reflect inadequate exposure rather than truly dense tissue. Troubleshoot underexposed images. It may require increases in kilovoltage or compression (in some patients, using the spot compression paddle may help). Verify photocell positioning to make sure the photocell is under glandular tissue and not fat.

tissue are critical. In most women, adequate exposure of the glandular tissue results in the burning out of skin and subcutaneous tissue. With an adequate exposure, trabeculae, small tubular structures, and vessels are seen through the glandular tissue (Figure 2.33).

ARTIFACTS

Artifacts are defined as density variations in an image that do not reflect true attenuation differences in the patient (Figures 2.34 to 2.40). Artifacts can originate from the x-ray

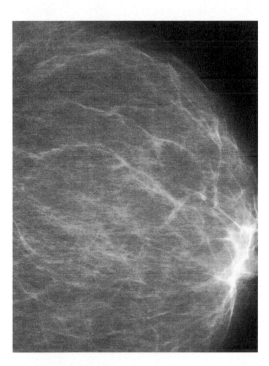

Figure 2.34 *Artifact. Grid lines.* Malfunction of the grid is depicted.

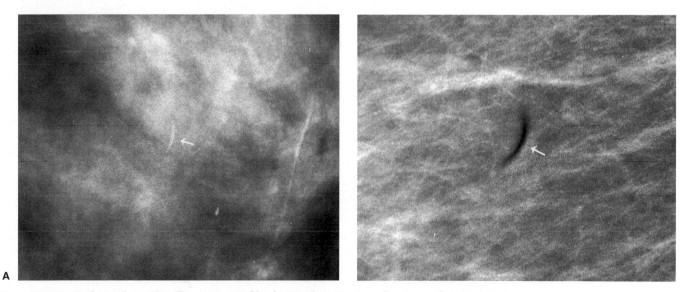

A   B

Figure 2.35 *Artifact. Film mishandling; crimp in film from nail.* A. Negative-density artifact (*arrow*) reflects improper film handling or pressure before exposure. The film is bent at this site. B. Positive-density artifact (*arrow*) usually reflects improper film handling or pressure after the latent image is taken but before the film is processed. The film is bent at this site.

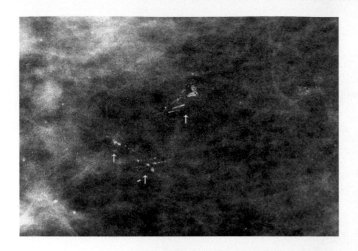

Figure 2.36 *Artifact. Moisture.* Negative-density artifact (*arrows*). The cassette was incompletely dried after cleaning.

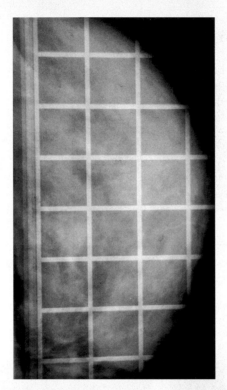

Figure 2.37 *Artifact. Upside-down cassette.* The cassette was incorrectly placed.

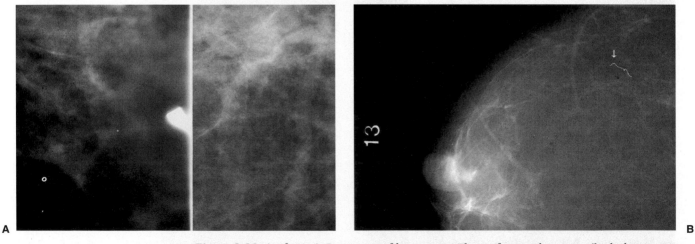

Figure 2.38 *Artifacts. A.* Poor screen-film contact. The artifact on the screen (high-density material) precludes good contact between the film and screen. Blurring around the artifact reflects the fact that the film is slightly lifted off the screen by the artifact. *B.* Lint (*arrow*) artifact on the screen. The cassette number (13) is helpful in identifying the cassette that needs to be cleaned.

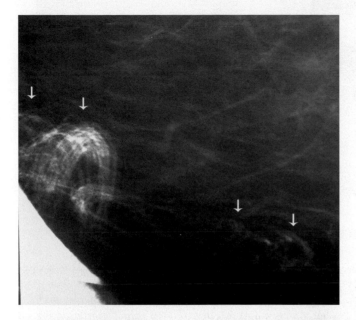

Figure 2.39 *Artifact.* Hair (*arrows*) commonly results in a swirl pattern, as seen in this patient.

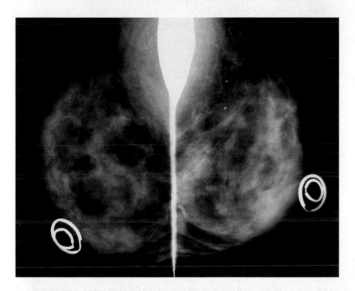

Figure 2.40 *Artifact.* Nipple rings and subpectoral implants are seen.

equipment (Box 2.9), cassette, film handling and screen (Box 2.10), processor (Box 2.11), and patient (Box 2.12) (8,9). Positive-density artifacts are dark and usually reflect improper film handling or pressure after exposure but before the film is processed. Negative-density artifacts are light (white) and commonly reflect improper film handling or pressure before the latent image is taken (e.g., before film exposure). These can also occur during processing (e.g., at pickoff) (8,9).

Box 2.9: X-ray Equipment–Related Artifacts

Filter (corrosion or damage)
Lip of compression paddle
Image receptor holder
Grid (Fig. 2.34)

Box 2.10: Cassette, Film Handling, and Screen-Related Artifacts

Film scratches
Nail dents (Fig. 2.35)
Finger pressure (fingerprints)
Moisture (Fig. 2.36)
Loading of film incorrectly (e.g., upside down) (Fig. 2.30)
Loading of cassette incorrectly (upside down) (Fig. 2.37)
Fog
Static
Foreign object on screen (poor film screen contact) (Fig. 2.38)

Box 2.11: Processor-Related Artifacts

Entrance roller marks (plus density; evenly spaced)
Guide shoe marks (plus or minus density; evenly spaced; leading or trailing edge of film)
Delay streaks (plus or minus density; random)
Stub or hesitation lines (plus density; $1\frac{5}{8}$ inch from leading edge of film)
Chatter (plus density; evenly spaced)
Slap lines (plus density, $2\frac{1}{8}$ to $2\frac{1}{4}$ inch from trailing edge of film)
Water spots
Wet pressure marks
Runback
Pick off

Box 2.12: Patient-Related Artifacts

Deodorant
Talc on skin
Hair, hair products (Fig. 2.39)
Jewelry (nipple rings) (Fig. 2.40)
Tattoos
Other body parts projecting on image

SCREENING

Screening and diagnostic studies should be approached differently and, ideally, should be spatially or temporally separated. Screening is for detection of potential lesions. Diagnostic studies are for characterization of lesions.

Screening and diagnostic studies should be approached differently. The purpose of screening is the detection of potential abnormalities, not characterization. There are different ways to increase the efficiency of the interpreting radiologist, maximize lesion detection, and minimize the number of women called back for additional studies. Although a discussion of all the viable strategies is beyond the scope of this text, we will discuss some of the issues to consider.

We have pulled all breast imaging studies out of the patient's master jacket. A separate file room for the Breast Center has been created for films, including breast ultrasounds (filmed on 8×10-cm film), are filed in a small jacket. This allows us more control over the breast imaging studies so that films and patient information are readily available for consultations. We have sign in and out methods in place to document the number of outgoing or incoming films. Having these films in a separate jacket is also helpful in handling film purging. Laws governing the purging of mammography films may vary compared with those for other x-rays. Under MQSA, facilities must keep medical records and films for 5 years, or 10 years if no additional mammograms are done, on a patient (1). This timeframe may be longer under state or local law.

Spatial separation, or if this not possible, temporal separation of screening and diagnostic studies should be undertaken; different tactics are used for each. One of the most critical, ongoing tasks is to educate referring physicians and patients about the differences between screening and diagnostic studies. Screening is undertaken in asymptomatic women. No radiologist need be on site when screening studies are done. Diagnostic studies are done in patients who have either an abnormal screening mammogram or signs and symptoms possibly indicating the presence of a cancer. A radiologist should always be available to monitor diagnostic studies. A set schedule with rapid throughput and minimal overhead costs is important for the screening program, particularly given the low reimbursement rates for this type of study. The configuration of the mammography and dressing rooms is important in obtaining these goals. Ideally, the mammography room is not used as the dressing room. Although discussed at greater length in Chapter 3, flexibility is critical for the diagnostic program.

With respect to interpretation, we interpret all of our screening studies in batches. The current study is loaded on high-luminance view boxes with the study from 2 years ago for comparison. The patient's jacket with other prior studies is available to us above the view box, organized in the same sequence used to load the studies. Current history forms are available, as are prior history forms and pathology reports on those patients who underwent a previous breast biopsy. The films are presented in a standardized manner on high-luminance view boxes that enable us to cone down around the films as needed to eliminate extraneous light. Ambient light and other distractions are eliminated. Paperwork is minimized, and only a few (less than 1%) of the screening studies are actually dictated. We use standardized ("canned") normal reports for about 93% of our patients, including women with implants. We also use standardized reports for those patients in whom a potential abnormality is seen and we are requesting additional views. A bar code on the requisition form for the study is used to bring up the patient's demographic information on a computer screen next to our view box. The report to be used is selected from the list of canned reports, and with one keystroke, that report is finalized and automatically faxed to the referring physician. This has allowed us to significantly reduce the need for transcription services and has decreased report turn-around times (reports do not go back to the radiologist for final approval).

Consider batch interpretation of screening studies.

EVALUATION OF IMAGES

In evaluating images, consider adopting two principles: develop a standardized way of approaching mammogram films, and prepare your brain to find abnormalities ("chance favors a prepared mind"), for many patients, in specific locations (9). Evaluate the current study fully before looking at prior films. Although prior studies can be extremely useful (Figure 2.41), they can sometimes create a false sense of security relative to findings that should be pursued (Figure 2.42), and would be pursued, if you did not have the previous films (e.g., stability does not ensure benignity).

As a starting point, evaluate the images for overall quality. Set the height of the quality bar at your center: the higher you set it, the better the quality of the images generated

In interpreting screening studies, consider developing a standardized approach, and send your brain out looking for specific abnormalities and evaluating specific locations.

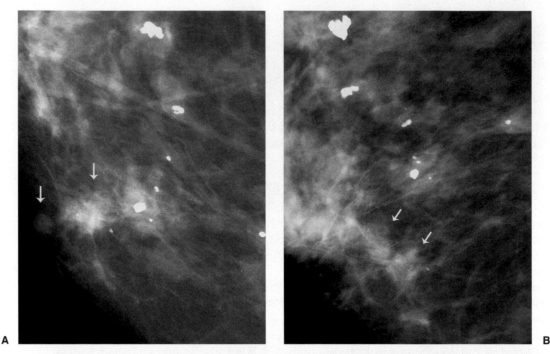

Figure 2.41 *Previous films. Invasive ductal carcinoma.* Craniocaudal (*A*) and mediolateral oblique (*B*) views show scattered benign, coarse calcifications consistent with hyalinized fibroadenomas. At least one mass is noted medially (*arrows*).

Before interpreting a study, assess image quality. Evaluate adequacy of positioning, compression, contrast, and exposure. There should be no blurring, nor a significant number of artifacts. Do not settle for suboptimal images.

Rather than looking at the entire image during interpretation, focus your evaluation by splitting the images into thirds and reviewing those areas where cancers are likely to develop or may be troublesome.

at your facility. Set it high and watch your technologist rise to the occasion time and time again. If you determine the films to be of interpretable quality, then evaluate the images for gross findings (e.g., breast size, parenchymal asymmetry, diffuse changes). Follow this with a closer inspection of the images. Using a magnifying lens, scrutinize the images, specifically looking for calcifications, masses, or distortion; do not sit passively waiting for abnormalities to jump out. Also, rather than viewing the entire image, systematically evaluate the upper, middle, and inferior portions of the breast on the MLO views and the lateral, middle, and medial portions on the CC views (Figure 2.43). Go back and forth from one side to the other. If there are obvious findings, do not focus on them to the exclusion of the remaining tissue and contralateral breast. Obvious findings serve as distracters that keep us from identifying the small, potentially curable cancers (Figure 2.44).

In addition to looking for specific findings, look at those areas that are particularly troublesome or in which cancers have a predilection for developing. On the MLO views, evaluate the upper cone of tissue, the lower fatty regions, and the usually fatty strip of tissue between pectoral muscle and glandular tissue (Figure 2.43). If the upper cone of tissue starts to round off (Figure 2.45), or densities begin to develop in these areas, additional views are warranted. On the CC views specifically, evaluate medial (Figure 2.46) and retroglandular tissue, particularly the fat–tissue interface (Figure 2.47). In most women, the medial portion of the breast is relatively fatty. Any developing densities in these areas warrant additional evaluation. Developing distortion or alteration in the contour of the fat–glandular tissue interface posteriorly likewise warrants evaluation. Scrutinize and focus your attention on the subareolar areas. Remember that these areas may be inadequately compressed and are the second most common place for breast cancers to develop (9).

In determining the appropriateness of calling a patient with vague densities (larger than 1 cm) back for additional evaluation, consider the position of the potential lesion and its apparent size (Figure 2.48). The location of a potential lesion on the CC view should be compatible with the location noted on the MLO view. If you see a potential abnormal-

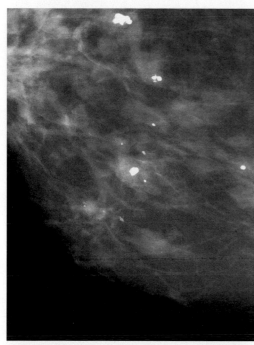

C

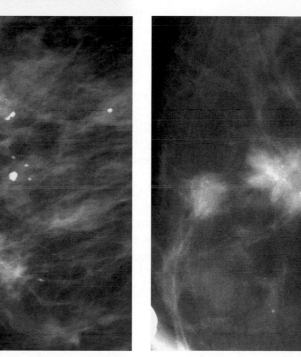

Figure 2.41 (continued) Craniocaudal (*C*) and mediolateral oblique (*D*) views from previous year. Finding represents an interval change. Category 0: incomplete, need additional imaging evaluation. *E.* Spot compression view confirms the presence of two spiculated masses. Imaging-guided biopsy was done.

D

E

ity within a centimeter of the nipple and what concerns you on the MLO is far posteriorly, it is unlikely that these two findings represent the same thing. Also, although there are exceptions (e.g., some invasive lobular carcinomas, complex sclerosing lesions), most lesions are three dimensional. If a 1.5-cm area of concern is noted on one of the screening views, and no comparably sized abnormality is identified on the other view (at the approximate distance from the nipple), it is unlikely to represent a significant finding (Figure 2.49).

On CC and MLO views, potential lesions should be similar in size, and the location of the potential lesion on the CC view should be compatible with the location noted on the MLO.

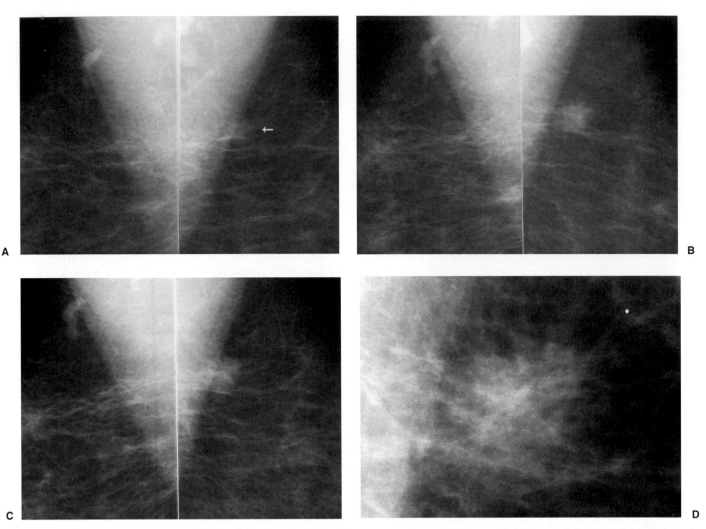

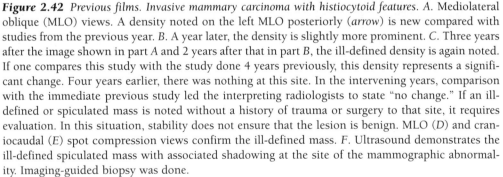

Figure 2.42 *Previous films. Invasive mammary carcinoma with histiocytoid features.* A. Mediolateral oblique (MLO) views. A density noted on the left MLO posteriorly (*arrow*) is new compared with studies from the previous year. B. A year later, the density is slightly more prominent. C. Three years after the image shown in part A and 2 years after that in part B, the ill-defined density is again noted. If one compares this study with the study done 4 years previously, this density represents a significant change. Four years earlier, there was nothing at this site. In the intervening years, comparison with the immediate previous study led the interpreting radiologists to state "no change." If an ill-defined or spiculated mass is noted without a history of trauma or surgery to that site, it requires evaluation. In this situation, stability does not ensure that the lesion is benign. MLO (*D*) and craniocaudal (*E*) spot compression views confirm the ill-defined mass. *F*. Ultrasound demonstrates the ill-defined spiculated mass with associated shadowing at the site of the mammographic abnormality. Imaging-guided biopsy was done.

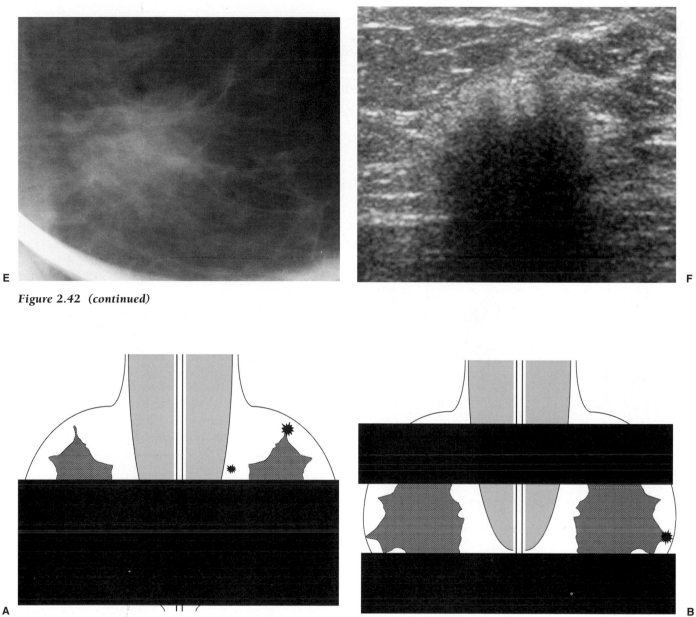

Figure 2.42 (continued)

Figure 2.43 *Image evaluation. A.* On the mediolateral oblique (MLO) views, evaluate the upper third of the images. Go back and forth from one breast to the other. By limiting your field of view in a consistent manner, you enhance the likelihood of detecting subtle changes. *B.* Evaluate the middle portion of the breasts.

(*continued on next page*)

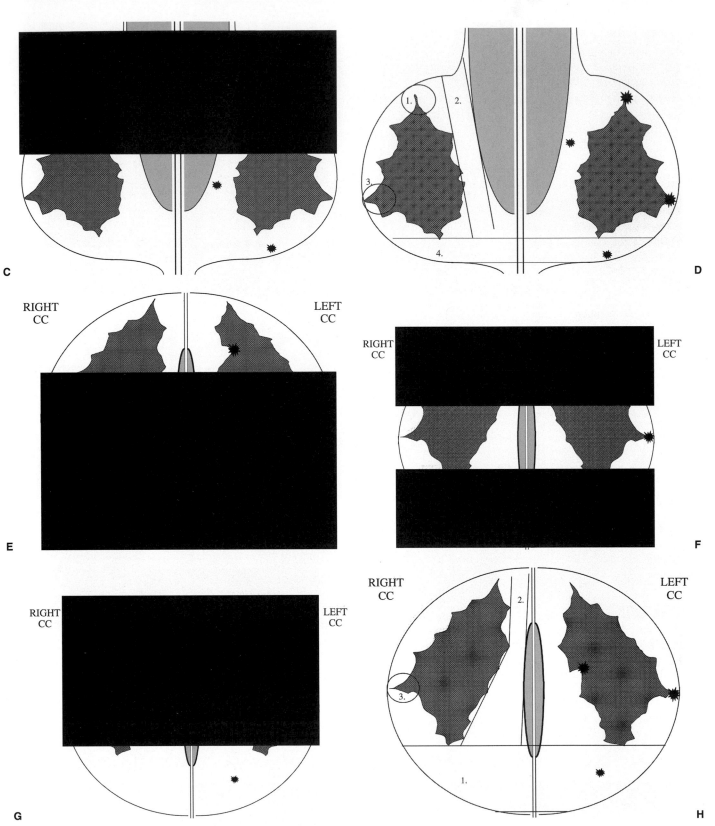

Figure 2.43 (continued)*. C.* Evaluate the lower portion of the breast. *D.* On MLO views, specifically evaluate the upper cone of tissue (1), the usually fatty stripe between glandular tissue and pectoral muscle (2), the subareolar area (3), and the usually fatty stripe inferiorly above the inframammary fold (4). Developing densities or asymmetries in these areas warrant additional evaluation. On the craniocaudal (CC) views, evaluate the lateral portions of the breasts (*E*), the middle portions of the breasts (*F*), and the medial quadrants (*G*). *H.* On the CC views, evaluate the medial quadrants (1) carefully, the retroglandular area, and in particular the fat–glandular tissue interface (2) and the subareolar areas (3).

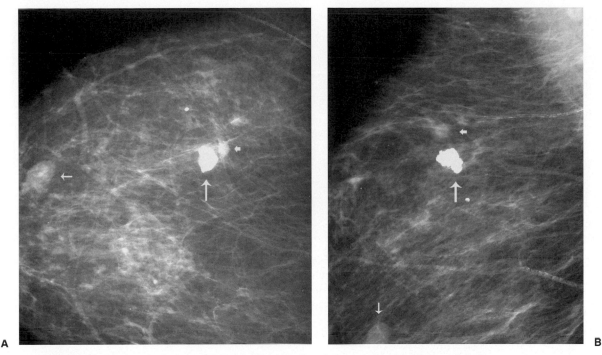

A   B

Figure 2.44 *Invasive ductal carcinoma.* Craniocaudal (*A*) and mediolateral oblique (*B*) views. In this "busy mammogram" bilaterally, only the right side is shown. Popcorn calcification (*long, thin arrow*), oval nodule (*short, thin arrow*), a smaller mass (*short, thick arrow*) adjacent to the popcorn calcification, and vascular calcification are seen. It is easy to be distracted and not notice that the mass (*short, thick arrow*) adjacent to the popcorn calcification has irregular borders and is relatively high in density. Compared with prior studies, this represents a change. When there are obvious benign mammographic findings or the patient presents with a specific concern, be careful not to focus on these to the exclusion of evaluating remaining tissue and the contralateral breast.

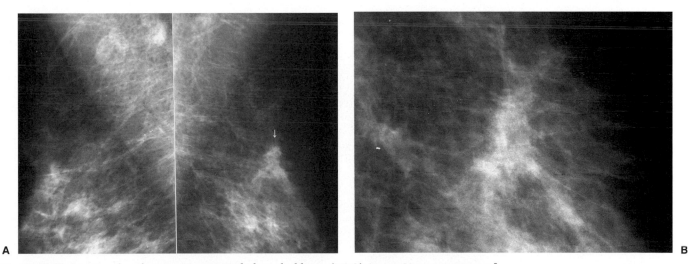

A   B

Figure 2.45 *Invasive ductal carcinoma. A.* Mediolateral oblique (MLO) views. Upper portions of breasts photographed. Notice that the upper cone of tissue on the left (*arrow*) is rounded compared with the right. This warrants additional evaluation. *B.* Spot compression view confirming the presence of an irregular, spiculated mass.

(*continued on next page*)

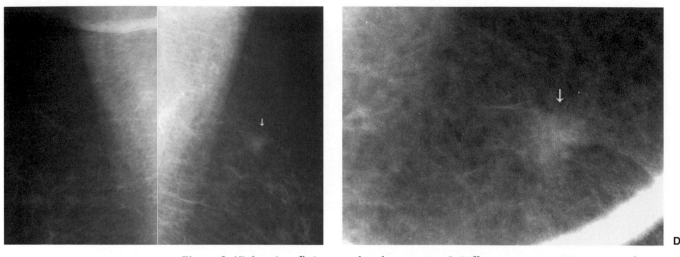

C   D

Figure 2.45 (continued) *Invasive ductal carcinoma. C.* Different patient; MLO views. In the upper portions of the left breast, developing density is seen just anterior to the pectoral muscle (*arrow*). Although it appears to be low density and relatively innocuous, developing densities in this area on MLO views warrant additional evaluation. *D.* Spot compression view confirms an ill-defined mass (*arrow*). Both patients underwent ultrasound-guided core biopsy to establish the diagnosis.

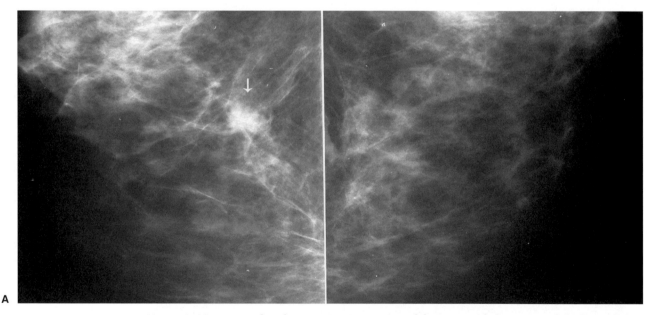

A

Figure 2.46 *Invasive ductal carcinoma. A.* Craniocaudal views; medial portions of the breasts photographed. In the medial portion of the breast, a mass is identified (*arrow*). Developing densities in the medial aspect of the breast usually require additional evaluation.

(*continued on next page*)

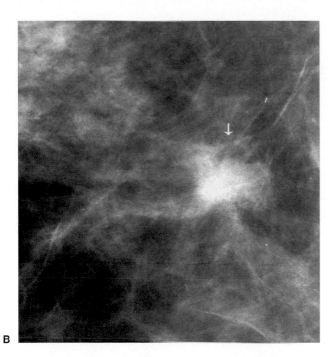

Figure 2.46 (continued) B. Spot compression view confirming the presence of a spiculated mass (*arrow*).

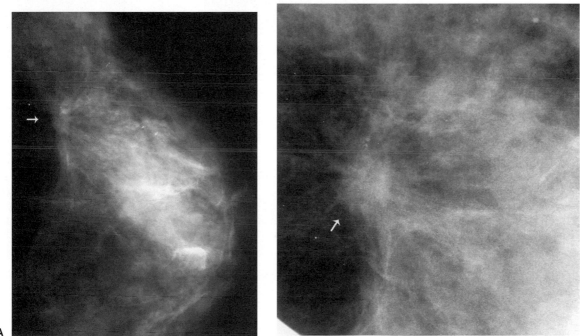

Figure 2.47 *Invasive ductal carcinoma.* A. Craniocaudal view. Always evaluate fat–glandular tissue interface. Tissue is drawn in (*arrow*) with associated straight lines (distortion). B. Spot compression view confirms the presence of a spiculated mass (*arrow*). Imaging-guided biopsy was done.

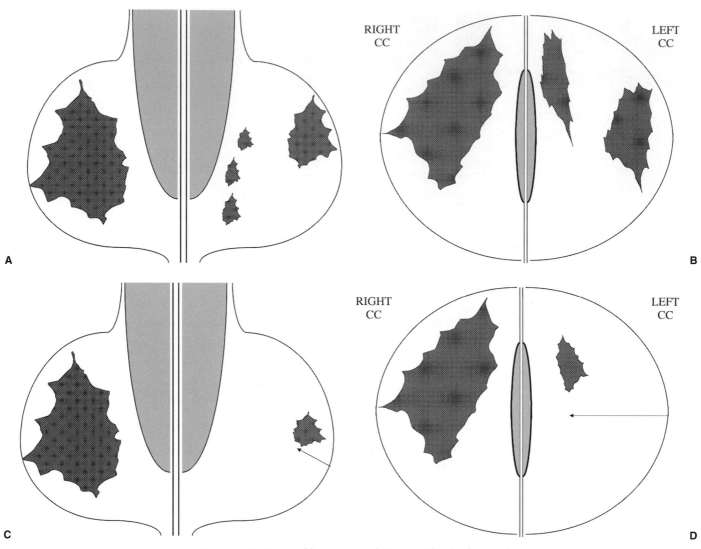

Figure 2.48 *Size and location correlation.* A. Islands of parenchymal asymmetry on the mediolateral oblique (MLO) view. B. On the craniocaudal (CC) view, these islands represent larger islands of parenchymal asymmetry (in summation) that spread out as expected with normal tissue. MLO (C) and CC (D) views. The location of the potential abnormality on the left MLO view does not match the location of what is seen on the CC view.

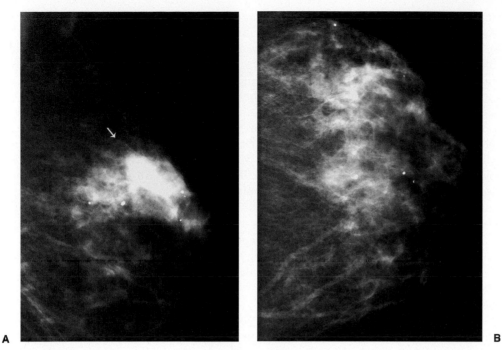

A   **B**

Figure 2.49 Pseudolesion. A. Mediolateral oblique (MLO) view. An area of increased density is noted, potentially representing a lesion (*arrow*). *B.* Craniocaudal (CC) view. The area seen on the MLO view represents the superimposition of tissue that is spread out on the CC view.

CALLBACKS

As mentioned previously, screening studies are for detection, not characterization. Consequently, the only assessment categories we use on screening studies are: 1, negative; 2, benign findings, negative; and 0, incomplete, additional imaging evaluation is needed. We assign category 0 to women in whom we are requesting prior films for comparison or in women in whom we are recommending additional studies. At the time of a screening study, the patient is informed by the technologist of the possibility of a callback for additional evaluation.

Our protocol relative to women in whom prior films are needed requires that these studies be dictated. We do not hold them aside without a dictation waiting for the old films to come in. In a busy practice, putting undictated films aside is fraught with potential problems. We dictate the study after it is hung and classify it as a category 0 study. This sets in motion attempts to procure prior studies and helps keep the referring physician informed. The steps we follow are listed in Box 2.13. Every step taken is documented to show that a reasonable effort has been made to locate prior studies. If prior films are not

---

Box 2.13: Steps Followed in Procuring Prior Studies

At the time of the study, patient signs a release form for outside film/report requests.
Contact the facility listed by the patient.
If unsuccessful, contact the referring physician for a prior film report; this provides the date and name of facility where prior study was done.
If necessary, the patient is contacted to verify site of prior study.

received within 2 weeks after the date of the study, we dictate an addendum and proceed with our recommendations as though the patient had no prior films.

For those women in whom a potential abnormality is identified, the interpreting radiologist qualifies the callback. This is used exclusively as an internal means to communicate with our schedulers about the time slot that should be assigned to that patient. Category 1 callbacks are assigned a 15-minute time slot. For these patients, the radiologist has a low level of concern and thinks that with one or two additional views, the issue will be resolved. Category 2 callbacks are assigned a 30-minute slot. For these patients, the interpreting radiologist believes that additional views and an ultrasound, or additional views and a ductogram, may be needed. Category 3 callbacks are patients for whom the radiologist considers an imaging-guided biopsy a likely possibility. An 1-hour time slot is provided for these patients. This system is not intended to be an exact science but rather an internal effort to control the diagnostic schedule and run it efficiently. The system actually works well and has eliminated bottlenecks as well as slow periods. Most important, it allows us to perform a biopsy at the time the patient returns for her evaluation. This helps expedite patient care by virtually eliminating the need for rescheduling a biopsy or ultrasound and yet does not generate significant delays for other patients. In addition, it helps lessen patient anxiety because most patients, when told of a possible abnormality, want a definitive answer as soon as possible.

As is done by many facilities now, we do our own callbacks. The benefits of the imaging facility scheduling callbacks are immeasurable (10–14). The reason for the callback is communicated appropriately to the patient; if this responsibility is relegated to individuals who do not understand the process, the patient is often misinformed about why more images are needed (e.g., "they didn't get it right and need to repeat your films"). These are not repeat images but rather additional views with special techniques to evaluate a specific area of concern. When we control the callbacks, patients are scheduled in a manner that is convenient for the patient and that allows us to assign appropriate time slots for the individual patient's potential problem. Handling the callbacks ensures that patients are scheduled promptly, often within 1 or 2 days of the screening studies. If a patient cannot be reached, steps are put in motion to attempt to communicate with the patient. If after three attempts within a 48-hour period we are unable to reach the patient, we send a letter (regular mail). If a week later we still have not heard from the patient, we mail a certified letter to the patient with a copy to the referring physician. Every effort made is documented. It is important to be able to show that a reasonable effort was made to communicate directly with the patient. The people who handle the callbacks need to be empathetic, compassionate, and considerate. The patient needs to be informed that, most of the time, nothing significant is found on the additional views. The patient is also told that she will be given her results by a radiologist at the time of her study.

We also print a bimonthly report of all unsettled category 0 patients from our data-tracking system. Each outstanding case is investigated, and a last effort is made to communicate with the patient.

REFERENCES

1. *Quality mammography standards, final rule.* Federal Register, October 28, 1997; 62:55852-55993. Department of Health and Human Services, Food and Drug Administration. 21 CFR, Pt 16, 900.
2. American College of Radiology. *Mammography quality control manual.* Reston, VA: American College of Radiology, 1999.
3. American College of Radiology. *Standard for screening mammography.* Reston, VA: American College of Radiology, 1995.
4. Eklund GW, Cardenosa G. The art of mammographic positioning. *Radiol Clin North Am* 1992; 30:21–53.
5. Eklund GW, Cardenosa G, Parsons W. Assessing adequacy of mammographic image quality. *Radiology* 1994;190:297–307.

6. Samuels TH, Haider MA, Kirkbride P. Poland's syndrome: a mammographic presentation. *AJR Am J Roentgenol* 1996;166:347–348.
7. Eklund GW, Busby RC, Miller SH, et al. Improved imaging of the augmented breast. *AJR Am J Roentgenol* 1988;151:469–473.
8. Widmer JH, Lillie RF, Jaskulski SM, et al. *Identifying and correcting processing artifacts.* Technical and Scientific Monogram 4. Rochester, NY: Eastman Kodak, 1994.
9. Tabar L, Dean PB. *Teaching atlas of mammography*, 3rd ed. New York: Thieme Verlag, 2001.
10. Cardenosa G, Eklund GW. Rate of compliance with recommendations for additional mammographic views and biopsies. *Radiology* 1991;181(2):359–361.
11. Robertson CL, Kopans DB. Communication problems after mammographic screening. *Radiology* 1989;172(2):443–444.
12. Meyer JE, Stomper PC, Lee RR. Pectoralis muscles simulating a breast mass. *AJR Am J Roentgenol* 1989;152:481–482.
13. Bradley FM, Hoover HC, Hulka CA, et al. The sternalis muscle: an unusual normal finding seen on mammography. *AJR Am J Roentgenol* 1996;166:33–36.
14. Haus AG, Jaskulski SM. *The basics of film processing in medical imaging.* Madison, WI: Medical Physics Publishing, 1997.

DIAGNOSTIC BREAST IMAGING

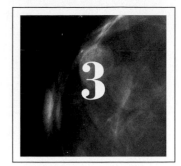

APPROACH TO DIAGNOSTIC BREAST IMAGING

The diagnostic patient population is composed of two groups of patients: those with abnormal screening mammograms requiring additional imaging evaluation, and those who have signs and symptoms of breast disease. Different approaches to diagnostic mammography are available. Our approach has been to develop a consultative breast service such that we run the center more like a clinical practice than a radiology service. We believe that as breast imagers, we are in a unique position to provide a desperately needed comprehensive breast health service. In many communities, breast care is disjointed and provided haphazardly with no standardization by general surgeons, gynecologists, family practitioners, and internists. Having someone who can put things together is quite helpful for patients. As radiologists, we have at our disposal all of the imaging modalities that are critical in the diagnosis and subsequent management of patients. If we complement this with clinical acumen, we can provide a much needed service. Functioning as a team member, we can serve as the pivotal patient care point. We have elected to develop our service with these concepts in mind. The radiologist is a clinical breast imager. Our approach to patients with possible breast cancer is to evaluate them as needed to reassure them of benign findings or low likelihood of malignancy, or to undertake the necessary procedures to establish a definitive diagnosis in a timely manner.

As discussed in Chapter 2, women with potentially abnormal mammograms are scheduled for diagnostic studies in 15-, 30-, and 60-minute slots, depending on the abnormality detected at screening. Our approach to these patients is to do whatever it takes, on their return trip, to arrive at a definitive, justifiable recommendation. In some patients, this may take 1 or 2 additional mammographic images, whereas in others, additional mammographic images, correlative physical examination, ultrasound, and an interventional procedure (e.g., cyst aspiration, ductogram, fine-needle aspiration, or biopsy) may be indicated. For those patients in whom a biopsy is indicated, we offer the patient the option of having it done immediately. Unless requested by the patient, we do not reschedule them for ultrasounds, aspirations, ductograms, or biopsies. About 99% of patients opt for having the biopsy done that same day. The referring physician is always contacted and informed of the patient's decision. Most patients appreciate being offered the option of having the biopsy done that same day.

The diagnostic patient population includes two major groups of women: those with potentially abnormal screening studies, and those with signs or symptoms of breast cancer.

> ### Box 3.1: Imaging Algorithms
>
> **Symptomatic patient** (30 years of age or older) ("lump," focal tenderness, dimpling, nipple retraction)
> - Metallic BB placed at site of concern
> - Craniocaudal views
> - Mediolateral oblique views
> - Spot tangential view at site of concern
> - Physical examination
> - Ultrasound (except if completely fatty tissue is present mammographically)
>
> **Symptomatic patient** (under 30 years of age; pregnant or lactating regardless of age) ("lump," focal tenderness, dimpling, nipple retraction)
> - Physical examination
> - Ultrasound
> - Full mammogram done if cancer is suspected

Our approach to patients presenting for diagnostic studies is to do whatever is needed to arrive at a definitive, justifiable impression and recommendation. In some women, this may require one or several interventional procedures.

Although there are many more projections available to us during diagnostic mammography (e.g., caudocranial, lateromedial oblique, and superolateral to inferomedial oblique views), I have purposely limited the discussion to those used most often. Having a handle on the material discussed in this chapter will enable you to evaluate most patients presenting to your diagnostic center in a logical and efficient manner. Appropriate and justifiable recommendations become self-evident, and confidence in your work is enhanced greatly.

SYMPTOMATIC PATIENTS: IMAGING ALGORITHMS

Our imaging algorithms are listed in Box 3.1. In women 30 years of age or older presenting with a lump, focal tenderness, skin dimpling, nipple retraction, or other focal symptom, a metallic BB is placed at the site of concern, and CC and mediolateral oblique (MLO) views are obtained bilaterally. A spot tangential view at the site of concern is obtained. Correlative physical examination and an ultrasound are done, unless the tissue is completely fatty and there is no possibility that the area of concern is excluded from the image. In women with spontaneous nipple discharge, a ductogram may be done. We do not consider diffuse, cyclical tenderness as an indication for a diagnostic study; these women are scheduled for screening mammography.

In symptomatic women younger than 30 years of age and those who are pregnant or lactating (regardless of age), a physical examination and ultrasound are undertaken (Figure 3.1). If cancer is suspected after this initial evaluation, a full mammogram is obtained.

SPOT COMPRESSION VIEWS

Spot compression views help minimize superimposition and geometric unsharpness and improve resolution by decreasing object-to-film distance.

Spot compression views are the most common additional view obtained in our practice. The area of concern is maximally compressed and immobilized. This minimizes superimposition and geometric unsharpness, while resolution is improved as the object to film distance is decreased. When evaluating spot compression views, it is important to ensure that the area of concern is included in the field of view. As focal compression is applied, lesions can "roll" or "squeeze" out of the field of view. For purposes of orienting ourselves on the spot compression views, we like to include surrounding tissue on the image. Consequently, we do not cone-down on spot compression views, and, although not compressed, surrounding tissue is evaluated and used to ensure inclusion of the area of concern.

Indications for spot compression views are listed in Box 3.2. As a general rule, if we are not sure a lesion is present, our starting point is spot compression (Figure 3.2). Spot

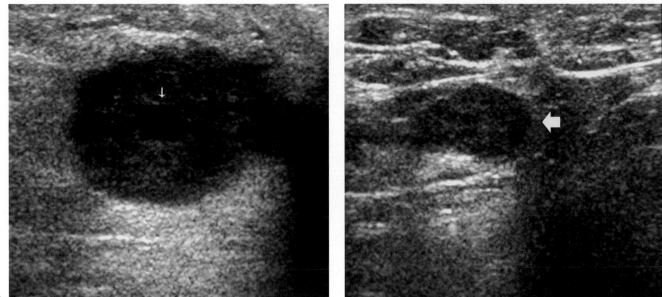

Figure 3.1 *Poorly differentiated, invasive ductal carcinoma (not otherwise specified) with metastatic disease to the axilla. A.* This 29-year-old patient presented describing a lump in the upper outer quadrant of her right breast. On physical examination, the upper outer quadrant of the right breast is hard and fixed (particularly compared with upper outer quadrant tissue on the left). Ultrasound is our starting point. An irregular, lobulated mass with a nearly anechoic central area (*arrow*) and posterior acoustic enhancement is imaged corresponding to the area of clinical concern. The consistency of this mass and surrounding tissue on palpation, coupled with the ultrasound features, suggest a rapidly growing, poorly differentiated invasive ductal carcinoma. *B.* Several hypoechoic masses (only one is shown) are also seen in the right axilla associated with posterior acoustic enhancement (*arrow*). The central echogenic focus one expects to see with lymph nodes is not seen in these masses. Their appearance suggests metastatic disease. Our starting point with symptomatic women younger than 30 years of age, or if pregnant or lactating regardless of age, is an ultrasound focused to the area of concern. As in this patient, if the clinical and ultrasound findings suggest the presence of breast cancer, a full, bilateral mammogram (not shown here) is obtained. This helps evaluate remaining tissue and the contralateral breast. In this patient, a core biopsy of the breast mass and fine-needle aspiration of one of the axillary lymph nodes confirmed the suspected diagnosis.

Box 3.2: Indications for Spot Compression Views

Evaluation of questionable areas
- Density
- Asymmetry
- Distortion

Evaluation of masses
- When surrounding tissue may obscure margins

Inclusion of tissue
- Posterior
- Axillary
- Upper inner quadrant

Technical issues
- Blurring
- Underexposure (focal)

Localizations
- See Chapter 11

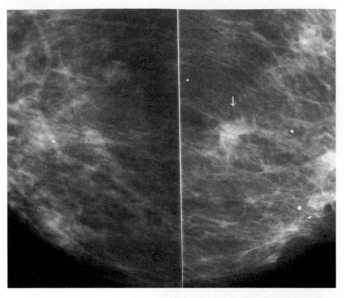

Figure 3.2 *Invasive ductal carcinoma, not otherwise specified.* Craniocaudal (CC) (*A*) and mediolateral oblique (MLO) (*B*) views from a screening study. An irregular density is seen in the retroglandular fat in the medial aspect of the left breast on the CC view (*arrow*). It is less apparent on the MLO view (*arrow*). Although this lesion is of concern, particularly because it represents an interval change from the prior study, it is inadequately characterized on screening views. Category 0: incomplete, requires additional imaging. CC (*C*) and MLO (*D*) spot compression views at the site of concern, left breast. A spiculated, irregular mass is imaged on the spot compression views. In an asymptomatic woman with no history of surgery or trauma to this site, this is considered breast cancer until proved otherwise. Making a specific, justifiable recommendation with confidence becomes significantly easier with appropriate evaluation. Category 4 or 5: Ultrasound-guided biopsy (not shown) is done.

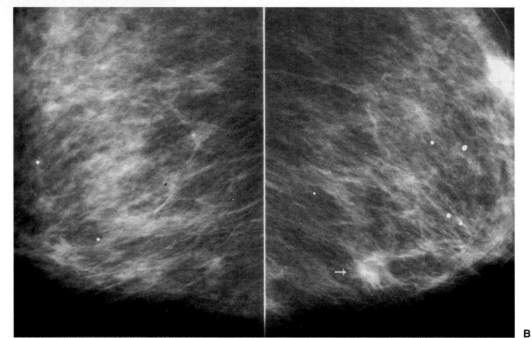

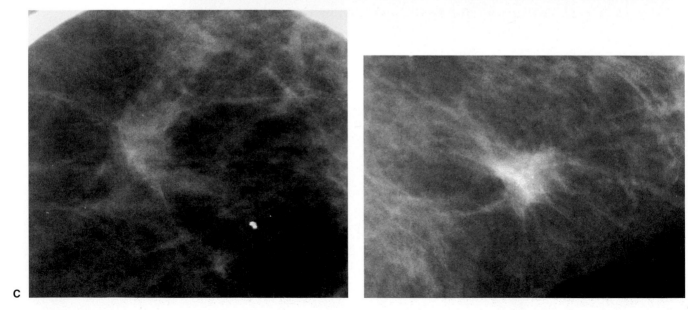

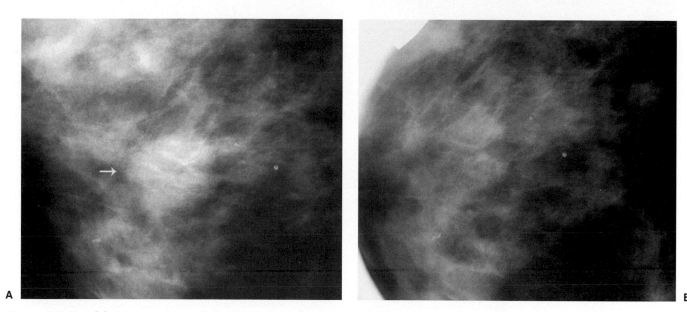

A   B

Figure 3.3 *Pseudolesion, superimposed glandular tissue.* A. Craniocaudal view. A round density (*arrow*), possibly representing a mass, is noted on the screening study. Time and time again, you will find that screening studies can be misleading. Lesions of concern on the screening study may turn out to be "imaginomas," and true lesions may look innocuous. Screening is for detection, not characterization. We make no attempt to describe features or arrive at any conclusion of possible lesions detected on a screening mammogram. Even in women who have an obvious cancer, additional views are helpful in characterizing the extent of the lesion, detecting additional unsuspected lesions, and allowing us to establish rapport with the patient and expedite her care by undertaking imaging-guided biopsy when she returns for additional views. Category 0: incomplete, requires additional imaging evaluation. B. Spot compression view. No abnormality is confirmed. Surrounding benign calcifications confirm that the right area of tissue has been evaluated on the compression view. The original density represents superimposition of normal glandular tissue (presumably tissue that is inadequately compressed).

compression views are used to evaluate densities (seen in only one view) (Figure 3.3), masses whose margins may be obscured by surrounding tissue (Figure 3.4), asymmetric tissue (Figure 3.5), and possible areas of distortion. Additionally, spot compression (Figure 3.6) can be used to reach and image lesions that are excluded from routine screening views: lesions close to the chest wall, in the axillary tail, or high in the upper inner quadrants (1–3). If there is blurring related to inadequate compression (e.g., subareolar or inframammary fold areas) or focal areas of underexposed tissue, spot compression can help overcome these technical limitations.

MAGNIFICATION VIEWS

Factors to consider associated with magnification views are listed in Box 3.3. Magnification views are obtained by moving the breast away from the image receptor (i.e., increasing the object-to-image distance and decreasing the source-to-object distance), thereby creating an air gap. A grid is not needed because scatter radiation is eliminated in the air gap. As the object-to-image distance increases, the amount of magnification increases (e.g., 1.5× and 1.8× common); however, this is associated with a loss of resolution from an increasing penumbra effect. The use of a small focal spot (0.1 mm) helps overcome the loss of resolution. With the small focal spot, however, exposure time is increased, leading potentially to motion. In an effort to obtain acceptable exposure times, the kilovoltage used to obtain magnification views can be increased by at least 2 from that used for routine views. Also helpful in shortening exposure times are magnification platforms made of

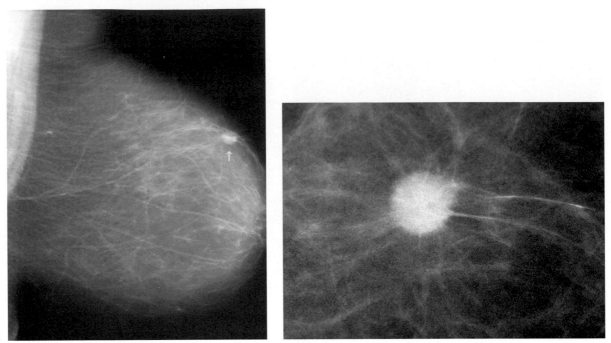

A   **B**

Figure 3.4 *Invasive ductal carcinoma, not otherwise specified. A.* Left mediolateral oblique view from a screening study (craniocaudal view not shown) in a 52-year-old patient. A round mass is identified (*arrow*). Category 0: incomplete, requires additional imaging evaluation. *B.* Spot compression view. A round, spiculated mass is confirmed. Margin evaluation is facilitated with spot compression views. With complete evaluation, it becomes relatively easy to make a specific, justifiable recommendation. By factoring clinical and imaging features, you can approximate a relatively specific diagnosis in most patients. Ultrasound-guided biopsy (not shown) is done at the time the patient returns for the additional views.

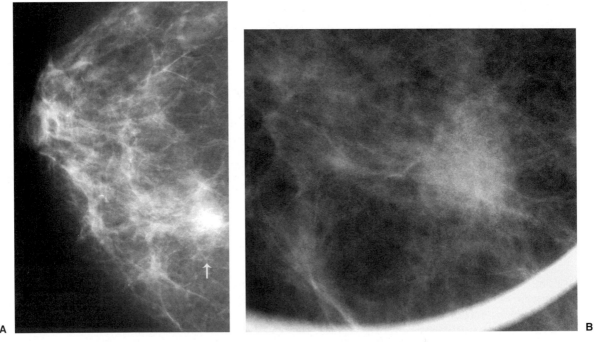

A   **B**

Figure 3.5 *Invasive ductal carcinoma, not otherwise specified. A.* Craniocaudal view from a screening study in a 60-year-old woman. An area of parenchymal asymmetry has developed in the medial aspect of the right breast. At this time, it is difficult to know the significance of this change—is it a screen-detected cancer or an area of developing tissue in a patient taking estrogen? With what degree of confidence can you make a recommendation? Do not make decisions with inadequate information. Category 0: incomplete, requires additional imaging evaluation. *B.* Spot compression view. A round, ill-defined mass in a 60-year-old patient, that develops in the medial aspect of the breast and is solid on ultrasound (not shown) is likely to represent breast cancer. Biopsy is done using ultrasound guidance.

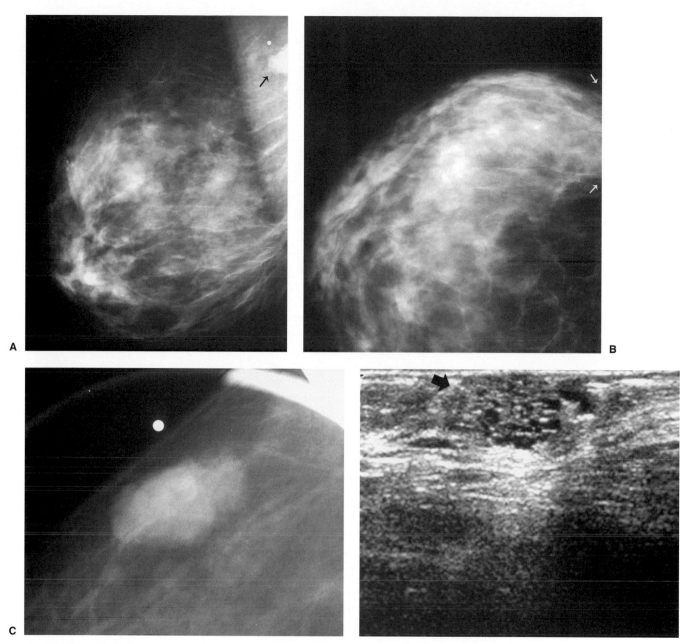

Figure 3.6 *Fibrocystic change with apocrine and epithelial lined cysts.* Mediolateral (MLO) (*A*) and craniocaudal (CC) (*B*) views in a 40-year-old patient who presents with a lump in the right breast. The lesion is partially seen on the MLO view superimposed on the pectoral muscle (*arrow*). It is not seen on the CC view; however, tissue is seen extending to the edge of the film (*arrows*). Spot compression views can be helpful in evaluating areas that may be excluded from the field of view (e.g., axillary tail, axilla, upper inner quadrant tissue). *C.* Spot compression view in an exaggerated craniocaudal (XCCL) projection. Mass is now seen surrounded by subcutaneous fat, so that margins can be characterized. *D.* Ultrasound demonstrates a hypoechoic mass with small, anechoic, round areas and posterior acoustic enhancement. The lesion decreased significantly in size after the first core sample and completely resolved after the second core sample, consistent with the findings described histologically.

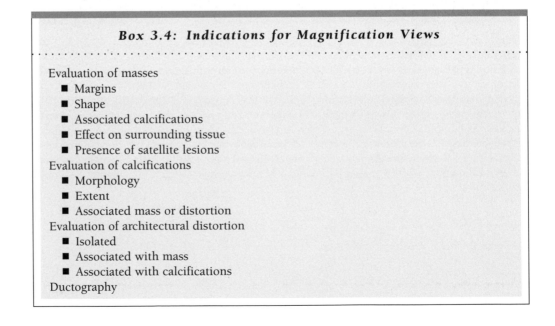

Box 3.3: Magnification Technique

Air gap
No grid used (scatter radiation eliminated in air gap)
Small focal spot (0.1 mm) to overcome loss or resolution resulting from the penumbra effect
Small focal spot increases exposure times
- Increase kV by factor of 2 from that used for screening images
- Lexan top absorbs 20% less radiation than carbon top
- Double spot compression to maximize compression
Spot compression paddle versus full paddle

For magnification views, consider increasing the kilovoltage used for routine views by at least 2. This helps minimize the effect of the lengthened exposure time that results from the use of a small focal spot (0.1 mm).

Lexan (e.g., Mammo Spot). The magnification stands made of Lexan absorb about 20% less radiation than magnification stands with carbon fiber tops. Optimal exposures are facilitated as exposure times are decreased by 33% to 40%. A spot compression device is built into the surface of the Lexan magnification stands. If this is combined with a spot compression paddle, double spot compression can be obtained, maximally reducing breast thickness and further improving image quality.

Magnification views can be done using the regular compression paddle or a spot compression paddle (1,4). With the regular compression paddle, a maximal amount of tissue is included on the image; however, compression may not be optimized. We use double spot compression for all of our magnification views (except those done for a ductogram). Using double spot compression at the site of mammographic concern maximizes compression and reduces exposure times, helping minimize the likelihood of motion. The disadvantages of using double spot compression relate to the smaller field of view and include the following:

- Positioning needs to be accurate so that the area being evaluated is included in the spot view.
- It can be difficult to orient the imaged area relative to the nonmagnified view; hence, making sure that the area of concern has been imaged can be a challenge.
- When dealing with a large area of calcifications, several images may be needed to evaluate the region of concern in its entirety.

Indications for magnification views are listed in Box 3.4. We use magnification views in evaluating masses (Figure 3.7) and calcifications (Figure 3.8) detected on screening

---

Box 3.4: Indications for Magnification Views

Evaluation of masses
- Margins
- Shape
- Associated calcifications
- Effect on surrounding tissue
- Presence of satellite lesions
Evaluation of calcifications
- Morphology
- Extent
- Associated mass or distortion
Evaluation of architectural distortion
- Isolated
- Associated with mass
- Associated with calcifications
Ductography

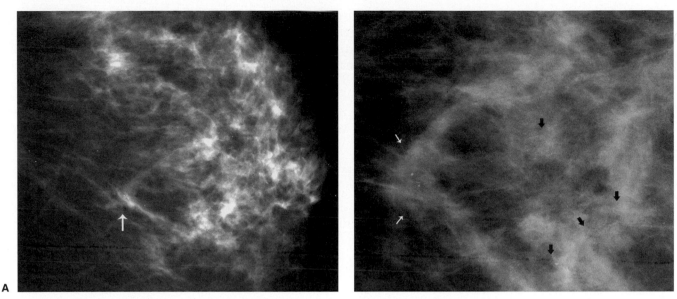

A   B

Figure 3.7 *Invasive ductal carcinoma with extensive ductal carcinoma* in situ. A. Mediolateral oblique (MLO) view from a screening study. A density is seen (*arrow*), possibly associated with calcifications. Category 0: incomplete, requires additional imaging evaluation. B. Double spot compression magnification view in the MLO projection demonstrates the presence of a spiculated mass (*white arrows*). Calcifications are present in the mass as well as extending about 2 cm beyond the mass (*black arrows*). The calcifications are pleomorphic with variable density and some linear forms.

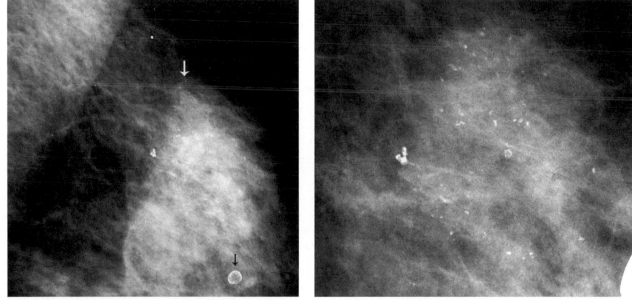

A   B

Figure 3.8 *Ductal carcinoma* in situ. A. Mediolateral oblique (MLO) view from the screening study on a 73-year-old woman. An area of calcifications is detected (*white arrow*); incidentally noted is a lucent-centered calcification (*black arrow*). Category 0: incomplete, requires additional imaging evaluation. B. Double spot compression magnification MLO view. The morphology and extent of the calcifications are readily appreciated on magnification views. These calcifications are pleomorphic, with linear, round, and punctate forms. The likelihood of ductal carcinoma *in situ* is high, and the differential for calcifications with these features is limited. Category 4: biopsy is indicated and undertaken using imaging guidance. Impression is confirmed histologically.

studies (refer to Chapters 5, 6, and 7 for additional examples). If there is architectural distortion in isolation or associated with masses or calcifications, magnification views are also helpful in further characterizing the lesion. When a mass is detected on screening images, double spot compression magnification views are done to evaluate the shape and margins of the mass and to establish the presence and morphology of associated calcifications or satellite lesions. When calcifications are detected on screening studies, magnification views are used to evaluate the morphology and extent of the calcifications. Every effort possible is made to obtain well-exposed, high-contrast images with no blur.

ROLLED OR CHANGE-OF-ANGLE VIEWS

Rolled or change-of-angle views are done to establish the presence of a lesion and are also used in triangulating the location of lesions. As with all additional views, we use the spot compression paddle for these views.

Rolled or change-of-angle views are commonly used in conjunction with spot compression views in establishing the presence of a lesion. These views are done using the spot compression paddle. Breast tissue is often planar, changing significantly in appearance as tissue is rolled or the angle of the incident beam is changed. In contrast, most breast cancers [except some invasive lobular carcinomas and small (less than 5 mm) invasive ductal carcinomas] are three dimensional. As tissue is rolled, the contour and appearance of most cancers does not change significantly. Rolled or change-of-angle views can also be used to triangulate the location of a lesion or to move a lesion away from glandular tissue so that it is surrounded by fat and evaluated more completely.

For triangulation purposes, rolled or change-of-angle views can give the approximate location of a lesion seen in only one view on the screening study. If there is a lesion on the CC view that cannot be identified with certainty on the MLO view, rolled views can be done. If the top of the breast is rolled medially while the lower part is rolled laterally and the lesion moves medially, this suggests that the lesion is in the superior portion of the breast. If the lesion does not shift in position significantly, the lesion is in the central portion of the breast; and if the lesion moves laterally, it is in the inferior aspect of the breast. This can be confirmed by repeating the image and rolling the upper portion of the breast laterally and the lower portion medially. Given an approximate location for the lesion, an MLO or 90-degree lateral view can now be reviewed, and additional workup of the upper, central, or lower portions of the breast is undertaken (Figure 3.9). Breast ultrasound can also be done at this time.

Rolled or change-of-angle views can also be used to move a lesion away from surrounding tissue so that it can be better evaluated. For example, if there is a lesion in the inferior and medial aspect of the breast that is partially visualized on the CC view medially, the lower portion of the breast can be rolled medially so that the lesion is moved away from surrounding glandular tissue into a fatty area (Figure 3.10).

Figure 3.9 *Use of rolled views for triangulation purposes.* A. Lesion seen on the craniocaudal view is not identified with certainty on mediolateral oblique or 90-degree lateral views. In scenario 1, the lesion is in the superior aspect of the breast. The lesion will move with superior tissue. If superior tissue is moved laterally and inferior tissue is moved medially, the lesion moves laterally. If superior tissue is moved medially and inferior tissue is moved laterally, the lesion moves medially. In scenario 2, the lesion is central in the breast. No significant shifts in position are noted when tissue is rolled. In scenario 3, the lesion is in the inferior aspect of the breast. If superior tissue is moved laterally and inferior tissue is moved medially, the lesion will move medially. If superior tissue is moved medially and inferior tissue laterally, the lesion will move laterally. B. Lesion seen on the lateral view, not identified with certainty on the craniocaudal view. In scenario 1, the lesion is lateral in the breast. If lateral tissue is rolled superiorly and medial tissue inferiorly, the lesion moves up on the rolled view. If lateral tissue is rolled inferiorly and medial tissue superiorly, the lesion moves inferiorly. When the lesion is central in the breast (scenario 2), no significant movement of the lesion is seen when tissue is rolled. In scenario 3, the lesion is in medial tissue. As lateral tissue is rolled superiorly and medial tissue inferiorly, the lesion moves down. As lateral tissue is rolled inferiorly and medial tissue superiorly, the lesion moves superiorly. M, medial; L, lateral; S, superior or cranial; I, inferior or caudal.

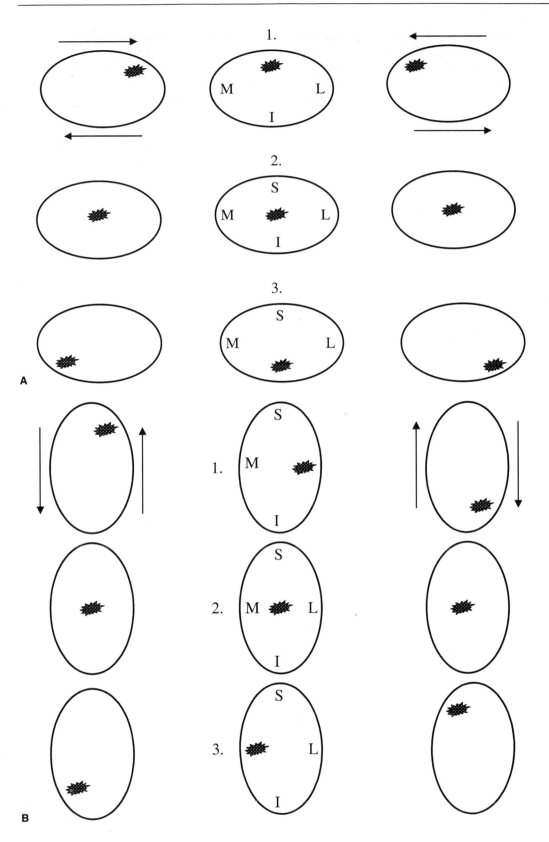

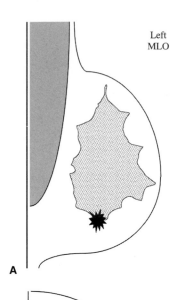

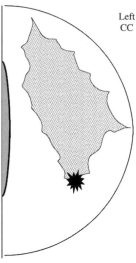

Left
MLO

Left
CC

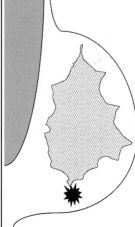

1.

2.

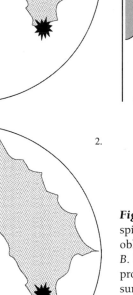

A

B

C

1.

2.

Figure 3.10 *Use of rolled views for better lesion visualization. A. A spiculated mass is partially seen inferiorly on the mediolateral oblique (MLO) view and medially on the craniocaudal (CC) view. B. In considering how to better visualize this lesion in the lateral projection, if medial tissue is rolled inferiorly, the lesion will be surrounded by fatty tissue (1). If medial tissue is rolled superiorly, the lesion will be moved into glandular tissue and will actually become less apparent (2). C. In considering how to visualize this lesion in the CC projection, if inferior tissue is moved medially (1), the lesion is surrounded by fatty tissue and better evaluated. If inferior tissue is moved laterally (2), the lesion will be thrown farther into glandular tissue and will become less apparent.*

TANGENTIAL VIEWS

Tangential views are used in evaluating women with palpable masses, focal tenderness, or a history of lumpectomy and radiation therapy for breast cancer, and in localizing lesions to the skin. We do all of our tangential views using a spot compression paddle.

Tangential views are done in women presenting with focal findings. As with all additional views, we use a spot compression paddle for the images.

For women presenting with a palpable abnormality or focal tenderness, a metallic BB is used to mark the location of the mass as CC and MLO views are done. Additionally, a tangential view of the area of concern is obtained (1) (Figure 3.11). This is particularly helpful in women with dense tissue (Figure 3.12). The purpose of the tangential view is to try to at least partially surround the area of concern with subcutaneous fat (Figure 3.13).

On any two views of the breast, only a small amount of skin is tangent to incident x-rays; most of the skin is superimposed on the breast parenchyma (in fact, most of the radiation used in exposing the breast on any given image is expended in penetrating the two layers of skin). Consequently, skin calcifications and masses are commonly superimposed on the breast parenchyma on screening views and mischaracterized as potential breast lesions. By placing a marker on the skin lesion, a tangential view is obtained to document that the lesion is on the skin rather than in the breast. With skin calcifications, you can follow some of the principles described for needle localizations (Chapter 11). Orthogonal

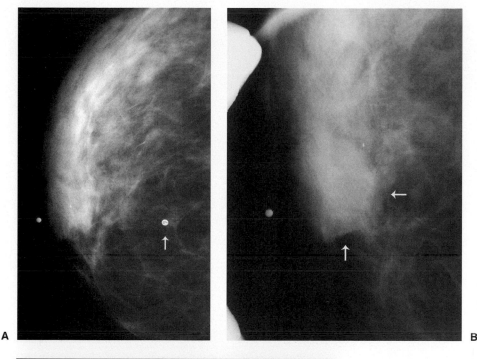

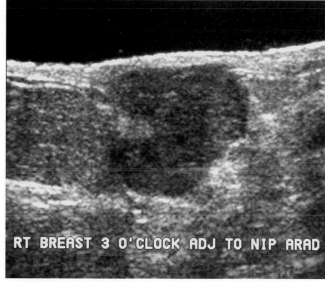

Figure 3.11 *Invasive ductal carcinoma, not otherwise specified. A.* Mediolateral oblique (MLO) view. Patient presents describing a lump adjacent to her right nipple. Metallic BB marks the lump. Dense tissue is present in the subareolar area. No definite abnormality is seen on the routine MLO and craniocaudal views. Lucent-centered calcification is noted (*arrow*). *B.* Spot tangential view of the area of clinical concern. Round mass is now apparent with partially well-circumscribed margins (*arrows*). If appropriate positioning technique is used in women with dense tissue, tangential views are often helpful by either partially or completely surrounding the lesion with subcutaneous fat. *C.* Ultrasound demonstrates a superficial, solid mass with well-circumscribed margins, a heterogeneous echotexture, and posterior acoustic enhancement. What is the differential diagnosis? What additional piece of information would you like on this patient? In formulating a differential for this lesion, the age of the patient is most helpful. In a young woman, a fibroadenoma would be a primary consideration. In an 88-year-old patient, however, a fibroadenoma is unlikely; a new palpable mass is likely to represent breast cancer.

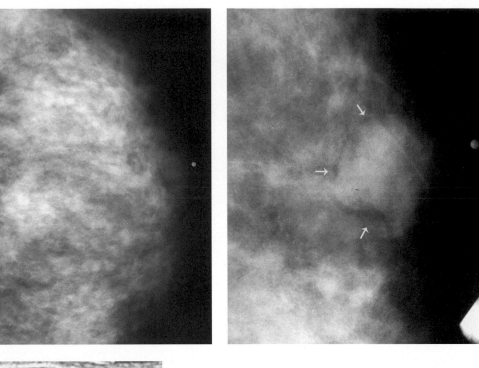

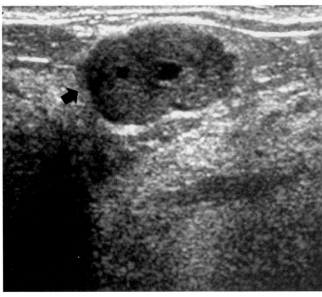

Figure 3.12 *Fibroadenoma. A.* Mediolateral oblique view in a 36-year-old patient who presents describing a lump in her left breast. Metallic BB marks the lump. Dense glandular tissue is present. No abnormality is apparent at the site of clinical concern. *B.* Spot tangential view demonstrates a macrolobulated, well-circumscribed mass. Although dense tissue is present, the mass is now seen, and the margins can be characterized. *C.* Ultrasound demonstrates a well-circumscribed, oval mass with two small central cystic areas, gentle macrolobulations, and posterior acoustic enhancement. A fibroadenoma is diagnosed after imaging-guided biopsy.

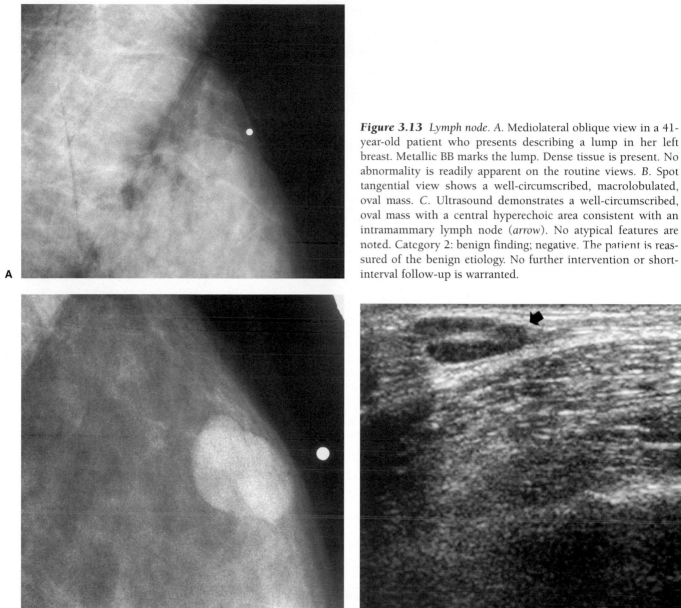

Figure 3.13 *Lymph node. A.* Mediolateral oblique view in a 41-year-old patient who presents describing a lump in her left breast. Metallic BB marks the lump. Dense tissue is present. No abnormality is readily apparent on the routine views. *B.* Spot tangential view shows a well-circumscribed, macrolobulated, oval mass. *C.* Ultrasound demonstrates a well-circumscribed, oval mass with a central hyperechoic area consistent with an intramammary lymph node (*arrow*). No atypical features are noted. Category 2: benign finding; negative. The patient is reassured of the benign etiology. No further intervention or short-interval follow-up is warranted.

views (CC and 90-degree lateral) of the breast are reviewed, and the shortest skin-to-calcification distance is established. The fenestrated alphanumeric compression paddle is used to compress the skin surface thought to contain the calcifications, and an image is obtained (e.g., a CC view, using the alphanumeric compression paddle, is done if the calcifications are closest to the superior skin surface on the 90-degree lateral view). A BB is then placed at the coordinates for the calcifications, and a tangential view of the BB is obtained to show that the calcifications are in the skin (Figure 3.14).

Skin thickening and distortion are seen in women after lumpectomy and radiation therapy. These skin changes can project on the lumpectomy site, thereby limiting the evaluation for recurrent disease. If the lumpectomy site is imaged tangent to the x-ray beam, skin changes can be separated from the underlying parenchymal changes (5). In these patients, the tangential views can be done using magnification technique (Figure 3.15).

Tangential views are done to demonstrate that a cluster of calcifications projecting on the breast parenchyma is actually dermal in location.

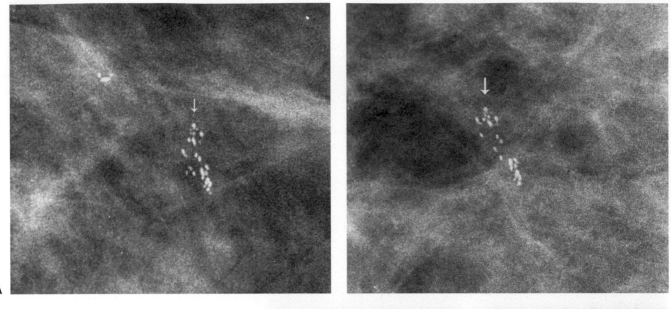

A

B

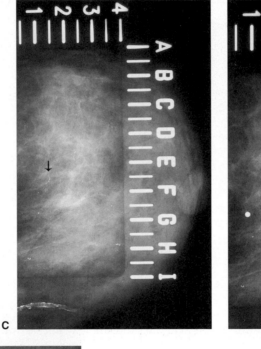

C

D

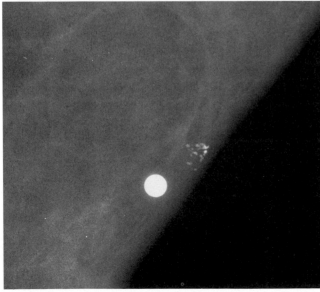

E

Figure 3.14 *Skin calcifications; skin localization.* Mediolateral oblique (*A*) and craniocaudal (*B*) views demonstrate a cluster of calcifications (*arrows*). These appear to be closest to the inferior aspect of the breast. *C.* A from below view (FB, caudocranial view) is done using the alphanumeric fenestrated paddle. The coordinates for the calcifications are determined (*arrow*) on this image, and a metallic BB is placed on the skin surface at the intersection of the coordinates. *D.* Follow-up image demonstrates the BB in close proximity to the calcifications. *E.* Tangential view is taken at the location of the BB. This confirms the dermal location for these calcifications. The patient is reassured of a benign finding. No further intervention is warranted. Screening mammogram is recommended in 1 year.

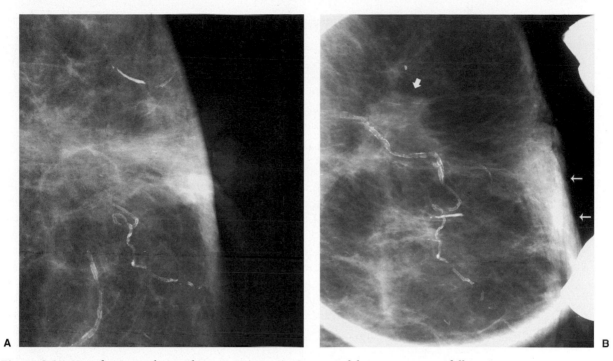

A   B

Figure 3.15 Use of tangential view, lumpectomy site. A. Craniocaudal view in patient following lumpectomy and radiation therapy. Skin thickening superimposed on the lumpectomy site may preclude good evaluation of the lumpectomy site. *B.* Spot tangential view at the lumpectomy site using magnification technique. Skin thickening (*thin arrows*) is now tangent to the x-ray beam and no longer superimposed on the lumpectomy site (*thick arrow*). Early changes of a local recurrence are easier to appreciate on spot tangential views such as these. Incidentally noted is extensive vascular calcification.

CLEAVAGE VIEWS

Cleavage views are used to evaluate medial and posterior tissue in the CC projection. The film holder is placed up against the chest wall while medial and posterior tissue is imaged. Manual timing is needed, or if phototiming is used, the technologist needs to offset the breasts so that the breast being evaluated is placed over the photocell (1). If the breasts are centered on the bucky and phototiming is used, the exposure may not be optimal because the phototimer sees air (Figure 3.16).

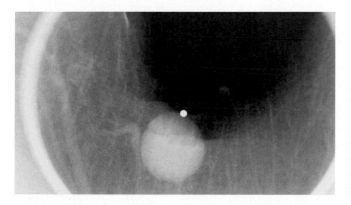

Figure 3.16 Cleavage view. Sebaceous cyst. Patient presents describing a lump medially on the right. A cleavage view is needed to image the lesion. This is a round, well-circumscribed mass (metallic BB). On physical examination, a readily mobile, superficial mass is palpated. On careful inspection of the overlying skin, a "black head" is noted overlying the lesion. With gentle pressure, a small amount of white, thick material can be expressed. Category 2: benign finding, negative.

90-DEGREE LATERAL VIEWS

Lateral views can be done in two different ways: lateromedial (LM) and mediolateral (ML) views. For the 90-degree LM view, the film holder is placed up against the sternum, so that medial tissue is closest to the film. For 90-degree ML views, lateral tissue is closest to the film.

90-DEGREE LATEROMEDIAL VIEW

Inclusion of medial tissue and the evaluation of medial lesions are the major advantage of 90-degree LM views. This view is also used in the localization of lesions closest to the lateral aspect of the breast and in triangulating the location of lesions. Unless we are evaluating a lateral lesion, we prefer LM views. The film holder is placed up against the sternum, and the patient is asked to lower the chin onto the film holder while compression is applied from the lateral aspect of the breast. By placing the film holder up against the sternum, it is unlikely that a medial lesion will be excluded from the image and, because the medial aspect of the breast is close to the film, resolution of medial tissue is optimized. In a small number of patients, medial lesions may be completely or partially excluded, even on 90-degree LM views. Breast ultrasound is particularly helpful in evaluating these patients (Figure 3.17).

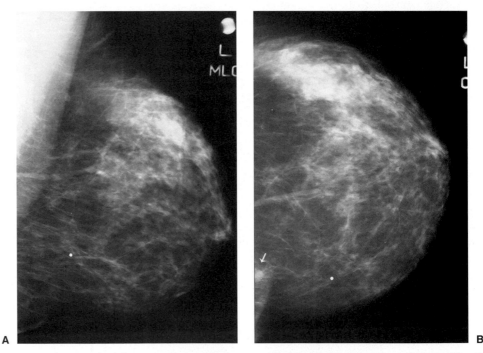

Figure 3.17 *Invasive ductal carcinoma, not otherwise specified.* Mediolateral oblique (MLO) (A) and craniocaudal (CC) (B) views in a 44-year-old patient presenting with a lump. Metallic BB purportedly marks area. The MLO is normal. On the CC view, a round density is partially seen posteromedially (*arrow*). Note that the BB is 2 to 3 cm anterior to the potential lesion. Because the lesion is on the medial aspect of the breast, the 90-degree lateral and cleavage views might be helpful. In selecting between the lateromedial (LM) and mediolateral (ML) 90-degree lateral views, the LM is selected because on this view, medial tissue is up against the film.

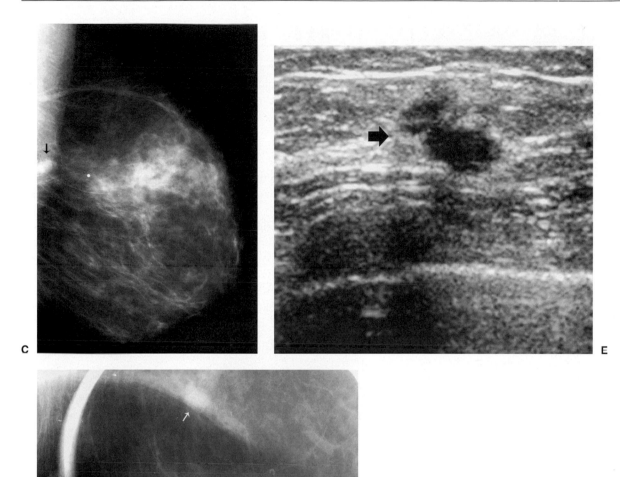

C

D

E

Figure 3.17 (continued) *C.* The 90-degree LM view. More of the lesion is seen on this view (*arrow*). *D.* Cleavage view. A round mass is seen (*arrow*) corresponding to the area of concern to the patient. *E.* Ultrasound demonstrates an irregular mass corresponding to the palpable area. Ultrasound is helpful in reaching areas that are difficult to image mammographically. This includes upper inner quadrant and axillary tissue. Ultrasound-guided biopsy was used to establish the diagnosis. Note the upward movement of the lesion and metallic BB as one goes from the MLO view to the LM view. Medial lesions move up as you go from MLO to LM views.

90-DEGREE MEDIOLATERAL VIEW

The evaluation of lateral lesions, localization of medial lesions, and lesion triangulation are done with the 90-degree ML view. The film holder is placed on the lateral aspect of the breast, and compression is applied from the medial side. Resolution of lateral tissue is maximized because lateral tissue is placed closest to the film (Figure 3.18).

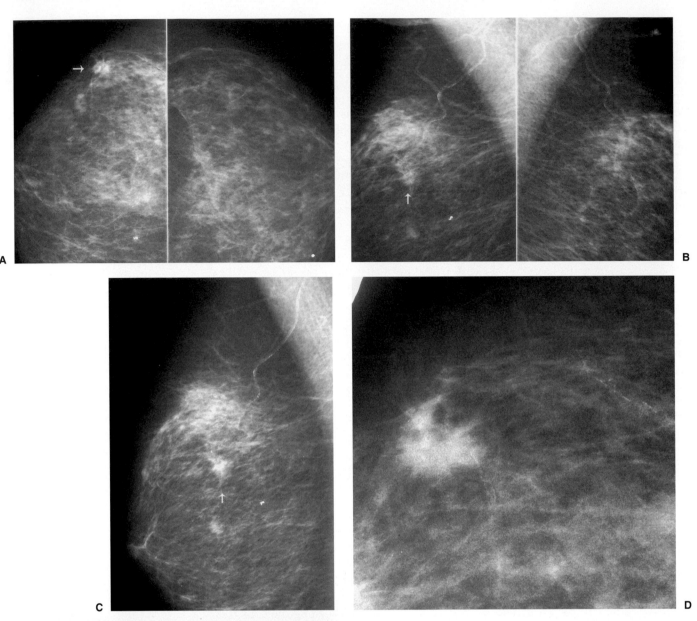

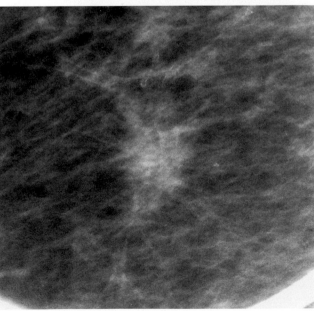

Figure 3.18 *Invasive lobular carcinoma.* Craniocaudal (CC) (*A*) and mediolateral oblique (MLO) (*B*) views from a screening study in a 74-year-old patient. A density is readily apparent on the right CC view (*arrow*). It is not as clearly seen on the MLO view; however, if one measures back from the nipple and scans the MLO at the expected location of the lesion, a potential corresponding abnormality is seen (*arrow*). Category 0: incomplete, requires additional imaging evaluation. *C.* Because the lesion is lateral in the breast, a mediolateral (ML) 90-degree lateral view is obtained. As expected, the potential lesion on the MLO moves inferiorly on the ML view (*arrow*). CC (*D*) and ML (*E*) spot compression views demonstrate a spiculated mass. A new spiculated mass in a 74-year-old woman is likely to be breast cancer, particularly if there is no history of surgery or trauma to this site. Ultrasound-guided biopsy (not shown) is done.

TRIANGULATION

The ability to establish the location of lesions is critical for breast ultrasound; correlation of clinical, mammographic, and ultrasonographic findings; imaging-guided biopsies; and preoperative wire localizations. Incomplete workups account for many of the lesions described as "seen in only one view." If a logical approach is taken in the evaluation of potential lesions seen in only one view initially, the location of the lesion in the orthogonal image can be established reliably in most patients.

Our approach to an area of concern seen in only one view is first to establish whether it represents superimposition of normal tissue on the view in which the abnormality is seen initially. For example, if a potential lesion is seen on an MLO view and not identified with certainty on the CC view, we first obtain a spot compression view (and sometimes rolled views) in the MLO projection to determine whether the lesion persists or represents the superimposition of normal parenchymal structures (Figure 3.19). If the abnormality is real, we need to establish its location on the CC view. Rolled views can be obtained to determine whether the lesion moves with lateral or medial tissue. Another crude way of establishing the approximate location of a lesion on the CC view is to make use of the movement of the lesion between MLO and 90-degree lateral views. If the lesion moves up from the MLO to the 90-degree lateral view, the lesion is in the medial aspect of the breast (Figure 3.20). If the lesion moves down ("down and out") between the MLO and 90-degree lateral views, the lesion is in the lateral aspect of the breast (Figure 3.21). If the location of the lesion does not change significantly between MLO and 90-degree lateral views, it is in the central area (e.g., deep to the nipple). In general, the more the lesion moves, the more peripheral the location of the lesion.

An approach described by Sickles (6) involves lining up CC, MLO, and 90-degree lateral views (nipple on the same horizontal plane for all three images) and drawing a line connecting the lesion in the two views in which the lesion is seen. If this line is extended onto the third image, the lesion will be found along the course of that line (Figure 3.22). The distance from the nipple to the lesion can be used to approximate the location of the lesion along the line on the third view.

Eklund (7) described a practical method that is useful in approximating the location of lesions when going from MLO and CC views to ultrasound (Figure 3.23). On MLO views, x-rays pass from upper inner to lower outer quadrants, so that some tissue in the lower outer quadrant of the breast projects above the nipple on the MLO view. Likewise, some tissue in the upper inner quadrant of the breast projects below the nipple. If one assumes that the MLO view has been taken at a 45-degree angle, lesions on the course of the x-ray beam will project behind the nipple on the MLO view along the course of the posterior nipple line (PNL). If a lesion is 1 cm above the PNL on the MLO view, a line drawn 1 cm above and parallel to the line of the incident x-ray beam on a frontal diagram of the breast will describe the possible locations of the lesion. In combination with the CC view, one can establish whether the lesion is in the upper inner quadrant at the 11-o'clock position (e.g., medial on the CC view), at the 12-o'clock position (e.g., retroareolar on the CC view), or at the 3:30 position (e.g., lateral on the CC view).

Finally, a stepwise approach can be taken to finding the lesion on an orthogonal view (8). If a lesion is confirmed to be real on the CC view and not identified with certainty on the MLO view, small amounts of angulation are incrementally added, and the lesion is followed (e.g., 0, 15, 30, 45, 60, 75, and 90 degrees).

Incomplete workups account for many of the lesions described as "seen in only one view." If a logical approach is taken, the location of many of these lesions can be reliably established on orthogonal views.

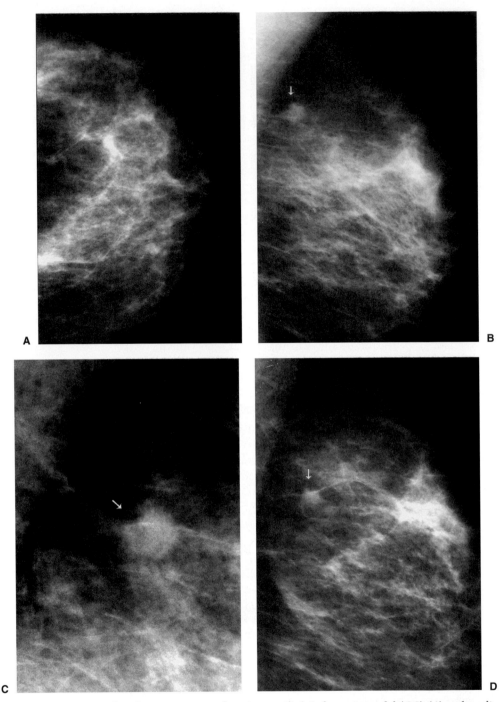

Figure 3.19 *Invasive ductal carcinoma, not otherwise specified.* Left craniocaudal (CC) (*A*) and mediolateral (MLO) (*B*) views from a screening study in a 45-year-old woman. The CC view is normal. In evaluating the strip of tissue anterior to the pectoral muscle, a density is detected (*arrow*). At this point, it is unclear whether this is a significant finding. Category 0: incomplete, requires additional imaging evaluation. When the patient returns for her diagnostic study, our approach is to first establish whether what we are seeing on the MLO view is real. *C.* Spot compression view in the MLO projection. A spiculated mass (*arrow*) persists on the spot compression view. The location of the abnormality now needs to be determined on the CC projection. Is this a lateral, medial, or central lesion? Instead of making any assumptions and blindly evaluating potential areas for the location of the lesion, a 90-degree lateral view is obtained. If the lesion moves down in going from the MLO to the lateral view, the lesion is in lateral tissue, and an exaggerated craniocaudal (XCCL) view would be appropriate. If the lesion moves up in going from the MLO to the lateral view, the lesion is in medial tissue, and a cleavage view would be appropriate. *D.* The 90-degree lateral view. The lesion moves down on the lateral view.

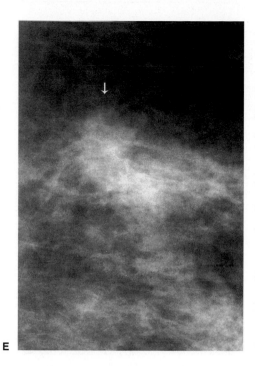

E

Figure 3.19 (continued) E. Spot compression view in the XCCL projection. The spiculated mass (*arrow*) is identified. The location of the lesion is now known precisely. Ultrasound-guided biopsy (not shown) is used to establish the diagnosis.

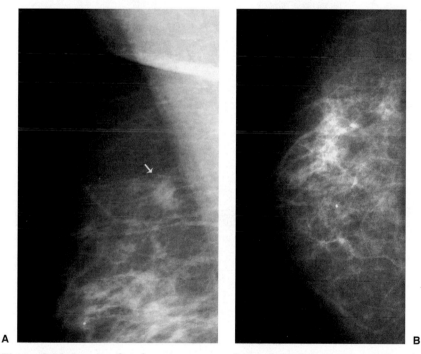

A   B

Figure 3.20 *Invasive ductal carcinoma, not otherwise specified.* Right mediolateral oblique (MLO) (*A*) and craniocaudal (CC) (*B*) views in a 61-year-old woman. A density (*arrow*) is perceived anterior to the pectoral muscle. The CC view is normal. This patient had been evaluated at two other facilities and both groups had obtained multiple views. The assumption was made that the lesion was in lateral tissue. The patient presents to us with a lesion that was purportedly seen in only one view. As discussed, we first establish whether the lesion is real.

(*continued on next page*)

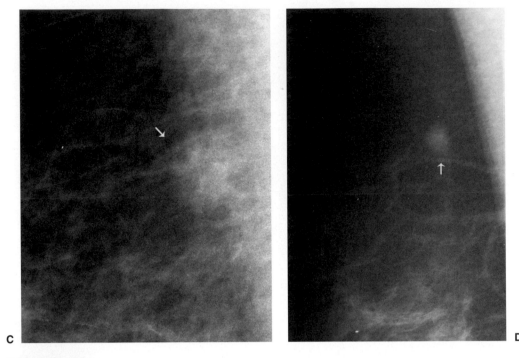

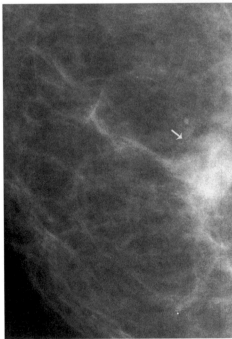

Figure 3.20 (continued) *C.* Spot compression view in the MLO projection. The lesion detected on the screening study persists (*arrow*). Instead of making any assumptions and blindly evaluating areas on the CC, a 90-degree lateral view is obtained. If the lesion moves down in going from the MLO to the lateral view, the lesion is in lateral tissue, and an exaggerated craniocaudal (XCCL) view would be appropriate. If the lesion moves up in going from the MLO to the lateral view, the lesion is in medial tissue, and a cleavage view would be appropriate. *D.* The 90-degree lateral view. The lesion moves up in going from the MLO to the 90-degree lateral view. The lesion is in the medial aspect of the breast. *E.* Spot compression view, CC projection. A mass with indistinct margins is imaged (*arrow*). Using the spot compression paddle enables us to include more tissue in the field of view compared with the regular CC view. With two additional views, the density detected on the screening study is confirmed to be real, and its exact location is established on orthogonal projections. Ultrasound-guided biopsy is done. Make no assumptions about the nature or location of a lesion during diagnostic studies; otherwise, you will overlook the obvious. If patients and workups are approached one step at a time, most things are easily resolved, appropriate recommendations become self-evident, and your confidence in them is increased greatly.

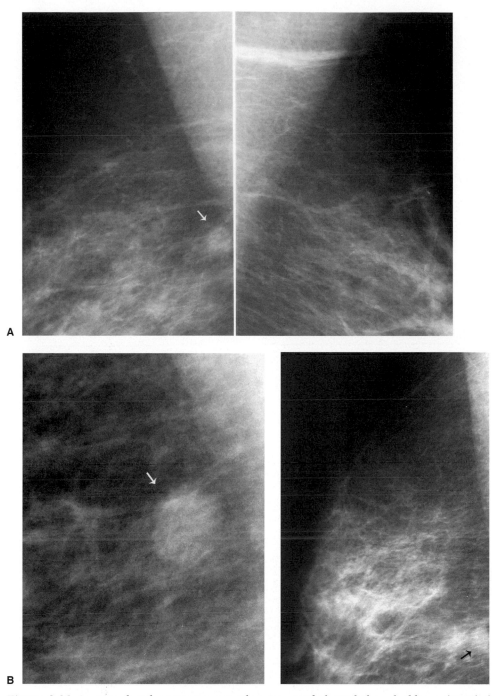

Figure 3.21 *Invasive ductal carcinoma, not otherwise specified.* Mediolateral oblique (MLO) (*A*) views from a screening study in a 70-year-old patient demonstrate a density anterior to the pectoral muscle (*arrow*). The craniocaudal views are normal. *B.* Spot compression in the MLO projection confirms the presence of a round, ill-defined mass. *C.* The 90-degree lateral view. The lesion (*arrow*) moves down compared with the MLO view. The lesion is in the lateral aspect of the breast.

(*continued on next page*)

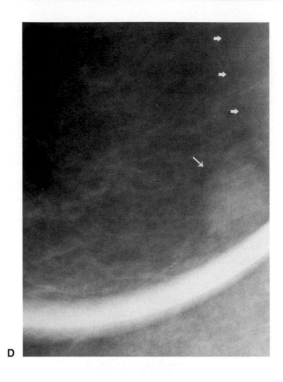

D

Figure 3.21 (continued) D. Exaggerated craniocaudal (XCCL) spot compression view. The mass (*thin arrow*) is now localized in the breast. A small amount of pectoral muscle is routinely seen on well-positioned XCCL views (*thick arrows*). Ultrasound-guided biopsy (not shown) confirms the diagnosis.

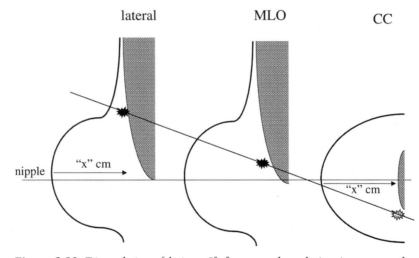

Figure 3.22 Triangulation of lesions. If, for example, a lesion is seen on the mediolateral oblique (MLO) view and not on the craniocaudal (CC) view, a lateral view can be done. The lateral, oblique, and craniocaudal views are lined with the nipple on the same horizontal plane. A line is drawn connecting the lesion on the lateral and MLO views and extended into the CC view. The lesion will be along the course of this line. The distance from the nipple to the lesion on the lateral view ("x" cm) is used to determine where along the course of the line the lesion is located on the CC view. Note that this is a medial lesion. In going from the MLO to 90-degree lateral view, the lesion moves up, as discussed earlier.

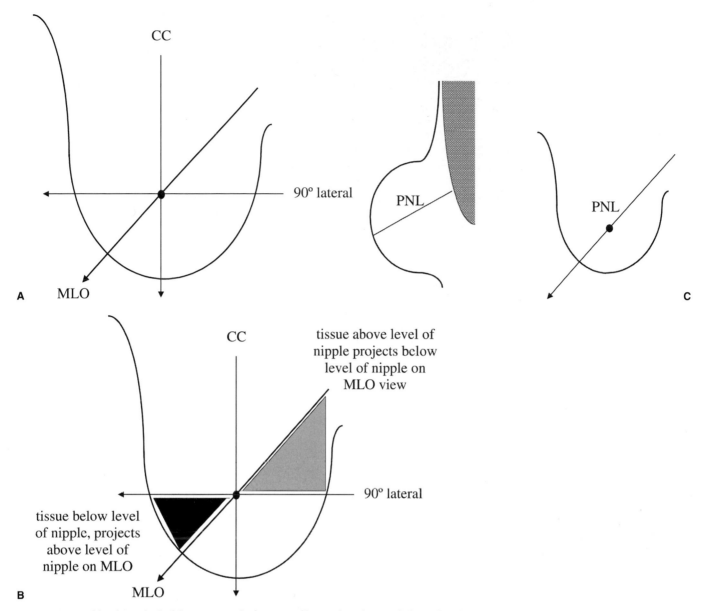

Figure 3.23 *Eklund's method of determining the location of lesions based on mediolateral and craniocaudal views. A.* On craniocaudal views, lateral tissue is lateral to the nipple, and medial tissue is medial to the nipple. On 90-degree lateral views, tissue projecting above the nipple is above the nipple and tissue projecting below the nipple is below the nipple. For the mediolateral oblique (MLO) view, the x-rays pass from the upper inner quadrant through the breast and out at the lower outer quadrant. *B.* Consequently, on a mediolateral oblique view, a small amount of tissue projecting above the nipple is really below the nipple (*black triangle*), and some tissue projecting below the nipple is really above the nipple (*gray triangle*). *C.* The posterior nipple line (PNL) can be used on the frontal view of the breast to establish the approximate o'clock position of a lesion for correlating and targeting ultrasound studies appropriately.

(*continued on next page*)

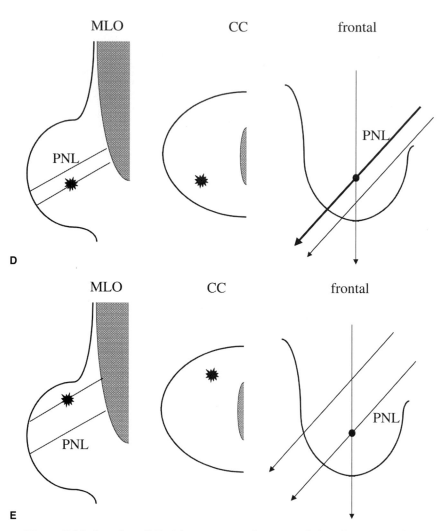

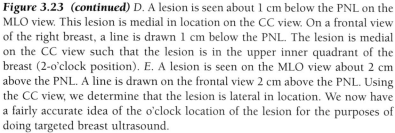

Figure 3.23 (continued) D. A lesion is seen about 1 cm below the PNL on the MLO view. This lesion is medial in location on the CC view. On a frontal view of the right breast, a line is drawn 1 cm below the PNL. The lesion is medial on the CC view such that the lesion is in the upper inner quadrant of the breast (2-o'clock position). E. A lesion is seen on the MLO view about 2 cm above the PNL. A line is drawn on the frontal view 2 cm above the PNL. Using the CC view, we determine that the lesion is lateral in location. We now have a fairly accurate idea of the o'clock location of the lesion for the purposes of doing targeted breast ultrasound.

REFERENCES

1. Eklund GW, Cardenosa G. The art of mammographic positioning. *Radiol Clin North Am* 1992;30: 21–53.
2. Berkowitz JE, Gatewood OMB, Gayler BW. Equivocal mammographic findings: evaluation with spot compression. *Radiology* 1989;171:369–371.
3. Logan WW, Janus J. Use of special mammographic views to maximize radiographic information. *Radiol Clin North Am* 1987;25:953.
4. Sickles EA. Combining spot compression and other special views to maximize mammographic information. *Radiology* 1989;173:571.
5. Karstaedt PJ, Jeske JM, Mendelson EB. *Tangential magnification view of lumpectomy site: should it be standard in mammographic follow up after breast conservation?* [Abstract] Society of Breast Imaging meeting, 1997.

6. Sickles EA. Practical solutions to common mammographic problems: tailoring the examination. *AJR Am J Roentgenol* 1988;151:31–39.

7. Eklund GW. Triangulation method. Personal communication, August 1998.

8. Pearson KL, Sickles EA, Frankel SD, et al. Efficacy of step-oblique mammography for confirmation and localization of densities seen on only one standard mammographic view. *AJR Am J Roentgenol* 2000;174:745–752.

BREAST ULTRASOUND

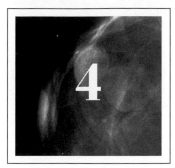

EQUIPMENT AND TECHNICAL ISSUES

Spatial resolution in ultrasound is defined as axial, lateral, and elevation resolution (Figure 4.1). Axial resolution is the ability to resolve two adjacent structures along the axis of the beam and is determined by the pulse length (wavelength times number of cycles per pulse). Pulse length decreases as the frequency of the transducer increases. Consequently, high-frequency transducers have greater axial resolution; however, the higher frequencies are attenuated more quickly. These characteristics make high-frequency transducers the choice for imaging breast tissue when maximal axial resolution is desired in relatively thin tissue. Determined by the width of the ultrasound beam, lateral resolution is the ability to resolve adjacent structures that are perpendicular to the beam, parallel to the long axis of the transducer. Focusing of the beam can alter the beam width at selected depths of interest. Elevation resolution is the ability to resolve adjacent structures in a plane perpendicular to the beam and long axis of the transducer. The thickness of the ultrasound beam, a factor not controlled by the operator, determines elevation resolution.

Contrast resolution refers to the ability of an ultrasound unit to resolve two objects with different but similar echogenicities; it is directly affected by the dynamic range setting on the ultrasound unit. When the dynamic range setting is too low, image contrast is increased, such that solid masses may appear cystic. Conversely, if the dynamic range is too high, there is little contrast in the image, and subtle solid masses are rendered indistinguishable from adjacent fat lobules (1).

Our dedicated ultrasound equipment is in immediate proximity to the mammography and stereotactic equipment. The units are equipped with 5- to 10-MHz and 6- to 13-MHz transducers. Doppler and tissue harmonic imaging are available on both units. The 6- to 13-MHz transducer is the most commonly used. However, the 5- to 10-MHz transducer is helpful in evaluating patients with larger breasts and lesions that are deep in the breast. This transducer is also helpful in women with dense tissue in whom we see significant amounts of artifactual shadowing when scanning with the higher-frequency transducer.

Optimization of the scanning parameters is critical. As discussed with mammographic image quality, it is important that you maximize ultrasound image quality. Set your quality standards high, and monitor image quality on a patient-by-patient basis. Do not settle for suboptimal equipment or images. Review and become familiar with the guidelines from the American College of Radiology (ACR) regarding breast ultrasound (2). Unfortunately, and somewhat reminiscent of the experience with mammography image quality in the 1980s and early 1990s, breast ultrasound image quality at many facilities may not be what is required for good diagnostic work. On a review of 152 breast ultrasound examinations from 86 different institutions, Baker and Soo reported noncompliance with at least

Axial resolution is greater for high-frequency transducers, making them optimal for imaging breast tissue.

Lateral resolution is determined by the width of the beam and can be altered by focusing the ultrasound beam.

The dynamic range setting on the ultrasound unit directly affects the ability to resolve objects with similar but different echogenicities (contrast resolution).

Optimized equipment, high image quality, and meticulous technique are critical for diagnostic ultrasound work in breast imaging. Set your quality standards high, and monitor image quality on an ongoing basis.

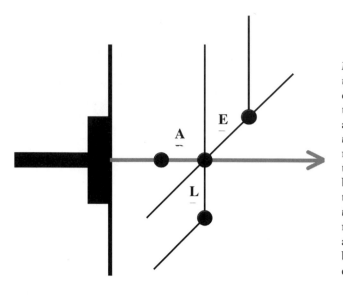

Figure 4.1 *Spatial resolution in ultrasound. Axial resolution* (A) *is defined as the ability to resolve two adjacent structures along the axis of the beam. Lateral resolution* (L) *is defined as the ability to resolve two adjacent structures that are perpendicular to the beam, parallel to the long axis of the transducer. Elevation resolution* (E) *is defined as the ability to resolve two adjacent structures in a plane perpendicular to the beam along the axis of the transducer.*

one of the ACR guidelines for breast ultrasound in 60.5% of studies (3). It is only when optimized equipment, image quality, and meticulous technique are used that ultrasound becomes an invaluable tool in the evaluation and management of women with breast-related diseases. Anything else is often misleading and may be worse than nothing.

The number and positioning of the focal zones need to be set appropriately. The focal zones should be at the level of the lesion or, at most, 1 cm superficial or deep to the anterior and posterior margins of the mass, respectively. Gain settings should enable the distinction between a simple cyst and solid mass. In the absence of a cyst, fat lobules should have varying shades of gray and not be so light as to be white or so dark as to be black. The field of view is adjusted so that an adequate amount of tissue is seen surrounding the lesion being evaluated. It should be possible to establish the distance from the skin to the mass, and there should be enough posterior tissue to assess any changes in the transmission of the ultrasound beam beyond or deep to the lesion (3). In patients with large masses, it may be difficult to image the entire lesion and surrounding tissue. With adjustments in technique as needed, evaluation of the lesion in segments may be indicated. Depending on the unit and transducer used, a standoff pad may be needed to evaluate superficial lesions. The standoff pad increases the distance from the transducer to the lesion, helping position the lesion at an appropriate depth of focus for the transducer. If the standoff pad is not used for superficial lesions, near-field artifacts may be created, leading to an inaccurate characterization of lesions.

Some minimal considerations when performing breast ultrasound examinations are listed in Box 4.1.

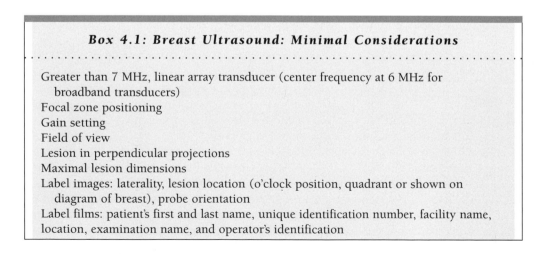

Box 4.1: Breast Ultrasound: Minimal Considerations

Greater than 7 MHz, linear array transducer (center frequency at 6 MHz for broadband transducers)
Focal zone positioning
Gain setting
Field of view
Lesion in perpendicular projections
Maximal lesion dimensions
Label images: laterality, lesion location (o'clock position, quadrant or shown on diagram of breast), probe orientation
Label films: patient's first and last name, unique identification number, facility name, location, examination name, and operator's identification

The use of film to display and store images from breast ultrasound studies is recommended. Some facilities print their images on strips of paper. For appropriate preservation of the images, quality paper and appropriate storage need to be used; otherwise, the images fade. Also, it is best if paper images are secured in plastic sleeves; otherwise, they can become mangled as the contents of the patient's film jacket are manipulated. If you are working in a Picture, Archiving and Comment section System (PACS) environment, these issues become secondary.

SCANNING TECHNIQUE

Breast ultrasound is an adjunctive method used to evaluate areas of mammographic or clinical concern. Although the entire breast can be scanned, studies limited to the area of mammographic or clinical concern are more common. The patient is positioned so that the tissue in the area of interest is thinned as much as possible. Supine positioning is used when evaluating the inner quadrants; decubitus positioning is used for far lateral tissue, and oblique positioning for tissue in the upper outer quadrants. In evaluating the lateral quadrants, having the patient raise the ipsilateral arm and place it comfortably under her head helps in further thinning the area to be scanned. One of the advantages of ultrasound is its real-time capabilities. Patients are positioned as needed to evaluate the area of concern. If the patient describes an abnormality as more apparent in the upright position, she is scanned upright. When there are significant physical limitations, however, patients can be scanned in a wheelchair or stretcher.

> Position the patient so that the area being evaluated is thinned as much as possible.

The reason for the study and how the study is done are explained to the patient. The coupling gel is prewarmed in commercially available warmers. If the gel is used at room temperature, it can be uncomfortably cold, particularly in the winter months. As with positioning for the mammographic study, it is important to consider the patient's modesty. Only the breast to be examined and scanned is exposed. The contralateral breast is kept covered unless a comparison needs to be done. At the completion of the study, the patient is provided a towel to wipe the coupling gel off her breast. A second staff person is always in the room when we scan patients.

Scanning by the radiologist is encouraged strongly. The breast imaging radiologists do all of the breast ultrasounds at our facility. We do not use an ultrasound technologist. A mammography technologist, or an assistant, helps us during diagnostic and interventional ultrasounds but does not perform the scan. We have several reasons for taking this approach. First, by having the radiologist do the ultrasound studies, we are able to examine the patient and correlate what is described or seen on the mammogram with our own physical exam. Real-time scanning and palpation are critical to our final impression. Second, ultrasound is an operator-dependent study. Normal tissue can be made to simulate a lesion, and true lesions can be easily overlooked. To establish the presence of a lesion, the transducer needs to be rotated over the potential lesion, using variable amounts of pressure to eliminate artifactual shadowing generated by ligaments. Third, as the physical examination is done, and an impression is generated during real-time scanning, selective images are taken to document the features of the lesion, leading us to make a specific recommendation (Table 4.1). We do not take images of normal tissue. Finally, by doing the ultrasound ourselves, we can establish rapport with patients. We can elicit pertinent history, reassure the patient that we are doing everything possible to take care of her, and discuss findings and recommendations. The patient's input is sought, and she is involved in the decision-making process. After discussing all reasonable alternatives, we provide the patient with a specific recommendation.

Correlative physical examination is done as the patient is scanned. The ultrasound coupling gel improves perception of palpable abnormalities. The transducer is moved in small increments over an area, while the index, middle, and ring fingers of the contralateral hand are placed at the leading edge of the transducer and used to palpate the area being scanned. If a possible abnormality is detected, the transducer is rotated 360 degrees over the area to help distinguish a mass from a fat lobule in cross-section. A mass main-

> As you are doing the study, undertake correlative physical examination by placing the pads of the index, middle, and ring fingers (dominant hand) at the leading edge of the transducer. This is the equivalent of having eyeballs on the tips of your fingers.

Table 4.1: Breast Ultrasound: Features of Lesions

Malignant	Benign	Indeterminate
Spiculation	Intensely hyperechoic, homogenous	Isoechoic
Angular margins	Oval, ellipsoid shape	Mildly hypoechoic
Marked hypoechogenicity	Gentle bilobulation or trilobulation	Heterogeneous echotexture
Shadowing	Thin, echogenic pseudocapsule	Homogeneous echotexture
Calcifications	No malignant features	Normal sound transmission
Duct extension		Posterior enhancement
Branch pattern		
Microlobulation		
Thickened, ill-defined margins		
Round or vertical orientation (taller than wide)		

tains a round, oval, or irregular shape as the transducer is rotated, whereas fatty tissue elongates and fuses with surrounding structures. Traditionally, transverse and longitudinal orientations are used for imaging, but because ductal structures radiate out from the nipple toward the chest wall, radial and antiradial scan orientations are recommended by some.

Images are not taken until a decision is made about the presence of a lesion. Making this determination involves correlation with mammographic and clinical findings, slow movements and rotations of the transducer over the area of concern, gradations in compression, time gain compensation (TGC) curve and power-setting manipulations, positioning of the focal zones, correct field of view, and if indicated, use of a standoff pad. If during real-time scanning it is determined that a lesion is present, images are then taken to document the presence and features of the lesion. Using whatever orientations demonstrate the features of the mass best, orthogonal images are taken with and without measurements for a total of four images per lesion. The images are annotated (2,3) to include the name of the patient, unique patient identifying number, date of study, name of facility, breast being imaged, o'clock location of the lesion (Figure 4.2A), distance of the lesion from the nipple, transducer orientation (radial/antiradial; transverse/longitudinal) (Figure 4.2B) and depth in the breast (retroareolar, anterior third, middle portion, posterior third, axillary tail, axilla). As the transducer is manipulated, the size of the lesion varies. In providing a measurement, an attempt is made to use the largest dimensions of the lesion (2,3). It is also useful to indicate on the film whether the lesion is palpable.

TERMINOLOGY

Several terms are used to characterize the appearance of tissue and lesions on ultrasound. In the breast, the echogenicity of an area of interest is compared to the appearance of subcutaneous fat. If the area contains fewer echoes (i.e., appears darker) compared with subcutaneous fat, it is hypoechoic; if it contains more echoes (i.e., appears whiter), it is hyperechoic; if it contains no echoes (i.e., it is black), it is anechoic; and if it is of the same echogenicity as subcutaneous fat, it is isoechoic. At the junction of tissues with significant acoustic impedance differences, variable amounts of the sound beam are reflected back, and a shadow is seen. The size of the shadow depends on the size of the interface. Shadowing is a feature of some lesions, and although more common with malignant lesions, it is also seen with some benign masses (Figure 4.3). In lesions associated with calcifications, shadowing is sometimes seen in association with the calcifications (Figure 4.4).

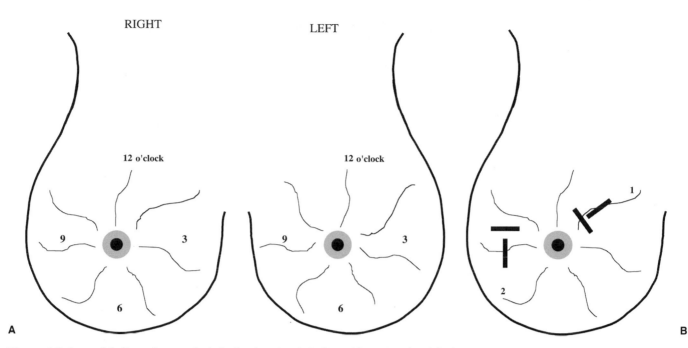

Figure 4.2 *Image labeling, ultrasound. A.* Lesion location is indicated by using the o'clock position of the lesion in the breast and the distance of the lesion from the nipple. *B.* Images are obtained in orthogonal projections. This includes radial and antiradial (1) or transverse and longitudinal (2).

Simple cysts do not attenuate sound energy. Consequently, a proportionately greater amount of sound energy reaches the tissues deep to a cyst. The TGC curve, however, is compensating for presumed decreases in echo strength as the distance from the transducer increases. The resulting effect is that tissue deep to cysts appears more echogenic than adjacent tissue. This increased echogenicity deep to fluid-filled structures is called *posterior acoustic enhancement* or *increased sound (through) transmission.* Enhancement is common with cysts; however, it can be seen with benign (Figure 4.4) and malignant solid masses.

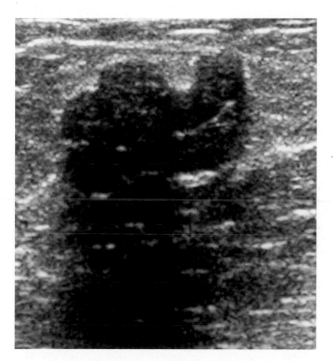

Figure 4.3 *Fibroadenoma, hyalinized.* Irregular, lobulated hypoechoic mass with shadowing. No calcifications are seen mammographically. Although more commonly associated with malignant masses, benign lesions, including hyalinized fibroadenomas, focal fibrosis, and masses with associated calcifications, can have shadowing.

BREAST ANATOMY ON ULTRASOUND

Understanding the anatomy of the breast on ultrasound is helpful in evaluating potential lesions. The pleural reflection, ribs, and pectoral muscles are deep to breast tissue and usually imaged during scanning. The pleural reflection is a hyperechoic band deep to the ribs. The tissue–air interface usually leads to shadowing deep to the pleural reflection. Simulating lesions, ribs in cross-section are well-circumscribed, oval structures (Figure 4.5A). Recognizing the relationship of the ribs to the pleural reflection and overlying pectoral muscles is important in distinguishing a rib in cross-section from a lesion. Longitudinally, ribs are echogenic bands of variable thickness with shadowing (Figure 4.5B). The pectoral muscles are hypoechoic with associated specular echoes that may be seen as bright spots in the muscle when in cross-section or as echogenic, parallel hyperechoic bands when imaged longitudinally (Figure 4.5C). The deep pectoral fascia is an echogenic line on the surface of the pectoral muscle that separates the muscle from overlying breast tissue.

Cooper's ligaments connect deep and superficial pectoral fascial layers, thereby providing a honeycomb-like structure or a "skeleton" for breast tissue. The ligaments are hyperechoic bands that crisscross the breast isolating oval and oblong areas of glandular and fatty tissues. Superficially, Cooper's ligaments extend to the superficial pectoral fascia in the deep dermis. Given the oval and oblong shape of breast tissue bundles, transducer movements and rotation over an area of concern are important. When breast tissue bundles are imaged in cross-section as round or oval structures, they can sometimes simulate a lesion. As the transducer is rotated 90 degrees, breast tissue bundles elongate and fuse with surrounding tissue; a lesion will maintain its round or oval shape (Figure 4.6). Breast tissue bundles also commonly have small, hyperechoic bands within them not typically seen in solid masses (Figure 4.7).

Dense glandular tissue is relatively hyperechoic (Figure 4.8). Because most breast lesions are hypoechoic relative to subcutaneous fat, lesions are identified more readily in women with dense tissue mammographically. Cooper's ligaments are not as apparent in

Rotation of the transducer (90 degrees) over the area being evaluated during real-time scanning is critical in characterizing lesions and distinguishing them from bundles of normal tissue.

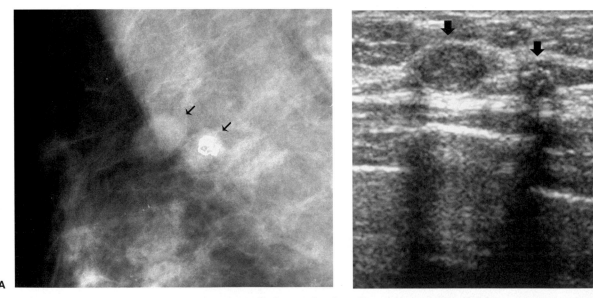

A   **B**

***Figure 4.4** Multiple, peripheral papillomas. A.* Mediolateral oblique view demonstrating two oval masses (*arrows*), new compared with the previous year's study. One of these is associated with a coarse calcification. *B.* Two solid masses (*arrows*) are seen on ultrasound corresponding to the areas of mammographic concern. The largest is oval and associated with posterior acoustic enhancement. The second, smaller mass, contains internal specular echoes reflecting the presence of calcifications with associated shadowing. Papillomas diagnosed on core biopsy and confirmed on excisional biopsy.

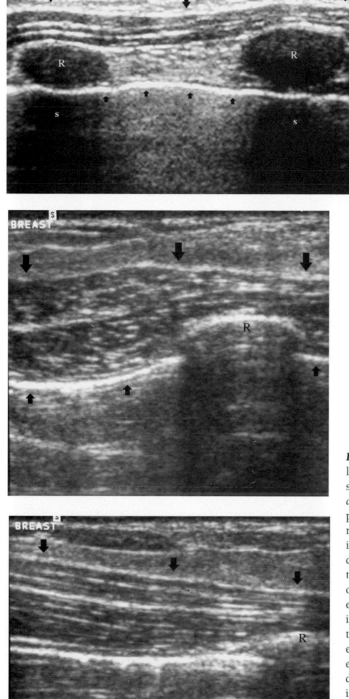

Figure 4.5 *Normal anatomy. A.* Ribs (R) in cross-section simulate an oval hypoechoic mass; these are often associated with shadowing (s). The echogenic line deep to the ribs (*short arrows*) is the pleural reflection. Two parallel echogenic lines are present in the body of the pectoral muscle, directly over the ribs. The echogenic line on the superficial surface of the muscle is the deep pectoral fascia (*long arrows*) and serves as the demarcation between breast tissue and chest wall structures. In this area, the pectoral muscle is thin, and there is not much overlying breast tissue. *B.* Different patient; longitudinally oriented rib (R) with associated shadowing. The pleural reflection is imaged as an echogenic line (*short arrows*) deep to the pectoral muscle. In this orientation, round and oval specular echoes are imaged in association with the pectoral muscle. The echogenic line (*long arrows*) on the surface of the muscle is the deep pectoral fascia. A small amount of overlying breast tissue is seen on this image. *C.* As the transducer is rotated, the specular echoes seen in the muscle in part *B* elongate and become parallel echogenic lines in the substance of the muscle. The pleural reflection is again seen as an echogenic line deep to the muscle; a portion of rib (R) with associated shadowing is also noted. The echogenic line associated with the surface of the muscle is the deep pectoral fascia (*arrows*) and separates the muscle from overlying breast tissue.

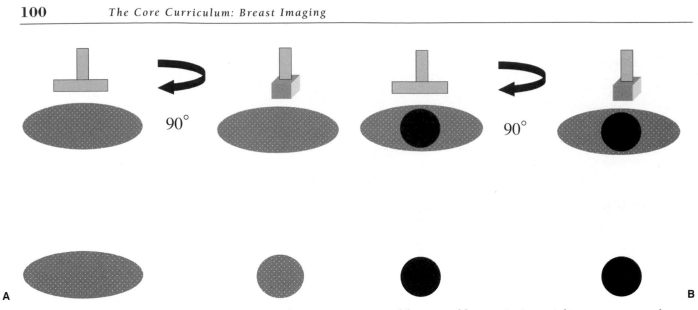

Figure 4.6 *Transducer orientation: pseudolesions and lesions. A.* Cooper's ligaments create a honeycomb-like "skeletal" framework for breast tissue. Oblong bundles of glandular and fatty tissues are found within the honeycombs created by the ligaments. When the tissue is imaged longitudinally, the oblong tissue bundles are easily detected as normal tissue. When viewed in cross-section, however, they can sometimes closely mimic a mass. Rotation and sometimes minor rocking of the transducer over a suspected mass is critical in determining the significance of any potential finding. *B.* If there is a mass present in the tissue bundles, it will be seen three dimensionally as the transducer is manipulated and rotated over the suspected mass.

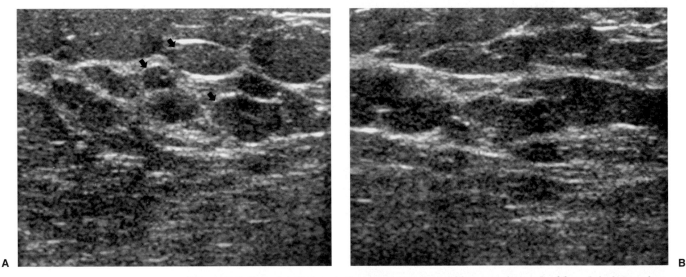

Figure 4.7 *Fatty lobulation. A.* Round and oval masslike areas (*arrows*) of fatty lobulation that can be mistaken for lesions. *B.* As the transducer is rotated 90 degrees, these areas fuse and elongate with surrounding tissue, consistent with normal fatty lobulation. A true mass will maintain its three-dimensional shape as the transducer is rotated.

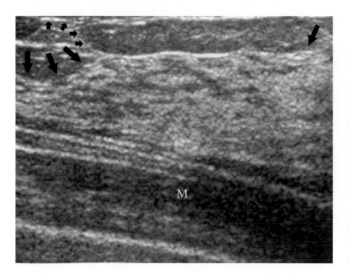

Figure 4.8 *Dense tissue.* Relatively hyperechoic tissue (*large arrows*) is seen, with visualization of Cooper's ligaments limited in this portion of tissue. Small, hypoechoic, round and oval areas are seen in the tissue, likely reflecting ducts and lobular units. Relatively hypoechoic fatty tissue is seen superficially (*small arrows*). Ligaments are sometimes apparent in this tissue type as echogenic lines. Muscle (M) is seen deep to the glandular tissue.

hyperechoic fibrous tissue because they are isoechoic with fibrous tissue. In women with predominantly fatty tissue, however, lesions may be isoechoic with surrounding tissue and not identifiable. In fatty tissue, Cooper's ligaments are identified more easily because they are hyperechoic relative to the surrounding tissue (Figure 4.9). In this patient population, however, mammography is reliable in depicting small water-density lesions. During pregnancy, breast tissue usually becomes more homogeneous with small round and oval anechoic spaces. Cooper's ligaments, fibrous ridges, and tissue bundles are not as readily apparent (Figure 4.10). Prominent ductal structures may be seen, particularly in the subareolar area.

Use of the standoff pad is often required for evaluation of the skin. Normally, skin measures 1 to 2 mm and is made up of a hypoechoic band sandwiched between two hyperechoic lines (Figure 4.11). Edema resulting from radiation therapy, congestive heart failure, benign inflammatory processes, or inflammatory carcinoma can present with skin thickening. The deep hyperechoic line may be disrupted, and there is thickening of the hypoechoic band. Small, anastomosing, serpiginous tubular structures, representing

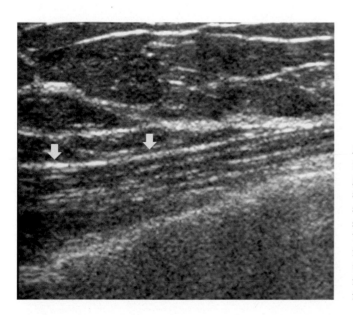

Figure 4.9 *Fatty tissue.* Relatively hypoechoic tissue. Echogenic lines crisscrossing tissue are ligaments. Muscle with parallel echogenic lines in its substance is seen deep to the tissue. The echogenic line on the surface of the muscle (*arrows*) is the deep pectoral fascia separating pectoral muscle from overlying breast tissue.

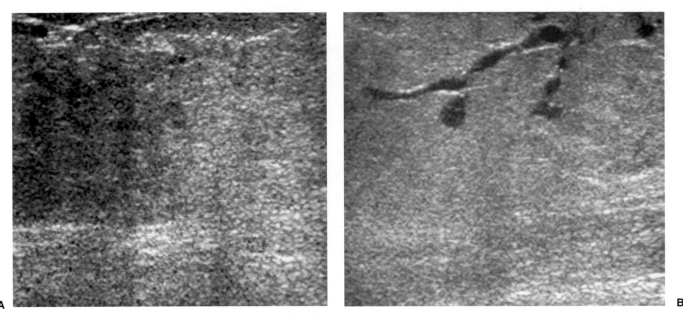

A   B

Figure 4.10 *Lactational changes. A.* During late pregnancy and lactation, breast tissue is more homogeneously hyperechoic, and demarcation of tissue bundles is less apparent. *B.* Mild to moderately dilated ducts with a somewhat beaded appearance can be seen coursing through the tissue for variable distances from the nipple. These can be more or less distended depending on when the last breast-feeding or pumping occurred.

dilated lymphatics, are sometimes seen deep to the thickened skin (Figure 4.12). Malignant and inflammatory processes arising in breast tissue can extend to involve the skin, with disruption of the deep hyperechoic strip and expansion in the hypoechoic band. Benign lesions (e.g., sebaceous cysts) involving the skin, and sometimes arising in the hypoechoic band, can be localized, and their connection to the skin surface through pores can sometimes be identified. Rarely, metastatic disease to the skin can be imaged as thickening of the hypoechoic band with disruption of the superficial echogenic line when there is associated skin ulceration (Figure 4.13).

The nipple contains connective tissue and smooth muscle. In some women, it can simulate a mass; in others, it produces intense shadowing (Figure 4.14A, B). To evaluate

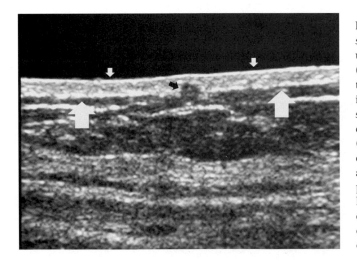

Figure 4.11 *Skin and developing skin lesion.* Spacer used to evaluate a superficial palpable mass (*black arrow*). Normal skin is 1 to 2 mm thick and is characterized by a hypoechoic band sandwiched between two echogenic lines. The superficial (*small arrows*) and deep echogenic (*large arrows*) lines are well seen in this patient. The palpable mass arises in the hypoechoic band, disrupts the deep echogenic line, and extends minimally into the subcutaneous fat of the breast.

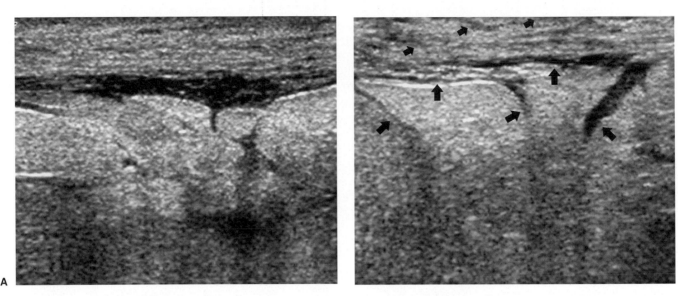

Figure 4.12 *Skin thickening and dilated subcutaneous lymphatics in a patient with congestive heart failure. A.* Skin thickening is noted in this patient with congestive heart failure. The superficial and deep echogenic lines are not apparent, and the hypoechoic band is thickened. Tubular, anastomosing, serpiginous structures deep to the skin are dilated lymphatics. The tissue is echogenic, and normal tissue planes are disrupted. *B.* Same patient, different area of the breast. In this area, thin lymphatic channels can be seen in the hypoechoic band of the skin (*arrows*).

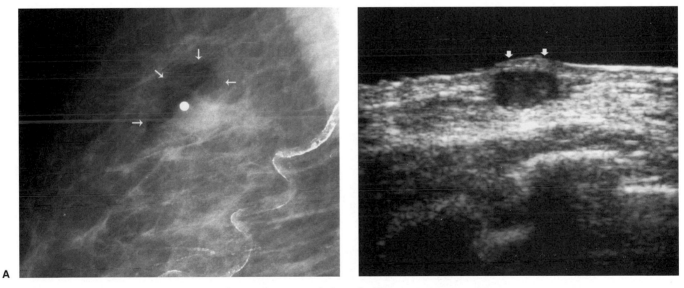

Figure 4.13 *Leiomyosarcoma, metastatic to breast skin. A.* Mediolateral oblique view in a patient with a history of leiomyosarcoma, presenting with a mass (metallic BB) in the right breast. Air (lucency) pocket (*arrows*) outlines the ulcerative portion of the mass. Vascular calcification is present. *B.* A standoff pad is used to evaluate superficial mass with ulceration. Mass in the hypoechoic band of the skin extending and disrupting both superficial (*arrows*) and deep echogenic lines.

the subareolar area, the transducer needs to be angled around the nipple. Ductal structures can be seen in the subareolar area coursing toward the nipple (Figure 4.14C, D). Intraductal lesions, such as papillomas, can sometimes be identified, particularly if the lesion is in the subareolar portion of the duct (Figure 4.15). Radial scanning is helpful in demonstrating the ducts coursing for variable distances away from the nipple.

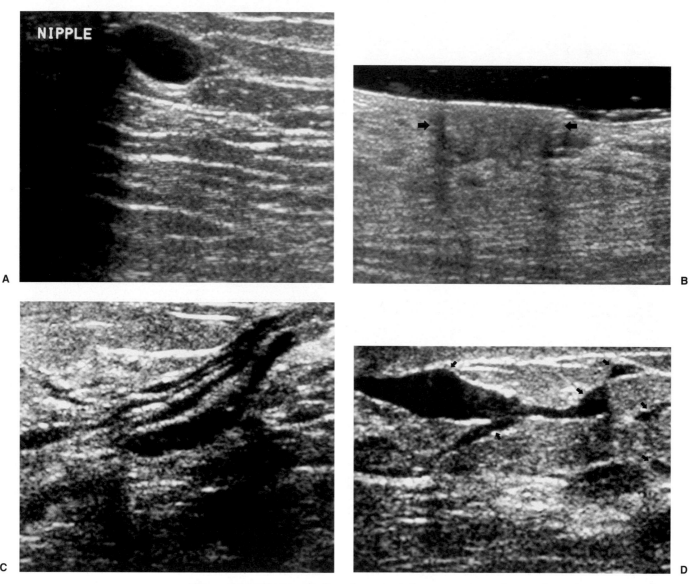

Figure 4.14 *Nipple and subareolar area.* A. In many women, the nipple produces a strong shadow that limits evaluation of the subareolar area. From the base of the nipple, the transducer needs to be angled into the subareolar area. B. In some patients, if generous amounts of coupling gel are put over the nipple and some pressure is applied to the nipple, an oval hypoechoic mass (*arrows*) is simulated that may be mistaken for a lesion. From the base of the nipple, the transducer is angled into the subareolar area to determine whether there is a lesion deep to the nipple. C. Several ducts are imaged coursing proximally from the nipple. Because ducts and their branches course in an out of the plane of the transducer, it can be difficult to follow and image them. D. Different patient. A duct with focal areas of dilation can be followed from the nipple proximally (*arrows*). During real time, it could be connected to some of the tubular structures in this image that appear separate from the main duct. This is common because ducts course in and out of the scan plane.

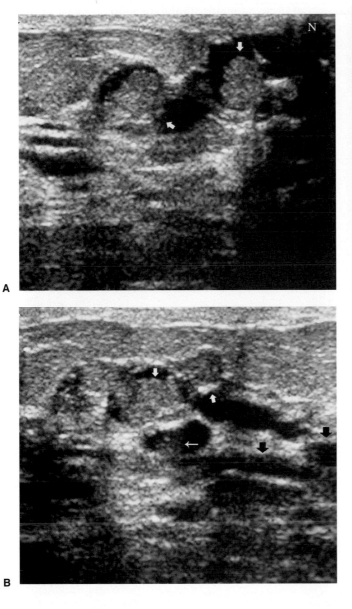

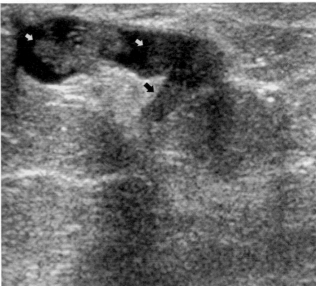

Figure 4.15 *Multiple papillomas in subareolar portions of ductal system.* A. Dilated duct with two intraductal lesions (*arrows*). These have some minimal posterior acoustic enhancement. The nipple (N) in this patient is generating a strong shadow. To evaluate the subareolar area, the transducer needs to be placed at the base of the nipple and angled toward the subareolar area. B. Different patient. A portion of the dilated duct is imaged in this scan. Two intraductal lesions are present (*white arrows*), one of which extends into one of the branches of the duct (*black arrow*). During real-time scanning, more portions of the duct could be seen as the transducer was gently manipulated. C. Different patient. Three intraductal lesions (*thick white arrows*) in a dilated duct. Although the smallest of these (*thin white arrow*) appears to be in a separate duct, during real-time scanning, this could be linked to the duct containing the two larger lesions. Other, seemingly isolated tubular structures on this image (*black arrows*) are also part of the duct containing the intraductal lesions. As the transducer is slowly manipulated during real-time scanning, the connections of this ductal system become apparent as branches of the duct come into and out of the plane being scanned.

Vascular structures can sometimes be seen in cross-section, less commonly longitudinally (Figure 4.16). Doppler is helpful in establishing the nature of the finding. In women with extensive, dense vascular calcification, the calcified vessels can sometimes be seen on ultrasound (Figure 4.17). Acutely, in women with Mondor's disease, the dilated thrombosed vein is often imaged subcutaneously (Figure 4.18); no flow is seen in the vein. Intramammary lymph nodes are well-circumscribed, hypoechoic masses with a central or eccentrically located hyperechoic hilar region (Figure 4.19). Bulging and thickening of a markedly hypoechoic cortical region and attenuation (mass effect) or complete loss of the hyperechoic fatty hilar region are nonspecific findings that may be related to metastatic disease (Figure 4.20), lymphoma, or benign reactive changes.

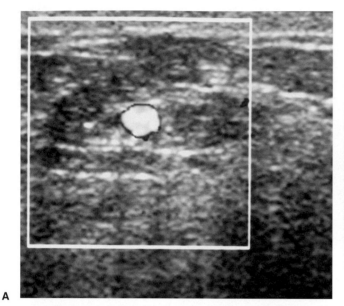

A

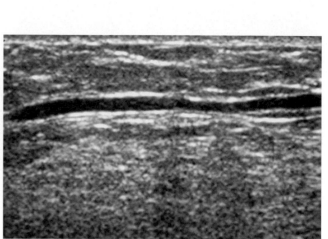

B

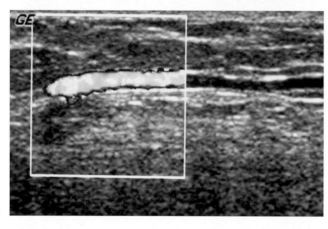

C

Figure 4.16 *Vascular structures. A.* Artery in cross-section with Doppler on. These vascular structures are imaged as anechoic, round structures that can simulate a cyst when imaged in cross-section. As the transducer is manipulated, they can sometimes be seen longitudinally. With careful observation, pulsations are evident during real-time scanning. Doppler is helpful in establishing the etiology. We routinely use Doppler on small, round, anechoic or hypoechoic structures to distinguish vessels from cysts. *B.* As the transducer is rotated over the round mass, the tubular nature of the structure is established. *C.* With Doppler, a vascular etiology is established.

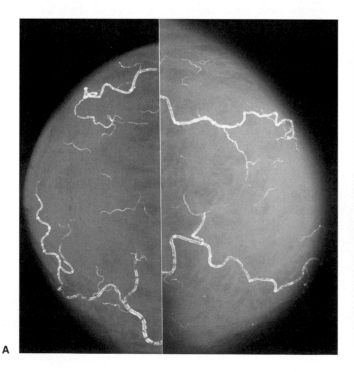

A

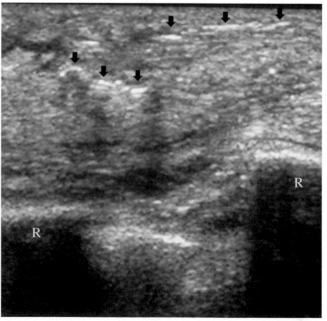

B

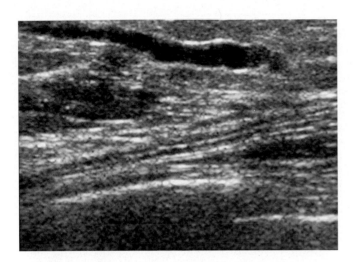

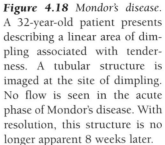

Figure 4.18 *Mondor's disease.* A 32-year-old patient presents describing a linear area of dimpling associated with tenderness. A tubular structure is imaged at the site of dimpling. No flow is seen in the acute phase of Mondor's disease. With resolution, this structure is no longer apparent 8 weeks later.

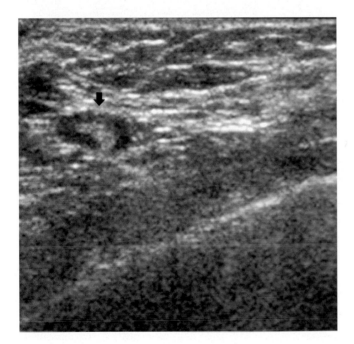

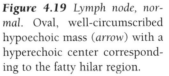

Figure 4.19 *Lymph node, normal.* Oval, well-circumscribed hypoechoic mass (*arrow*) with a hyperechoic center corresponding to the fatty hilar region.

Figure 4.17 *Vascular calcification.* A. Craniocaudal views in a 77-year-old patient. Dense tissue. Extensive vascular calcification is present. B. Irregular, linear areas of echogenicity (*arrows*) can rarely be seen when the vascular calcification is extensive, as in this patient. Shadowing is seen associated with some of the calcifications. Longitudinally oriented ribs (R) can be seen.

INDICATIONS FOR ULTRASOUND

For many years, ultrasound was used sparingly and almost exclusively to characterize breast masses as cystic or solid. Although this remains an important use, improvements in equipment have led to increases in the indications for breast ultrasound. It is now an important tool in evaluating women with mammographically or clinically detected abnormalities. The indications include (a) matrix characterization of palpable or mammographically detected masses; (b) characterization of solid masses; (c) evaluation of nonspecific mammographic findings (e.g., developing parenchymal asymmetry); (d) evaluation of tissue or lesions potentially excluded on routine mammographic views (e.g., upper inner quadrants, axillary tissue); (e) evaluation of women with inflammatory symptoms to distinguish mastitis from an abscess or an underlying advanced breast cancer or inflammatory carcinoma; (f) in conjunction with ductography, evaluation of women presenting with spontaneous nipple discharge (Chapter 11), and (g) guiding of interventional procedures (Chapter 11).

The use of ultrasound for screening purposes is controversial. As ultrasound units improve and we continue to learn, a role for screening women with dense tissue and who are at high risk for cancer is likely to develop. Data in support of screening are emerging (4–7). Kolb and colleagues reported a 42% increase in the detection of breast cancer with screening ultrasound in women with dense tissue mammographically (5). In this study, the cancers detected with screening ultrasound were similar in size and stage to those detected with screening mammography. The false-positive screening ultrasound rate was reported as 2.4% by these investigators (5).

Screening ultrasound in women with predominantly fatty tissue adds very little and may be misleading. In these patients, however, mammography is an excellent screening tool, with a sensitivity of 98% (5). The most likely and appropriate role for screening ultrasound would be to evaluate women with dense tissue mammographically in whom we know that breast cancers are missed; the sensitivity of mammography in women with dense tissue may be as low as 48% (5). Limitations of ultrasound and arguments against its routine use for screening relate to the inability to detect calcifications reliably and to the operator dependence of the study. As with mammography, quality issues and standardization of techniques and equipment would seem appropriate before widespread use. Also, it should be made clear to patients, referring physicians, and third-party payers that screening ultrasound would be used in conjunction with mammography, not as a replacement.

MATRIX DETERMINATION

One of the most important roles of breast ultrasound is to help establish whether a clinical or mammographically apparent mass is cystic or solid. Breast ultrasound is 96% to 100% accurate in the diagnosis of cysts when appropriate criteria are used (8). Simple cysts are anechoic, well-circumscribed masses with sharp anterior and posterior walls, thin edge shadows, posterior acoustic enhancement (Figure 4.21), and compressibility. Slight movements or changes in the orientation of the transducer may be needed to demonstrate posterior acoustic enhancement. Also, with small (less than about 5 mm) or deep cysts, posterior acoustic enhancement may not be demonstrable. Unless the cyst is under tension, pressure applied with the transducer leads to compression and elongation of the cyst. Reverberation artifacts can involve the anterior wall of some cysts (Figure 4.22). If the criteria for a simple cyst are fulfilled and the patient is asymptomatic, we do not recommend aspiration. We try to educate and reassure the patient that cysts are common, benign masses that fluctuate in size and tenderness with the menstrual cycle, may regress spontaneously, and often recur if aspirated. It the patient is symptomatic, aspiration is undertaken. Likewise, if we are not sure the finding is a cyst because atypical features are seen on the ultrasound, aspiration and sometimes pneumocystography are undertaken (Chapter 11).

In the early phases of cyst formation, as acini begin to distend with fluid, tightly clustered, round, 1- to 2-mm anechoic areas are seen on ultrasound. The microcysts are separated by thin, echogenic septations (Figure 4.23). Posterior acoustic enhancement may be

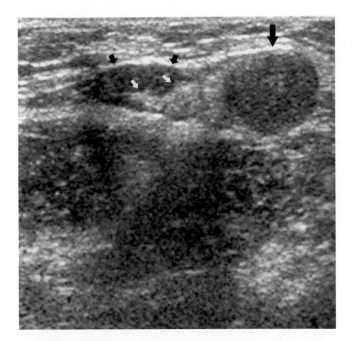

Figure 4.20 *Lymph node, metastatic disease.* Scan through axilla in a patient with a mass associated with malignant-type calcifications (ultrasound of breast lesion shown in Figure 4.37). Two lymph nodes are present. One of these (*small black arrows*) appears oval and retains the echogenic hilar area (*white arrows*). The second (*large black arrow*) is round, and no echogenic central or eccentric area is identified. Fine-needle aspiration of this node confirms the presence of metastatic disease. Bulging and thickening of the cortical region and attenuation, mass effect, or loss of the fatty hilum suggests metastatic disease.

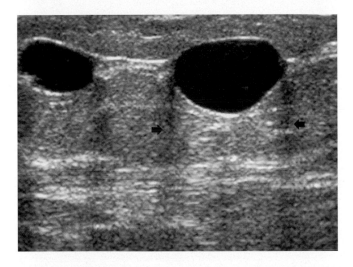

Figure 4.21 *Simple cysts.* Two adjacent, simple cysts. Well-circumscribed, anechoic mass with thin edge shadows (*arrows*), sharp anterior and posterior walls, and posterior acoustic enhancement. The enhancement is seen best in the larger of the two cysts.

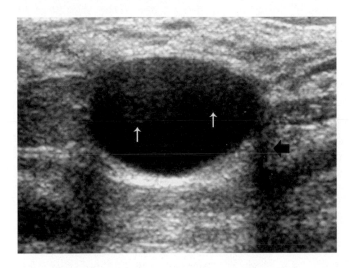

Figure 4.22 *Simple cyst, reverberation.* Oval, well-circumscribed mass with thin edge shadows (*black arrow*) and enhancement. Echoes in the superficial aspect of the cyst (*white arrows*) reflect reverberation artifact.

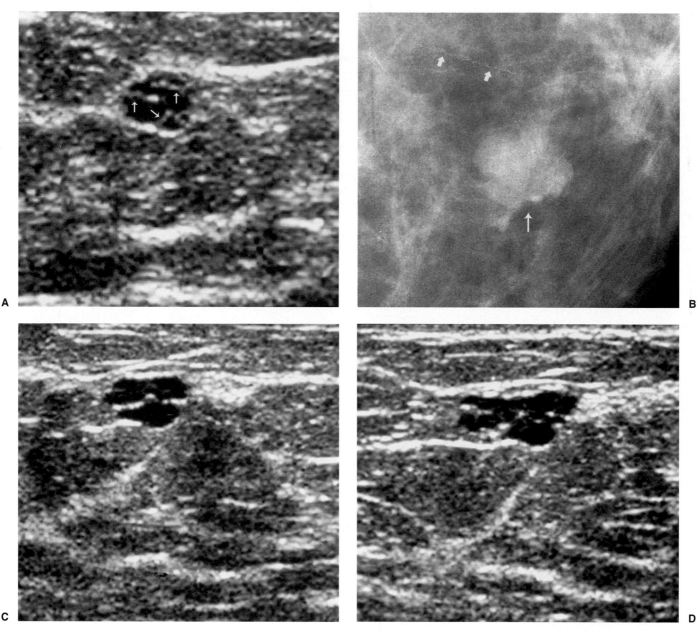

Figure 4.23 *Microcysts. A.* Clustered, small, round and oval anechoic masses. The thin walls of the distending acini are evident (*arrows*). During core biopsy, these tend to disappear after the first or second pass of the needle. Epithelial and apocrine-lined cysts are reported histologically. *B.* Different patient. Spot compression view of a new finding on screening mammography demonstrates a mass with partially well-circumscribed and indistinct margins (*thin arrow*). Incidentally noted is nail polish artifact (*small, thick arrows*). *C* and *D.* Ultrasound images corresponding to the area of mammographic concern demonstrating a cluster of anechoic, oval masses. The thin walls of the distending acini are evident as thin, echogenic lines separating the anechoic components. Epithelial and apocrine-lined cysts are reported histologically. As we have acquired experience, and with our medical audit data to support our approach, we no longer routinely biopsy patients with lesions having these mammographic and ultrasonographic features.

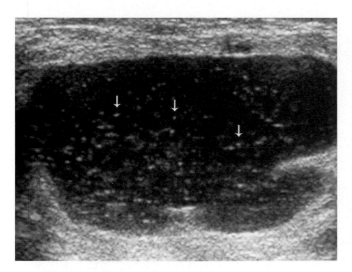

Figure 4.24 Gurgling cyst. Many specular echoes (few marked with *arrows*) in otherwise anechoic mass associated with posterior acoustic enhancement. During real-time scanning, these echoes can be seen moving and sometimes swirling in the fluid. Unless the patient is symptomatic or requests an aspiration, we do not routinely intervene when this feature is seen during real-time scanning.

present. Although initially described as apocrine-lined cysts (9), histologically, these areas are commonly a combination of small cystic spaces lined with either epithelial cells or cells characterized by apocrine metaplasia. As the acini continue to distend with fluid, clusters of small cysts may be seen. As these small cysts coalesce, the more characteristic appearance of the single cyst is seen.

The presence of internal echoes that move in the fluid (Figure 4.24) during real-time scanning (gurgling, swirling) and septations (Figure 4.25) are common variants. Nondependent, nongurgling internal echoes that partially or completely fill the cyst (Figure 4.26) and irregular or thickened walls when inflamed are atypical features of cysts. If not all of the criteria for the diagnosis of a cyst are present, there are atypical features, or the diagnosis of a cyst is otherwise in question, aspiration should be undertaken. Cysts should

Consider cyst aspiration when atypical imaging features are seen and when the patient is symptomatic.

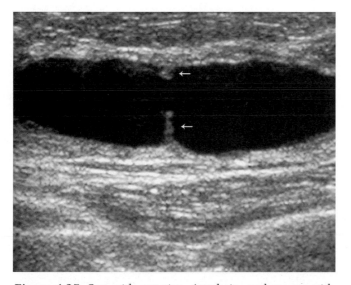

Figure 4.25 Cyst with septation. Anechoic, oval masses with well-circumscribed margins and posterior acoustic enhancement. Thin edge shadows are seen during real-time scanning as the transducer is manipulated over this area. Thin septations (*arrows*) such as these are common normal variations. Unless the septation is thickened or irregular, we do not intervene when these are seen on ultrasound.

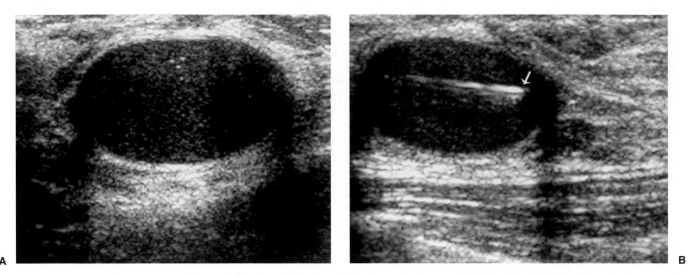

Figure 4.26 *Cyst. A.* Oval, well-circumscribed mass with thin edge shadows and posterior acoustic enhancement. Internal echoes make distinction from a solid mass difficult. However, when masses with these types of internal echoes (you can almost identify the individual echoes) are seen in the subareolar area, they are commonly cysts. *B.* Needle (*arrow*) in cyst. During the aspiration, the echoes are seen being sucked into the needle along with the fluid. No residual abnormality is seen after aspiration, and thin walls are seen in these patients when pneumocystography is done. On visual inspection of the fluid, the fluid in these types of cyst appears no different from that in cysts with no internal echoes. Unless we can unequivocally call a mass a cyst, we undertake aspiration to establish the diagnosis.

collapse completely, and no residual abnormality should be seen after aspiration. If an intracystic or mural lesion is suspected, pneumocystography is done (Chapter 11). Cyst fluid is not routinely submitted for cytologic evaluation unless the fluid is bloody. Galactoceles are cysts that contain milky fluid. They present in women during lactation but may be diagnosed several years after the cessation of breast-feeding. Ultrasound findings in women with galactoceles are variable. They are often indistinguishable from simple cysts, but they can be associated with atypical features, including significant shadowing (Figure 4.27).

Complex cystic masses can be seen in a variety of circumstances. Although there can be significant overlap in the diagnostic considerations, we characterize these masses as predominantly cystic with solid components or predominantly solid with cystic components (Table 4.2). Included in the first group are postoperative or traumatic fluid collec-

Table 4.2: Breast Ultrasound: Complex Cystic Masses

Cystic with Solid Elements	Solid with Cystic Features
Postoperative fluid collections	Complex fibroadenomas
Posttraumatic fluid collections (hematoma)	Pseudoangiomatous stromal hyperplasia
Abscess	Fat necrosis
Papilloma (solitary, multiple)	Phyllodes
Oil cyst (fat necrosis)	Invasive ductal carcinoma
Galactocele	Mucinous carcinoma
Papillary carcinoma (central, solitary)	Metastatic disease

tions. After surgery, particularly in women undergoing a lumpectomy and radiation therapy or trauma, fluid collections may develop. In some patients, these may appear indistinguishable from a cyst. In other patients, these fluid collections have a variable ultrasound appearance, including mural nodules, intracystic septations, or a combination of these. The walls may be irregular, lobulated, and thickened (Figure 4.28). It is important to recognize the benign nature of these collections. Unless an infection is suspected, these should be left alone. Aspiration often leads to reaccumulation of fluid, and rarely, aspiration may lead to the development of draining sinuses than can be difficult to treat (Figure 4.29). Papillomas are most commonly imaged as either intraductal lesions (Figure 4.15), particularly if solitary, or as intracystic masses of variable sizes (Figures 4.30 and 4.31). In some women, they may be solid or predominantly solid with cystic components (Figure 4.32). Oil cysts and evolving areas of fat necrosis may have stages characterized ultrasonographically as cystic lesions with mural and solid-appearing intracystic nodules (Figure 4.33). Papillary carcinomas presenting centrally as solitary lesions are often characterized as a complex cystic mass (Chapter 7).

Benign complex cystic masses that are often predominantly solid with cystic components include complex fibroadenomas (Figure 4.34), pseudoangiomatous stromal hyperplasia, and phyllodes tumors. Fat necrosis in the acute setting is often imaged as a hyperechoic mass with cystic components (Figure 4.35). Malignant lesions presenting with complex cystic masses include invasive ductal carcinomas associated with necrosis (Figure 4.36), malignant phyllodes, metastatic lesions, and rarely, mucinous carcinomas (Chapter 7).

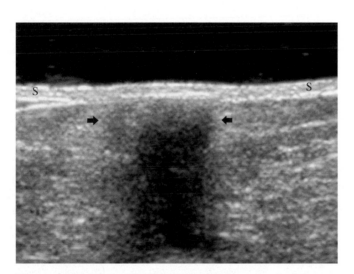

Figure 4.27 *Galactocele.* This 28-year-old patient who is breast-feeding presents with a lump. She thinks it might fluctuate in size. An oval mass is seen with indistinct margins and a heterogeneous echotexture. A portion of the mass is nearly isoechoic with surrounding tissue. Another portion of the mass is hypoechoic, and this is associated with a strong shadow (*arrows*). Thick, milky fluid is obtained on aspiration. Galactoceles are variable in their presentation. In our experience, the appearance presented here is not uncommon. Normal skin (S) is seen well because the standoff pad was used to evaluate the patient. Also note the appearance of the tissue, which is homogeneous and relatively hyperechoic, a common appearance during lactation.

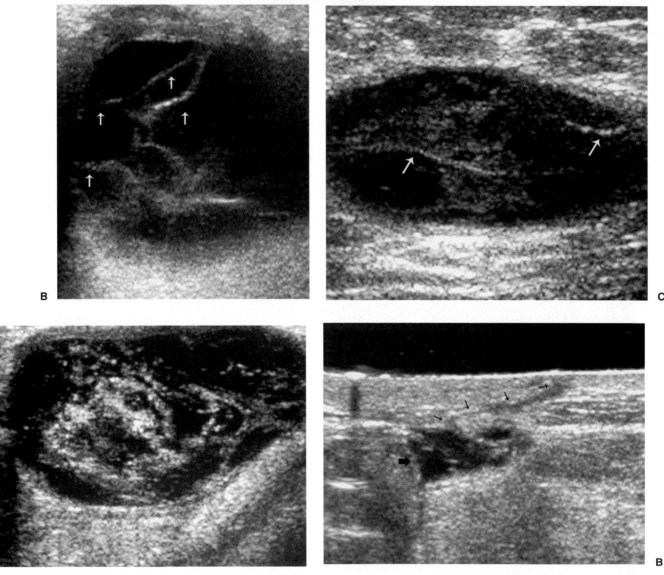

Figure 4.28 *Postsurgical fluid collections. A.* Cystic mass with mural nodules (*arrows*) corresponding to lumpectomy site. These nodules simulate intracystic masses; however, if these correlate to the lumpectomy site, no intervention is warranted unless an infection is suspected. *B.* Complex cystic mass with irregular, thick walls, septations (*arrows*), and posterior acoustic enhancement at the lumpectomy site. During real-time scanning, septations are seen "flapping" in the fluid and shifting position. Unless an infection is suspected clinically, no intervention is warranted in these patients. *C.* Complex cystic mass with solid-appearing components, septations (*arrows*), and posterior acoustic enhancement corresponding to the lumpectomy site.

Figure 4.29 *Development of a draining sinus in patient with a postoperative fluid collection. A.* Complex cystic mass at lumpectomy site. For unclear reasons, because superimposed infection was not suspected, the patient underwent aspiration, with rapid reaccumulation of fluid. A second aspiration was undertaken, after which the patient described a slow, continuous drainage of fluid. *B.* A residual complex cystic mass is present (*thick arrow*). When pressure is applied to this area, fluid drains just inferior to the nipple. Tract to the surface of the breast is evident (*thin arrows*). When these sinuses develop, they can be difficult to eradicate, often requiring surgical intervention. Unless superimposed infection is suspected, postoperative fluid collections do not require any intervention.

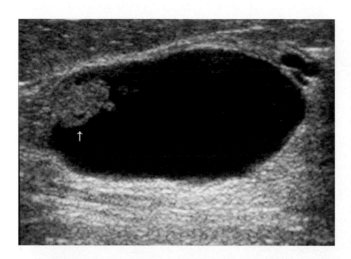

Figure 4.30 *Solitary intracystic papilloma.* Mass detected on screening mammogram (not shown). A predominantly cystic mass is seen corresponding to the area of mammographic concern (*arrow*). Well-circumscribed, sharp margins with posterior acoustic enhancement indicate that an intracystic mass is present. Papilloma is diagnosed on excisional biopsy.

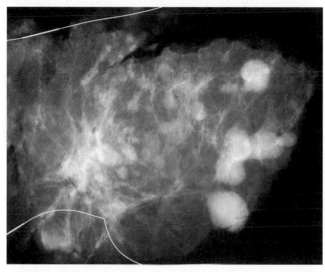

A

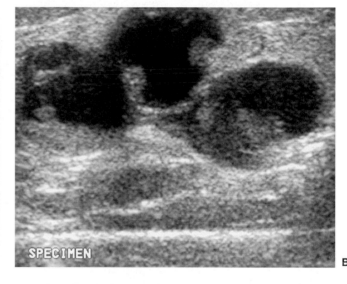

B

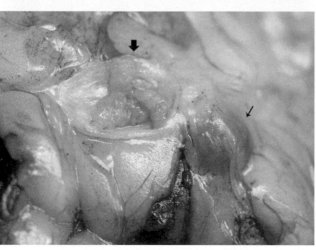

C

Figure 4.31 *Multiple peripheral papillomas.* A. In this 32-year-old patient, the specimen radiograph demonstrates multiple masses of varying density throughout the specimen. B. Ultrasound evaluation of the specimen demonstrates multiple complex cystic masses. In this area, three predominantly cystic masses with solid components are imaged. C. Correlation between gross pathology and ultrasonographic images is undertaken. As many of these masses are dissected, fluid is released. In some of these lesions, the fluid is bloody. With sectioning, a complex cystic mass is seen with a partially smooth wall and an irregular solid component (*thick arrow*) adjacent to a "blue-domed" cyst (*thin arrow*). When this second lesion is sectioned, fluid is obtained, and an intracystic mural lesion is identified. Multiple peripheral papillomas, some with associated low-grade ductal carcinoma *in situ*, are diagnosed histologically. In our experience, about 43% of patients with multiple peripheral papillomas have associated high-risk lesions, including low-grade ductal carcinoma *in situ* and lobular carcinoma *in situ*.

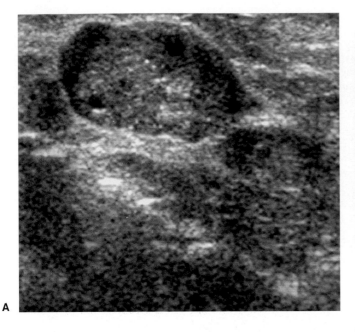

A

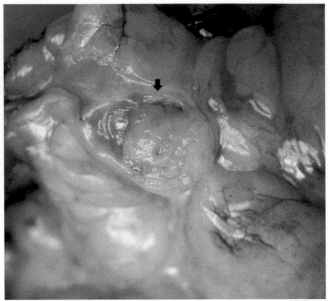

B

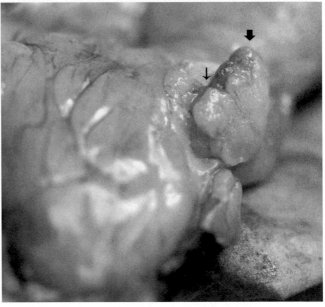

C

Figure 4.32 *Multiple peripheral papillomas. A.* Same patient as shown in Figure 4.31 with complex cystic masses. A predominantly solid mass with small cystic spaces and posterior acoustic enhancement is seen. *B.* Specimen with lesion sectioned. On one half of the specimen, the papilloma almost completely fills the cyst; however, only a small portion of it is actually attached to the wall of the cyst. *C.* On the other half, you can see the lesion in profile (*thick arrow*) and its point of attachment to the cyst (*thin arrow*). Multiple peripheral papillomas, some with associated low-grade ductal carcinoma *in situ*, are diagnosed histologically. In our experience, about 43% of patients with multiple peripheral papillomas have associated high-risk lesions, including low-grade ductal carcinoma *in situ* and lobular carcinoma *in situ*.

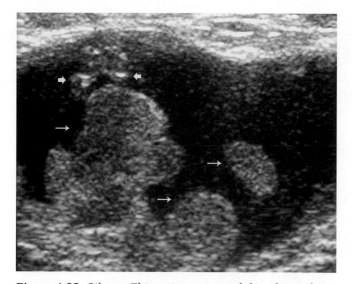

Figure 4.33 *Oil cyst.* This patient presented describing a lump in the left breast. A complex cystic mass is seen with solid-appearing intracystic nodules (*thin arrows*), some with associated calcifications (*thick arrows*). The diagnosis in this patient is made mammographically (Figure 6.18A in Chapter 6). An oil cyst is imaged at the site of concern to the patient. Although the ultrasonographic appearance is concerning, the diagnosis is made based on the presence of a lucent mass on the mammogram. No intervention is indicated. The patient needs to be reassured of the benign etiology of the lump, and the mammography report needs to be definitive. Category 2.

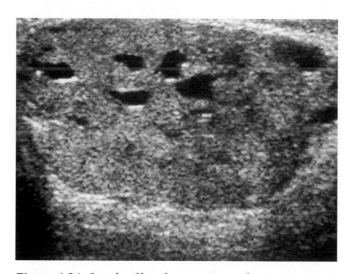

Figure 4.34 *Complex fibroadenoma.* A complex cystic mass is seen that is predominantly solid with associated cystic spaces. Posterior acoustic enhancement is noted. Complex fibroadenomas are fibroadenomas with superimposed fibrocystic changes, including cysts measuring at least 3 mm (Chapter 6).

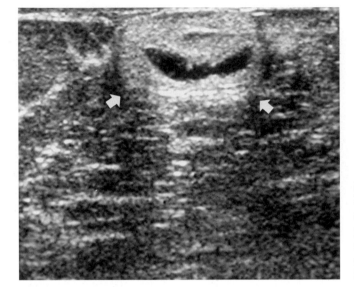

Figure 4.35 *Fat necrosis.* Oval, hyperechoic mass (*arrows*) with cystic spaces and minimal, focal posterior acoustic enhancement. In our experience, this is a common appearance for acute fat necrosis.

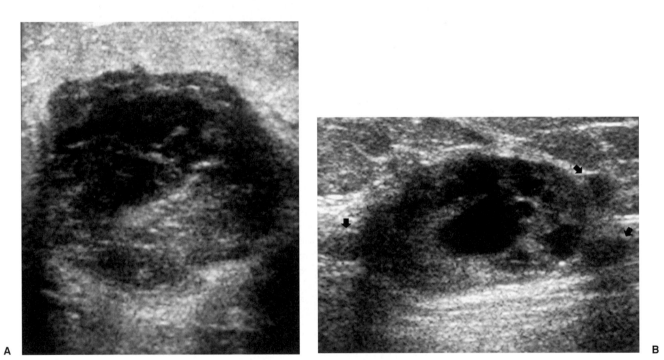

Figure 4.36 *Invasive ductal carcinoma, not otherwise specified.* A. Complex cystic mass in a 46-year-old patient. Predominantly solid mass with cystic areas, heterogeneous echotexture, irregular margins, and posterior acoustic enhancement. Imaging-guided biopsy is done. *B*. Different patient; 49 years old. Solid mass with heterogeneous echotexture, cystic spaces, irregular margins with nodular projections (*arrows*), and posterior acoustic enhancement is seen. Imaging-guided biopsy is done.

CHARACTERIZATION OF SOLID MASSES

With a solid mass, features that suggest a benign lesion include oval or ellipsoid shape, gentle bilobulation or trilobulation, hyperechogenicity, and a thin, echogenic pseudocapsule (10) (Figure 4.37). The presence of a complete pseudocapsule may only be demonstrable during real-time scanning. Characteristics of malignant lesions include spiculation, angular margins, microlobulation, shadowing, marked hypoechogenicity (Figure 4.38), calcifications (Figure 4.39), duct extension, and branch pattern (10). Malignant lesions usually demonstrate several of these characteristics in addition to being longer than they are wide and having a thickened border. Duct extension and branch pattern are determined during real-time scanning (10). Duct extension refers to tubular extension of the lesion toward the nipple, presumably within a duct (Figure 4.40). Branch pattern refers to tubular extension of the lesion away from the nipple, presumably within ducts (Figure 4.41). Posterior acoustic enhancement may be seen with malignant lesions. These lesions are often round and, in our experience, are commonly poorly differentiated, rapidly growing invasive ductal carcinomas or mucinous carcinomas (Figure 4.42). If any malignant feature is identified in a mass, a biopsy is done. As discussed in Chapter 7, when a malignancy is suspected based on clinical, mammographic, and ultrasonographic findings, we scan the ipsilateral axilla. In patients with potentially abnormal lymph nodes, imaging-guided sampling is undertaken at the same time the lesion in the breast is sampled.

Scrutinize lesions carefully; biopsy is indicated even if only one malignant feature is seen.

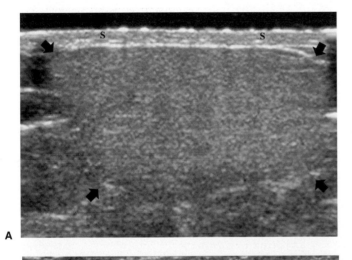
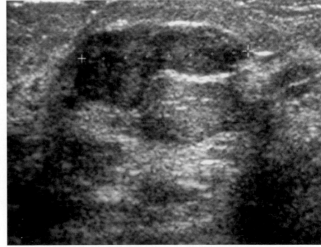

Figure 4.37 *Benign lesions.* A. Homogeneously hyperechoic mass (*arrows*) in a patient with a lipoma. Hyperechoic masses are usually benign. Normal skin (S) is noted. B. Oval, well-circumscribed hypoechoic mass with thin edge shadows and posterior acoustic enhancement. During real-time scanning, an echogenic pseudocapsule could be traced around the mass. Fibroadenoma. C. Oval, well-circumscribed hypoechoic mass with gentle macrolobulation. Fibroadenoma.

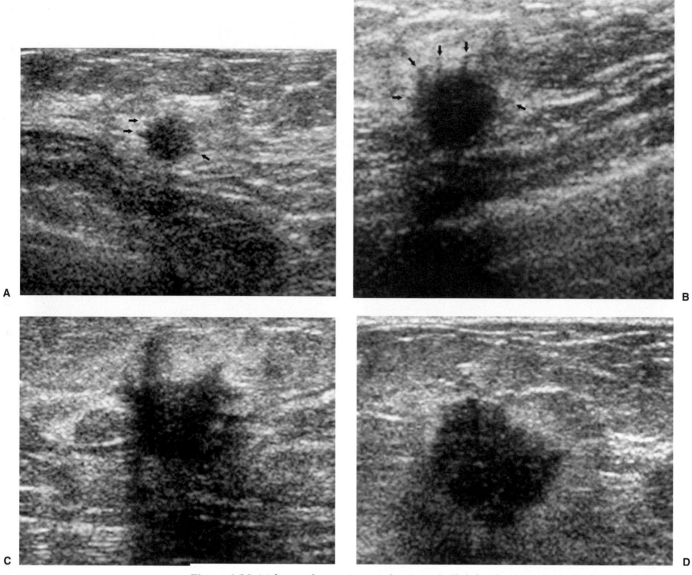

Figure 4.38 *Malignant lesions A.* Round mass with ill-defined margins and spiculations (*arrows*). *B.* Round, markedly hypoechoic mass with ill-defined margins, spiculations (*arrows*), and shadowing. *C.* Irregular hypoechoic mass with angular margins, spiculations, and shadowing. *D.* Round mass with microlobulations and shadowing.

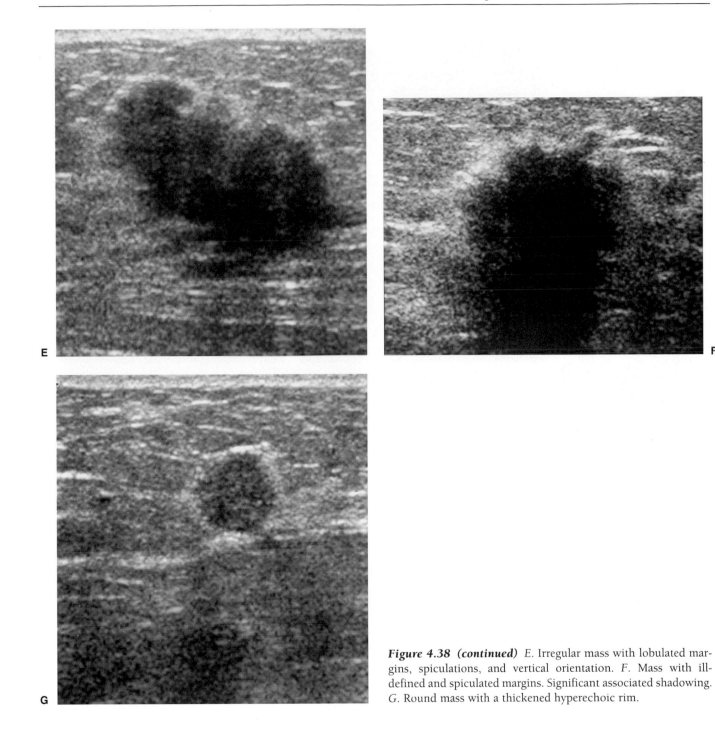

Figure 4.38 (continued) *E.* Irregular mass with lobulated margins, spiculations, and vertical orientation. *F.* Mass with ill-defined and spiculated margins. Significant associated shadowing. *G.* Round mass with a thickened hyperechoic rim.

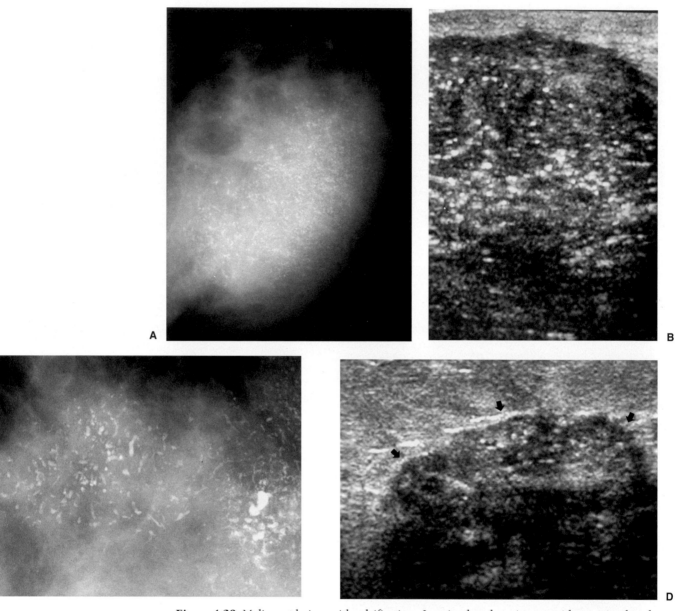

Figure 4.39 *Malignant lesions with calcifications. Invasive ductal carcinomas with extensive ductal carcinoma* in situ. *A. Dense mass with malignant calcifications. B. Round mass studded with high specular echoes consistent with calcifications. These are not associated with shadowing. C. Different patient. Large area of pleomorphic, linear, casting-type calcifications. D. Hypoechoic mass (arrows) with irregular shadowing. High specular echoes consistent with calcifications are seen mammographically.*

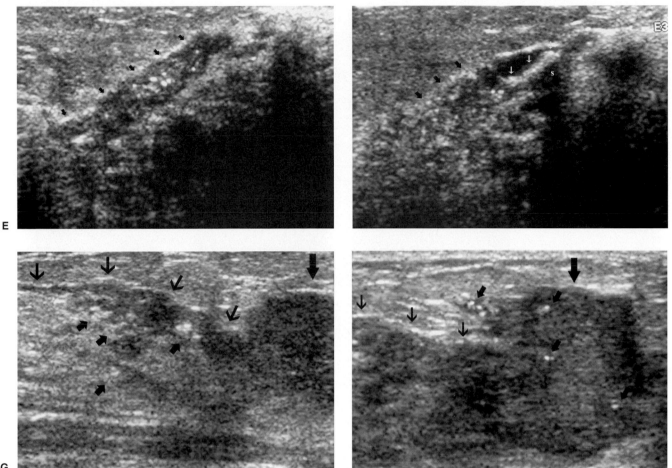

Figure 4.39 (continued) E. Scan through a different plane demonstrates a dilated ductal structure (*arrows*) with associated luminal calcifications. F. Scan through another plane. Dilated duct (*black arrows*) with associated high specular echoes in the lumen. A dense cluster of these is present (*white arrows*), generating a focal area of shadowing (S). G. Different patient. A round, hypoechoic mass with posterior acoustic enhancement is present (*long, thick arrow*). Extension of tumor into a dilated ductal structure (*thin arrows*) is noted, associated with luminal calcifications (*short, thick arrows*). The duct tapers distal to the mass. H. Scan through a different plane. Round mass with posterior acoustic enhancement (*long, thick arrow*). High specular echoes within mass and extending into a small spiculation (*short thick arrows*), consistent with calcifications. Extension of the tumors into a dilated ductal structure is also present (*thin arrows*).

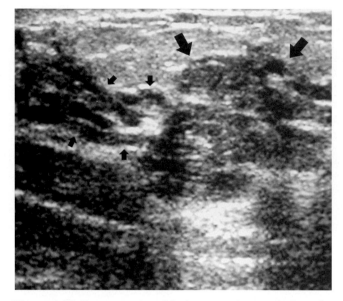

Figure 4.40 *Duct extension. Mucinous carcinoma.* A. Irregular mass (*long arrows*) with heterogeneous echotexture, ill-defined margins, and posterior acoustic enhancement. Extension of the tumor into dilated ductal structures (*short arrows*) coursing toward the nipple, consistent with extension of tumor. Ductal structures pointing toward the nipple indicate is ductal extension.

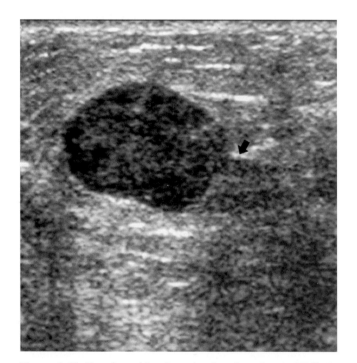

Figure 4.41 *Duct branching. Invasive ductal carcinoma.* Well-circumscribed mass with posterior acoustic enhancement. Extension of tumor into a dilated ductal structure coursing away from the nipple is present, consistent with ductal branching (*arrow*).

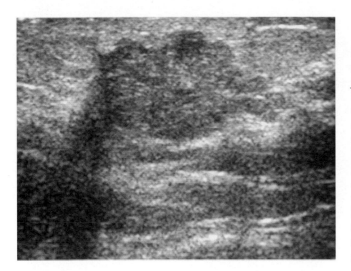

Figure 4.42 *Invasive ductal carcinoma with prominent mucinous features.* Mass with irregular and lobulated margins associated with some posterior acoustic enhancement. Enhancement is more commonly associated with benign lesions; however, it can be seen with malignant lesions. Although enhancement is seen with a variety of malignant lesions, in our experience, it is more common in poorly differentiated, rapidly growing tumors and mucinous carcinomas.

To classify a lesion as benign, a combination of features is sought (i.e., oval shape and thin pseudocapsule; gentle lobulations and thin pseudocapsule; intense and homogenous hyperechogenicity). Indeterminate features include isoechogenicity, mild hypoechogenicity, normal or enhanced sound transmission, and homogeneous or heterogenous echotexture (Table 4.2). In the absence of a malignant feature or a combination of benign features, the lesion is considered indeterminate, and biopsy is recommended (10).

If the lesion is likely benign, options discussed with the patient include ultrasound and clinical follow-up in 6 months, imaging-guided biopsy, or excisional biopsy. Depending on the physical attributes of the lesions, imaging features, patient history, and input, we will make a specific recommendation from among these three choices. It is critical, however, that before a recommendation for follow-up in 6 months is made, the lesion is scrutinized carefully for any malignant features (Figure 4.43). If at least one feature malignancy is present, a biopsy needs to be done.

EVALUATION OF NONSPECIFIC MAMMOGRAPHIC FINDINGS AND POTENTIAL AREAS OF TISSUE EXCLUSION

Breast ultrasound is well suited for the evaluation of mammographically detected masses, developing densities, and asymmetric tissue. With ultrasound, cysts can be diagnosed with a high degree of accuracy. Solid lesions can be separated into those likely to be benign or malignant and those that represent normal fibrous tissue or a fibrous ridge.

Ultrasonographic imaging of mammographic abnormalities requires knowledge of the approximate location of the lesion in the breast. Based on the mammographic images, the approximate o'clock position is established before starting the ultrasound (Figure 4.44). If there is any uncertainty about the ultrasonographic and mammographic correlation of a lesion, the abnormality seen on the ultrasound is marked with a metallic BB, and follow-up mammographic images are obtained. Alternatively, if biopsy of the lesion is to be undertaken, a needle can be placed through the presumed lesion under ultrasound, and a follow-up mammographic image is used to confirm mammographic correlation (Chapter 11).

Breast ultrasound is also useful in imaging areas that may be difficult to evaluate mammographically (Figure 4.45). Even when using the spot compression paddle, the margins of lesions deep in the breast, close to the chest wall, may be difficult to image mammographically. Superior, medial, axillary, and far lateral tissue may be excluded from mammographic images. With ultrasound, these areas are readily amenable to evaluation and imaging-guided biopsy procedures.

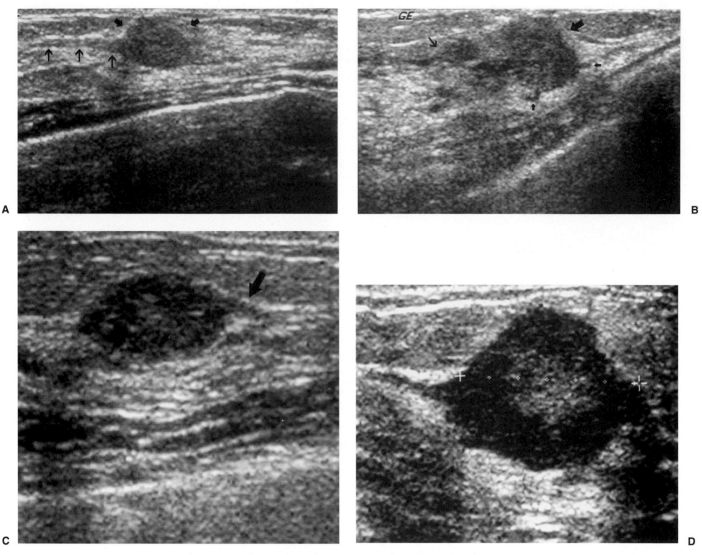

Figure 4.43 *Invasive ductal carcinomas, initially classified as likely benign. A.* A 44-year-old patient with hypoechoic, oval mass (*thick arrows*) described as probable fibroadenoma. Follow-up in 6 months is recommended. Retrospective review of the images demonstrates duct branching (*thin arrows*) not noted during the initial evaluation. *B.* Six months later, mass is enlarged (*thick arrows*), with irregular margins and spiculation (*thin arrow*). *C.* Different patient, 36 years old, with a hypoechoic, oval mass with posterior acoustic enhancement described as probable fibroadenoma. Follow-up in 6 months is recommended. Retrospective review of the images demonstrates duct branching (*arrow*). Also, note irregularity of margins. *D.* Six months later, mass is enlarged, with heterogeneous echotexture and posterior acoustic enhancement. Margins are irregular, and duct branching is again noted. It is important to evaluate masses carefully for any malignant feature. Even if only one malignant feature is seen, a biopsy is indicated.

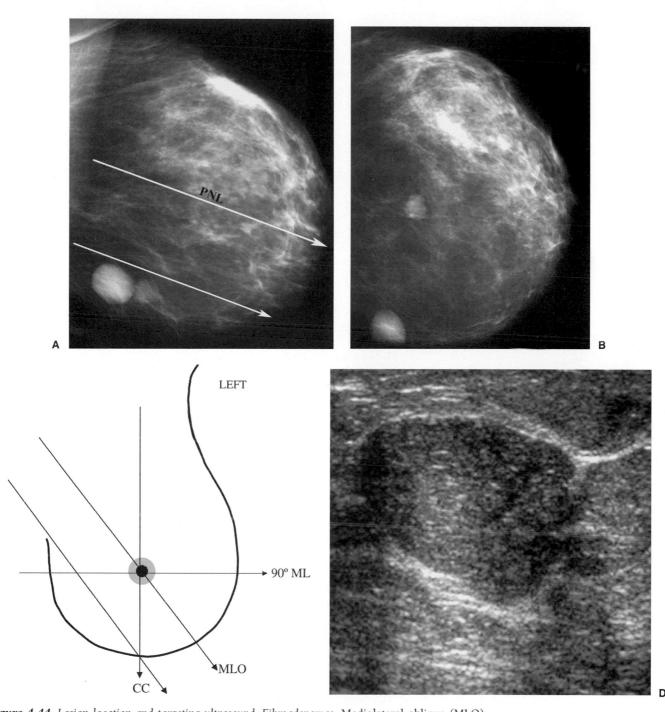

Figure 4.44 *Lesion location and targeting ultrasound. Fibroadenomas.* Mediolateral oblique (MLO) (*A*) and craniocaudal (*CC*) (*B*) views demonstrating two round masses in the left breast. *C.* Use of Eklund's method (see Chapter 2) for determining the o'clock position of lesions seen mammographically. On the MLO view, both masses project inferior to the posterior nipple line (PNL). On the CC view, the largest of the two is medial, and the other is directly behind the nipple. Based on the frontal diagram, the lesions will be found along the line drawn below the PNL. The largest lesion should be found at the 10-o'clock position (above the level of the nipple) and the second mass at the 6-o'clock position. For the ultrasound, the transducer is positioned at these o'clock positions as the starting points. *D.* The largest of the two masses is found at the 10-o'clock position, 12 cm from the nipple. A well-circumscribed, hypoechoic, oval mass is present.

(*Continued on next page*)

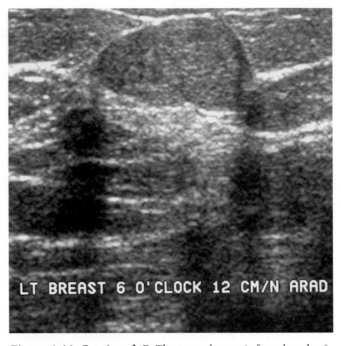

E

Figure 4.44 Continued E. The second mass is found at the 6-o'clock position, 12 cm from the nipple. A hypoechoic, oval mass is imaged. It is important to correlate mammographic and ultrasonographic findings. Our approach is to walk into the ultrasound room with the expected o'clock position of the lesion based on the mammographic findings.

EVALUATION OF CLINICAL FINDINGS

As described in Chapter 3, an ultrasound targeted to the area of concern is our starting point in patients younger than 30 years of age and in those who are pregnant or lactating, regardless of age, presenting with a focal symptom. In all other patients with a focal finding, a bilateral mammogram and spot tangential view at the site of concern are done to determine whether an ultrasound is indicated. Ultrasound is undertaken unless the area of clinical concern is completely fatty and there is no chance the lesion has been excluded from the field of view. During the ultrasound, the area of concern is palpated, and correlation is made with any imaging findings. If on palpation the finding is not impressive, and the imaging studies are negative, the patient is reassured that what she is feeling is benign breast tissue. Sometimes it helps reassure the patient to show her the appearance of the area of concern, comparing it to a rib in cross-section as a reference for what a lesion would look like. If a cyst is imaged at the site of concern, the patient is reassured that cysts are benign, fluctuate in size relative to the menstrual cycle, are associated with cyclical tenderness, and are common. If the lesion is of concern clinically and ultrasonographically, a biopsy is recommended and usually undertaken.

Cooper's ligaments and associated fibrous tissue can be palpated as a discrete mass, particularly if outlined by fat lobules. If, on imaging, the palpable mass is correlated directly to a fibrous ridge or fibrocystic area, biopsy is averted. Given the current state of technology, women should not undergo blind aspirations or excisional biopsies without an imaging evaluation. Ultrasound provides useful information, including the identification of unsuspected lesions within or adjacent to the palpable abnormality or mural abnormalities in an otherwise normal-appearing cyst. In many patients with palpable findings, ultrasonography reliably identifies a benign etiology, including fibrous ridges, fatty lobulation, and cystic changes. When benign changes are correlated directly to the clinical finding, attempts at blind aspiration and excisional biopsy can be averted (11–13).

It is important to emphasize that clinical and imaging findings need to be considered as equally important pieces of information. Overreliance on (or exclusion of) one or the other modality is no longer appropriate. In some patients, the physical examination may be unimpressive or normal in the presence of suspicious imaging findings. Conversely, in other patients, the physical examination is highly suggestive of a malignancy, and yet the imaging findings are normal (Figure 4.46). All information available needs to be factored into the decision-making process.

In evaluating patients and establishing appropriate recommendations, be sure to correlate clinical, mammographic, and ultrasonographic findings.

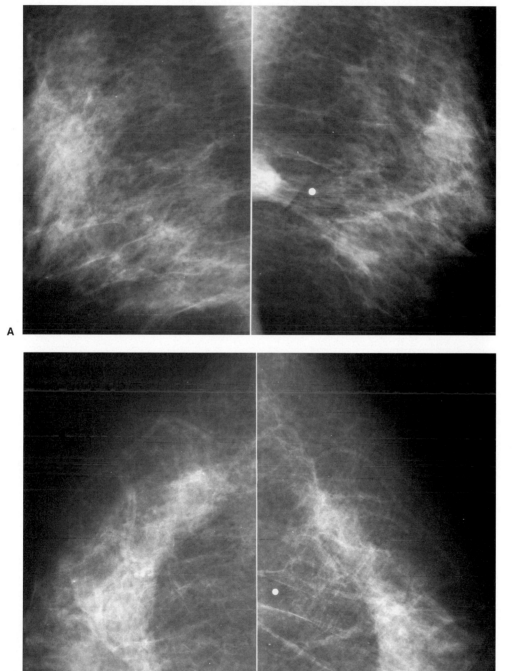

Figure 4.45 *Invasive ductal carcinoma* Mediolateral oblique (A) and craniocaudal (B) views in a patient presenting with a lump. Metallic BB marks the location of the lump. The mass is partially visualized on the left MLO view but is not seen on the CC view. When the metallic BB is seen close to the edge of the film (as seen on the CC view in this patient) in patients presenting with a focal area of concern, consider the possibility that the lesion has been excluded from the field of view.

(*continued on next page*)

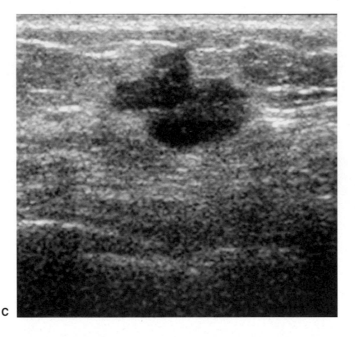

Figure 4.45 Continued *C.* Irregular, hypoechoic mass with angular margins. Ultrasound is helpful in evaluating areas that might be totally or partially excluded from the field of view, including lesions peripherally in the breast close to the chest wall as in this patient.

INFLAMMATORY PROCESSES: MASTITIS VERSUS ABSCESS

In women with an inflammatory process, ultrasound is useful in distinguishing those with mastitis from those with an abscess that may require drainage. Mastitis produces diffuse changes in the ultrasonographic appearance of breast tissue (Figure 4.47). The normal architecture is disrupted, and tubular areas of hyperechogenicity are intermingled with hypoechoic areas and shadowing (Figure 4.48). Cooper's ligaments may not be readily identifiable. With an abscess, a complex cystic mass or tubular area is imaged, sometimes with focal areas of marked hyperechogenicity possibly representing air (Figure 4.49). Drainage under ultrasound guidance is helpful in targeting pockets of purulent material.

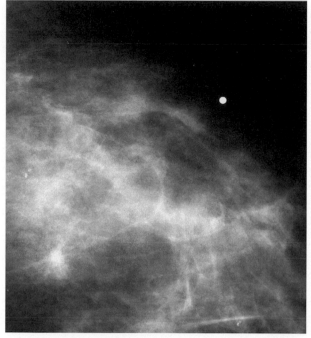

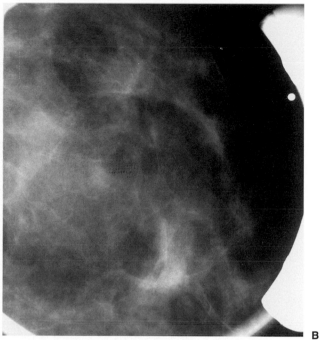

A

B

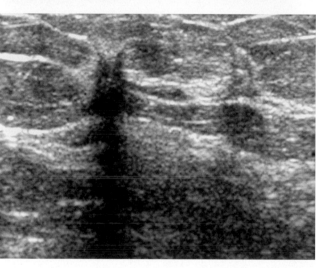

C

Figure 4.46 *Invasive ductal carcinoma, not otherwise specified.* A. A 62-year-old woman presents with a lump. Metallic BB marks the area of the lump. *B*. Spot tangential view at the site of clinical concern. Normal glandular tissue is imaged on all three views (mediolateral oblique view not shown). The area of concern is anterior, such that it is unlikely that it has been excluded from the field of view. *C*. On physical examination, a hard mass with little mobility is palpated at the site of concern to the patient. An ill-defined, spiculated mass with associated shadowing and vertical orientation is imaged, corresponding to the site of concern. Clinical, mammographic, and ultrasonographic findings are factored in making a recommendation. Given the clinical and ultrasonographic findings, a biopsy is indicated in this patient, although the mammogram is seemingly normal. Ultrasound is indicated in patients who present with a focal symptom and in whom glandular tissue is imaged mammographically at the site of the symptom.

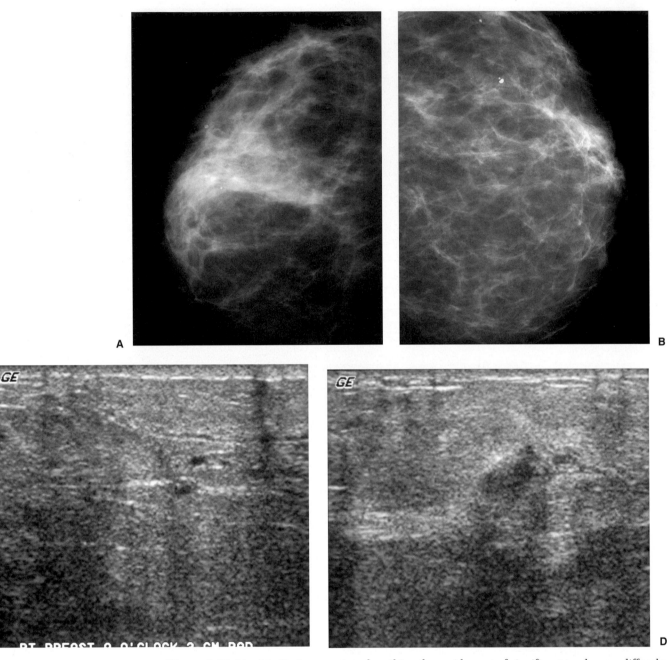

Figure 4.47 *Mastitis.* Patient presents describing the rapid onset of significant tenderness diffusely involving the right breast; there is associated edema and erythema. Right (*A*) and left (*B*) craniocaudal views. The overall density of the breast parenchyma is increased on the right when compared to the left breast. This may be partially related to suboptimal compression because of the discomfort experienced by the patient when the right breast is compressed. *C.* Diffusely increased echogenicity of the tissue with associated loss of normal architecture. Small tubular structures are noted within the tissue. *D.* Ultrasound image through another area of the right breast demonstrates similar appearance of tissue as well as some relatively hypoechoic nodularity. Symptoms and findings resolved completely following a 10-day course of antibiotics.

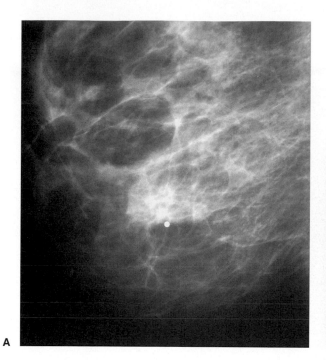

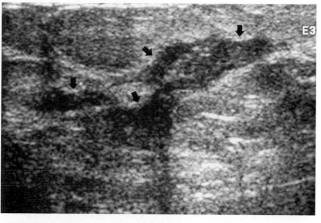

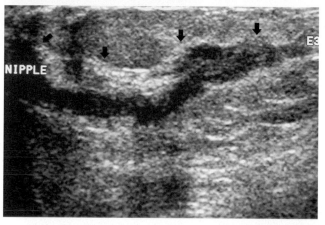

Figure 4.48 *Granulomatous mastitis. A.* This patient presented describing a tender lump in the right breast. Metallic BB marks the area of concern. Parenchymal asymmetry and increased density are noted at this site. *B.* Irregular tubular structure (*arrows*) is imaged at the site of clinical concern and extending beyond the palpable area to the subareolar area. *C.* Portions of the tubular structure closest to the nipple are surrounded by echogenic tissue. (Chapter 6).

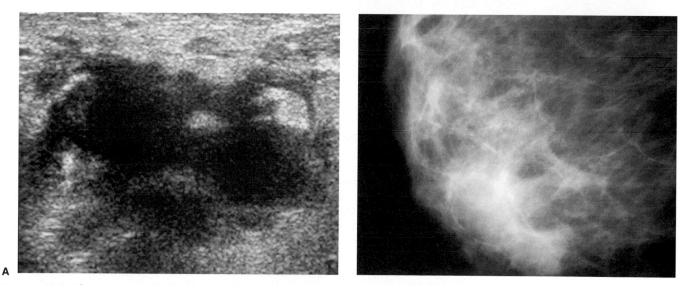

Figure 4.49 *Abscess. A.* Ill-defined mass with a heterogeneous echotexture including areas of marked hyperechogenicity. Pus was obtained during aspiration. No residual abnormality was noted 2 months after antibiotic therapy. *B.* Different patient. Right mediolateral oblique (MLO) view. Increased density is seen anteriorly in a patient with the rapid onset of tenderness and erythema.

(continued on next page)

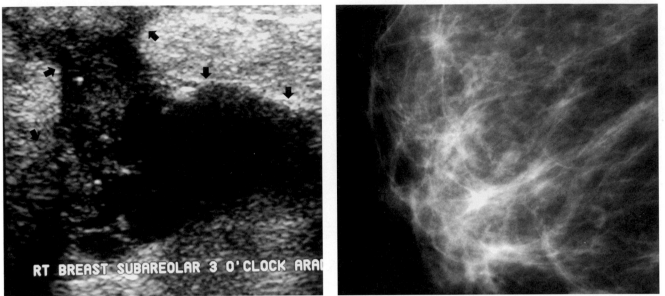

C

D

Figure 4.49 (continued) *C.* Tubular structure (*arrows*) with a cystic component extending to sub-areolar area. Nipple is seen directly over the tubular structure. Pus was obtained on aspiration. *D.* Repeat MLO view after resolution of symptoms. Overall density is decreased; trabecular markings are now apparent.

REFERENCES

1. Baker JA, Soo MS, Rosen EL. Artifacts and pitfalls in sonographic imaging of the breast. *AJR Am J Roentgenol* 2001;176:1261–1266.
2. American College of Radiology. *ACR standards 2002–2003.* Reston VA: American College of Radiology, 2002.
3. Baker JA, Soo MS. Breast US: assessment of technical quality and image interpretation. *Radiology* 2002;223:229–238.
4. Kolb TM, Lichy J, Newhouse JH. Occult cancer in women with dense breasts: detection with screening US—diagnostic yield and tumor characteristics. *Radiology* 1998;207:191–199.
5. Kolb TM, Lichy J, Newhouse JH. Comparison of the performance of screening mammography, physical examination, and breast US and evaluation of factors that influence them: an analysis of 27,825 patient evaluations. *Radiology* 2002;225:165–175.
6. Moon WK, Noh DY, Im JG. Multifocal, multicentric and contralateral breast cancers: bilateral whole breast US in the preoperative evaluation of patients. *Radiology* 2002;224:569–576.
7. Kaplan SS. Clinical utility of bilateral whole-breast US in the evaluation of women with dense breast tissue. *Radiology* 2001;221:641–649.
8. Feig S. Breast masses: mammographic and sonographic evaluation. *Radiol Clin North Am* 1992; 30:67–92.
9. Werner JK, Kumar D, Berg WA. Apocrine metaplasia: mammographic and sonographic appearances. *AJR Am J Roentgenol* 1998;170:1375–1379.
10. Stavros AT, Thickman D, Rapp CL, et al. Solid breast nodules: use of sonography to distinguish between benign and malignant lesions. *Radiology* 1995;196:123–134.
11. Soo MS, Rosen EL, Baker JA, et al. Negative predictive value of sonography with mammography in patients with palpable breast lesions. *AJR Am J Roentgenol* 2001;177:1167–1170.
12. Dennis MA, Parker SH, Klaus AJ, et al. Breast biopsy avoidance: the value of normal mammograms and normal sonograms in the setting of a palpable lump. *Radiology* 2001;219:186–191.
13. Moy L, Slanetz PJ, Moore R, et al. Specificity of mammography and US in the evaluation of a palpable abnormality: retrospective review. *Radiology* 2002;176–181.

CALCIFICATIONS

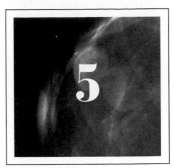

Calcifications developing in the breast are variable in number and appearance. Most calcifications detected in patients on screening mammograms reflect a benign etiology. A small percentage develop in association with ductal carcinoma *in situ* (DCIS) or, less commonly, the invasive component of ductal carcinomas. It is incumbent on the radiologist to detect, evaluate, classify, and make appropriate recommendations for calcifications perceived on mammograms.

Complete mammographic workups (Chapter 3), coupled with a knowledge of breast anatomy, histology, and histopathology, are critical in understanding the mammographic appearance of breast calcifications and establishing appropriate and justifiable recommendations. Calcifications developing in a space (i.e., ducts or acini) are molded by that space. Calcifications arising in ducts are tubelike or linear and may demonstrate linear distribution. If they develop in subsegmental ducts, they are large, rodlike, and dense compared with the smaller calcifications of variable density that develop in terminal ducts. When the epithelial lining is attenuated or denuded, the borders of the calcifications are smooth (Figure 5.1) compared with the irregular margins that may be seen when there is active cellular proliferation and necrotic debris in the lumen of the duct (Figure 5.2). Calcifications forming in acini are round or punctate (Figure 5.3). If the normally round acini are compressed, elongated, or deformed by proliferation of the surrounding perilobular stroma, the calcifications may demonstrate pleomorphism, including round, punctate, oval, and comma-shaped forms.

As discussed in Chapter 2, establishing optimal film quality is one of the initial steps in reviewing screening and diagnostic mammograms. Well-exposed, high-contrast images with optimal positioning and no blurring are essential in maximizing our ability to detect microcalcifications and small spiculated masses. The acceptance and interpretation of suboptimal films can result in a delay in the diagnosis of breast cancer.

When evaluating calcifications, consider the following characteristics: What is the *form* of the calcifications? Is it round or linear, coarse or fine (granular), monomorphic or pleomorphic within a cluster? What is the *size* of the calcifications? Is it large or small, and if in a cluster, are the individual calcifications homogeneous in size? What is the *density* of the calcifications? Is the density high or low? In a given cluster, is there homogeneity in density among the individual calcifications? What is the *distribution* of the calcifications? Is the distribution unilateral or bilateral, single cluster or multifocal, diffuse, regional, segmental, or linear? Diffuse bilateral calcifications, scattered in dense tissue, are typically benign, in contrast to linear calcifications in a segmental distribution.

Although some emphasis has been placed previously on the number of calcifications in a given cluster, we do not find this to be a particularly helpful characteristic. One or two linear calcifications with irregular margins may be related to the presence of DCIS and

Image quality is particularly critical in our ability to detect (screening) and characterize (magnification views) microcalcifications.

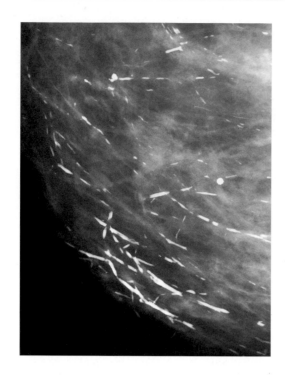

Figure 5.1 Large, rodlike calcifications. Forming in subsegmental ducts, these calcifications are large, dense, rodlike, and linearly oriented toward the nipple. The smooth border of the calcifications reflects a denuded or attenuated epithelial lining in the ducts. Category 2.

require a biopsy. Conversely, a tight cluster of many round, pearl-like calcifications of homogeneous density do not typically require a biopsy.

The presence of linear calcifications with irregular borders, variable density, and linear orientation that are haphazardly or segmentally distributed needs to be considered significant (Figure 5.4). The likelihood of an underlying DCIS (low, intermediate, or high

In evaluating a cluster of calcifications ask yourself: are there linear forms with irregular borders, or is there a linear distribution of round, oval, punctate calcifications?

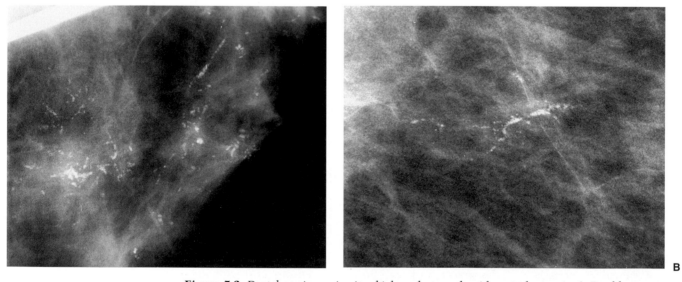

Figure 5.2 Ductal carcinoma in situ, *high nuclear grade with central necrosis. A.* Double spot compression magnification view (1.8×) demonstrates linear (casting-type) calcifications with clefts and irregular margins. These calcifications are molded actively by the proliferating epithelial cells lining the distended ducts. The calcifications are linearly oriented and show a regional distribution. Category 5. *B.* Double spot compression magnification view (1.8×) on a different patient. Linear calcifications with branching, clefts, and irregular margins reflecting the proliferative intraductal process. The calcifications are focal with a linear distribution. Category 4.

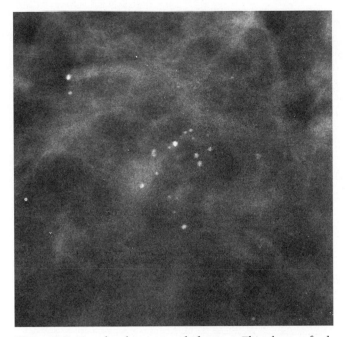

Figure 5.3 *Round and punctate calcifications.* This cluster of calcifications is characterized by well-circumscribed, high-density, round calcifications. No linear form or linear distribution is seen. These commonly form in the acini. Category 2.

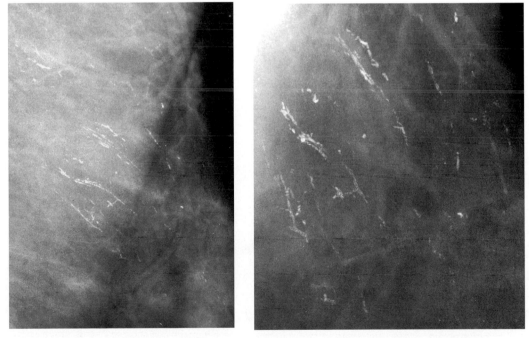

A
B

Figure 5.4 *Ductal carcinoma in situ (DCIS), intermediate and low nuclear grade solid growth pattern with necrosis. A.* Mediolateral oblique, screening view. Linear calcifications with irregular borders and linear orientation. *B.* Double spot compression magnification view (1.8×). Linear calcifications (casting-type) with clefts, irregular borders, and variable density. Round and punctate calcifications are also seen, demonstrating linear orientation. These types of calcifications are almost pathognomonic of DCIS. Category 5.

> ### Box 5.1: Linear, Casting, Branching, and Pleomorphic Calcifications
>
> Ductal carcinoma *in situ* (with central necrosis; commonly high nuclear grade but can also be seen in about 20% of low- or intermediate-grade cases)
> Fat necrosis (in the early stages of calcification)—rare
> Fibroadenoma—rare
> Dystrophic, fibrosis—rare
> Autoimmune disorders (dermatomyositis, scleroderma, lupus)—rare

nuclear grade) associated with central necrosis, is high; biopsy is indicated in these patients. These types of calcifications are rarely associated with benign processes including those listed in Box 5.1. We also consider the linear distribution of round, oval, punctate, or amorphous calcifications, with variable density, an indication for biopsy (Figure 5.5). However, in the absence of linear calcifications or a linear distribution, the likelihood of DCIS drops significantly and, when diagnosed, is usually, although not exclusively, low- or intermediate-grade DCIS with no central necrosis. Benign diagnostic considerations for clusters composed of round, oval, punctate (Figure 5.6), or amorphous calcifications include those listed in Box 5.2.

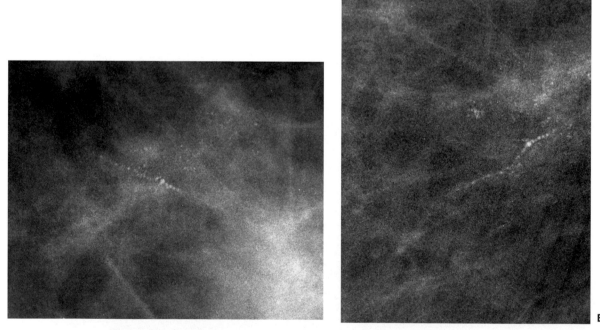

A   B

Figure 5.5 *Ductal carcinoma* in situ, *low and intermediate nuclear grade, with no necrosis.* Double spot compression magnification (1.8×). Craniocaudal (A) and mediolateral oblique (B) views show a cluster of round, punctate and amorphous calcifications, some demonstrating a linear distribution that has developed in the upper inner quadrant of the left breast. These calcifications are nonspecific and may be related to fibrocystic changes, focal fibrosis, fibroadenomas, and papillomas. Their interval development, linear distribution, and upper inner quadrant location, however, warrant a biopsy recommendation. Category 4.

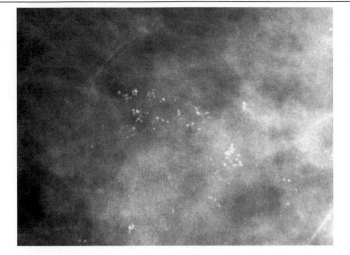

Figure 5.6 *Round and punctate calcifications.* The clusters are composed of tightly grouped, round, well-circumscribed calcifications of about equal density. No linear orientation is noted. These commonly develop in the acini, composing individual lobules. Although assigned as category 3, our follow-up for most of these patients is annual.

Box 5.2: Cluster of Punctate, Round Calcifications

Lobular calcifications
Sclerosing adenosis
Fibroadenoma
Fibrocystic change (hyperplasia, atypical ductal hyperplasia)
Papilloma
Ductal carcinoma *in situ* (more commonly low or intermediate cribriform, micropapillary cases without central necrosis)

BENIGN BREAST CALCIFICATIONS

For didactic purposes, I take an anatomic approach in describing breast calcifications. However, the terms provided in the American College of Radiology (ACR) BIRADS lexicon (1) are presented in Table 5.1 and Box 5.3 and used throughout the text.

As mentioned previously, when thinking about breast calcifications, consider the anatomic structures available for breast calcifications to develop and the potential pathologic processes associated with these structures. This becomes helpful when analyzing calcifications and determining appropriate diagnostic considerations and management. Include the following tissue types: skin, fibrous stroma, ducts (large and small), acini grouped into lobules and arteries. Calcifications developing in masses may be associated with the wall (mural) of the mass, if one is present (e.g., cysts, oil cysts), or with the epithelial or stromal elements of the mass. If the mass contains fluid, the calcifications may be in suspension (e.g., milk of calcium). Rarely, calcifications develop in association with foreign bodies, such as suture material and parasites.

In thinking about breast calcifications, consider the anatomic structures available in breast tissue within which calcifications can develop and the potential (pathologic) processes involving these structures.

Table 5.1: American College of Radiology Lexicon, Descriptive Terms for Calcifications

Typically Benign	Intermediate Concern	Higher Probability of Malignancy
Skin (dermal)	Amorphous or indistinct	Pleomorphic or heterogenous (granular)
Vascular		fine linear or fine linear branching
(casting)		
Coarse or popcorn-like		
Large rodlike		
Round		
Lucent-centered		
Eggshell or rim (<1 mm thick)		
Milk of calcium		
Suture		
Dystrophic		
Punctate (<0.5 mm)		

Box 5.3: American College of Radiology Lexicon, Distribution Modifiers for Calcifications

Group or clustered (neutral terms)
Linear
Segmental
Regional
Diffuse, scattered

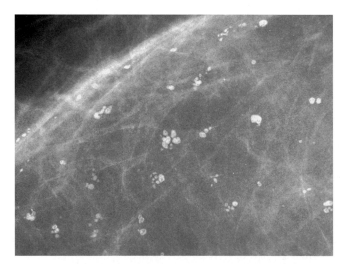

Figure 5.7 *Skin calcifications.* Screening view. Multiple clusters of round and oval, lucent-centered calcifications. Category 2.

SKIN (DERMAL) CALCIFICATIONS

Skin calcifications (Figure 5.7) form in dermal sweat glands after low-grade folliculitis and inspissation of sebaceous material. Consequently, they are:

- Round or oval
- Lucent centered
- Isolated, or more commonly, multiple clusters bilaterally
- Lacelike pattern when associated with moles

Commonly, skin calcifications are seen posteromedially projecting on the pectoral muscle on the mediolateral oblique (MLO) view and medially, at the cleavage, on cranio-caudal (CC) views; they can involve the skin diffusely.

On any two views, much of the skin projects superimposed on the breast parenchyma; only a small amount of skin is ever tangent to the x-ray beam, enabling distinction between skin and associated lesions from underlying breast tissue. Although the appearance of most skin calcifications is distinctive, if lucent centers are not readily apparent, definitive diagnosis is made when the skin surface containing the calcifications is imaged tangent (Figure 5.8) to the x-ray beam (2–4) (Chapter 3).

In some patients, calcifications develop in association with moles or other skin lesions (e.g., sebaccous cysts). These can outline the crevices of the mole, creating semicircular, lacelike calcifications (Figure 5.9); or, in some patients, they may be pleomorphic (Figure 5.10). In some women, talc, zinc oxide ointment (Desitin), or other high-density products deposited in the crevices of moles, can simulate calcifications. The overall density of these particles, their morphology and distribution are usually pathognomonic (Figure 5.11); alternatively, either placing a metallic BB on the skin lesion and demonstrating that the BB moves with the lesion on two views or obtaining a tangential view of the skin lesion provides definitive diagnosis.

Radiolucent-centered calcifications are benign.

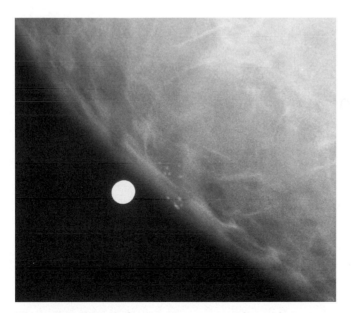

Figure 5.8 *Skin calcifications.* Spot tangential view demonstrating the dermal location of a cluster of round and oval calcifications, lacking a lucent center. Category 2.

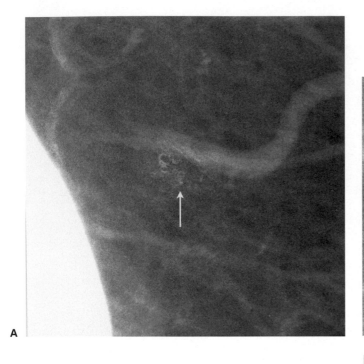

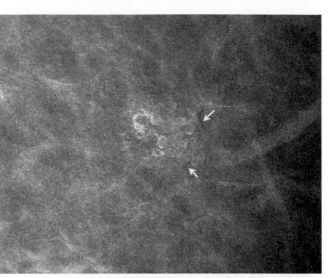

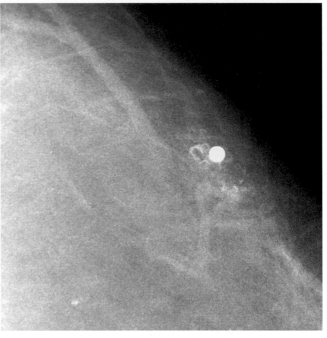

Figure 5.9 *Skin calcifications.* A. Implant-displaced view demonstrates a cluster of calcifications (*arrow*). B. Magnification view of the calcifications. Patient referred for stereotactically guided biopsy. On further review, the calcifications are curvilinear, and some have lucent centers. Additionally, a sharp curvilinear lucency is seen partially outlining the area of the calcifications (*arrows*). This is consistent with air partially outlining a skin lesion. On careful physical examination, a mole is noted. A metallic BB is placed on the mole. C. A spot tangential view confirms that the calcifications are associated with the skin lesion. Category 2.

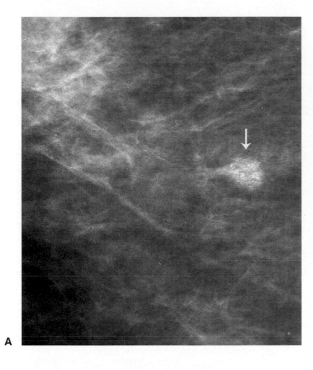

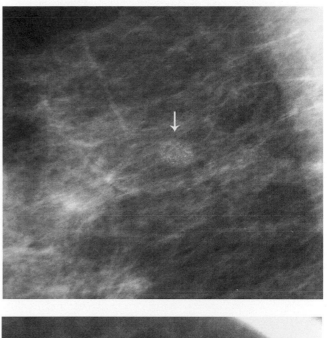

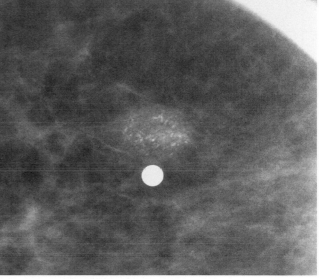

Figure 5.10 *Skin nodule with associated pleomorphic calcifications.* Craniocaudal (A) and mediolateral oblique (B) screening views show a mass with indistinct margins and associated calcifications (*arrows*). On careful physical examination, a skin lesion is seen corresponding to the expected location of the mammographic finding. A metallic BB is placed on the skin lesion. C. Follow-up spot compression views demonstrate that the BB moves with the skin lesion (only one view is shown). No further intervention is warranted. Category 2.

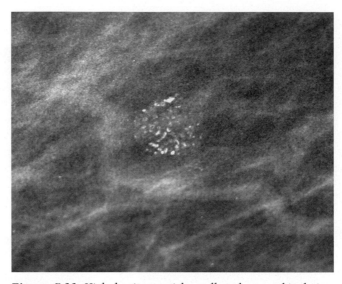

Figure 5.11 *High-density particles collected on a skin lesion.* Central lucencies are evident. The density of the particles and their morphology and distribution are helpful in establishing etiology. If concerns remain, follow-up images with a metallic BB marking the skin lesion can be done. Alternatively, if the skin is wiped clean, follow-up films demonstrate elimination of the high-density material.

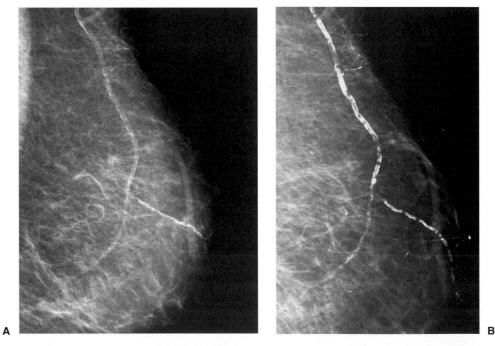

Figure 5.12 *Vascular calcifications.* A and B. Mediolateral oblique views obtained 4 years apart demonstrating progressive development of vascular calcifications. These linear, parallel, tram-track–like calcifications are pathognomonic. If present, and extensive, they may correlate with underlying coronary artery disease and should be described in the mammographic report.

VASCULAR CALCIFICATIONS

Deposition of calcium in the media, at the perimeter of the elastic fibers of arterial walls, results in dense, linear, parallel, or tram-track–like calcifications, most commonly in post-menopausal women with arteriosclerotic heart disease (Figure 5.12). When seen in younger, premenopausal women, it is often in patients with diabetes. When only a portion of the arterial wall is affected, or when small vessels are involved, the calcifications can simulate those occurring in DCIS because at this stage, the calcifications may be linear, irregular, variable in density, and have a linear orientation (Figure 5.13). In these patients spot compression magnification views demonstrate the contralateral uncalcified vessel

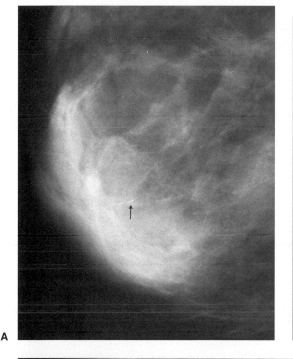

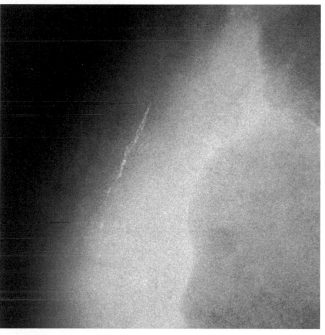

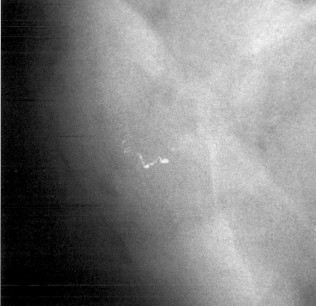

Figure 5.13 Vascular calcifications. A. Mediolateral oblique view. A linear calcification is perceived (*arrow*) on the screening views (craniocaudal view not shown). Category 0. Magnification views are recommended for further evaluation. Mediolateral oblique (*B*) and craniocaudal (*C*) double spot compression magnification views (1.8×) demonstrate "quirky" serpiginous calcifications with a central lucency consistent with vascular calcifications. Category 2.

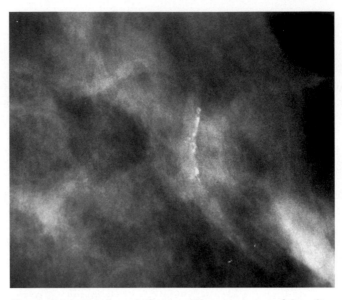

Figure 5.14 *Vascular calcifications.* The association of these linear calcifications with an artery is easily established on this view. The contralateral vessel wall and other portions of the vessel are identified easily. Category 2.

wall, the uncalcified portion of the vessel coming into and going out of the area of the calcifications, or an accompanying vein (Figure 5.14).

Occasionally, smaller vessels calcify, leading to the appearance of "quirky" types of calcifications. The borders of these calcifications are well defined, and a lucent center is often seen when evaluated closely with a magnifying lens (Figure 5.15). In our experience, these smaller arterial calcifications tend to be more common in premenopausal women with

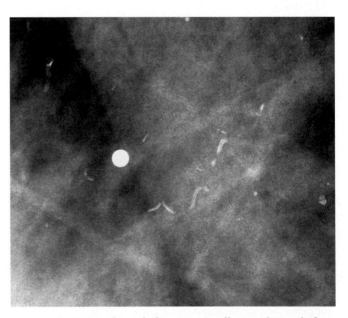

Figure 5.15 *Vascular calcifications.* Small, "quirky" calcifications are identified. Smooth margins and central lucencies are evident, consistent with arterial calcifications. Similar calcifications are diffusely scattered bilaterally. Category 2.

dense tissue and can fluctuate from year to year; in some patients, they resolve completely. These patients do not usually have a history of diabetes or arteriosclerotic heart disease.

It has been reported by several investigators that there may be a correlation between the extent of arterial calcifications seen on a mammogram and underlying coronary artery disease. The presence of extensive arterial calcifications should be described in mammographic reports (5–7). Rarely, tortuous and serpiginous calcifications associated with a venous structure, may be seen as a long-term sequela of Mondor's disease (8).

Consider describing the presence of extensive, bilateral vascular calcification in the mammography report.

DYSTROPHIC CALCIFICATIONS

Dystrophic calcifications form in stromal fibrous tissue, not in predefined anatomic spaces; consequently, they vary in size, shape, and density; no two of these calcifications are alike. They are coarse, dense, large, and irregularly shaped and may have associated areas of lucency (Figure 5.16). These are associated with benign conditions, such as fat necrosis related to prior trauma (Chapter 6), burns or surgery, radiation therapy (Chapter 9), a healed abscess, or hematoma. When diffuse and bilateral, they may reflect the presence of an underlying inflammatory, degenerative, or metabolic process (e.g., renal disease, hyperparathyroidism). Dystrophic calcifications can also be seen in the fibrous capsule that forms around implants or in conjunction with the granulomatous response elicited by foreign bodies, such as silicone or paraffin injections.

Some dystrophic calcifications demonstrate a linear appearance (Figure 5.17). These are commonly found in areas of dense stromal fibrosis (Figure 5.18). The margins are irregular and jagged, with some of the calcifications forming acute angles. In a given cluster, some of the linear calcifications are well defined with central lucencies (Figure 5.19).

Popcorn-like calcifications (Figure 5.20) are dystrophic, developing in the hyalinized fibrous stroma of fibroadenomas. They are dense and coarse and can be unifocal or multifocal, unilateral or bilateral. In the initial stages of hyalinization with calcification, pleo-

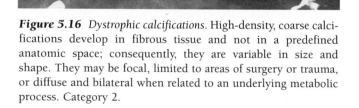

Figure 5.16 *Dystrophic calcifications*. High-density, coarse calcifications develop in fibrous tissue and not in a predefined anatomic space; consequently, they are variable in size and shape. They may be focal, limited to areas of surgery or trauma, or diffuse and bilateral when related to an underlying metabolic process. Category 2.

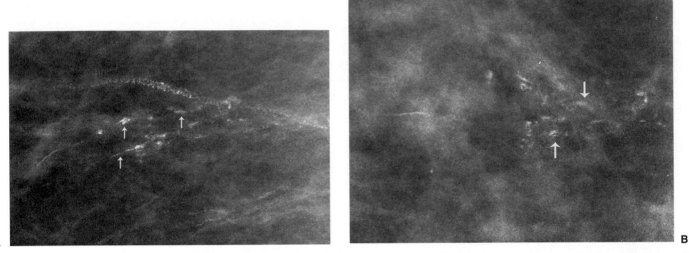

Figure 5.17 *Dystrophic calcifications in hyalinized breast tissue; vascular calcifications.* Mediolateral oblique (MLO) (*A*) and craniocaudal (*B*) spot magnification views. Linear calcifications demonstrating a linear orientation. On careful evaluation with a magnification lens, some appear to have a central lucency (*arrows*). Although the diagnosis was suspected based on the mammographic appearance, given linear forms with linear orientation, a biopsy is done. Category 4. Arterial calcifications are incidentally noted on the MLO view.

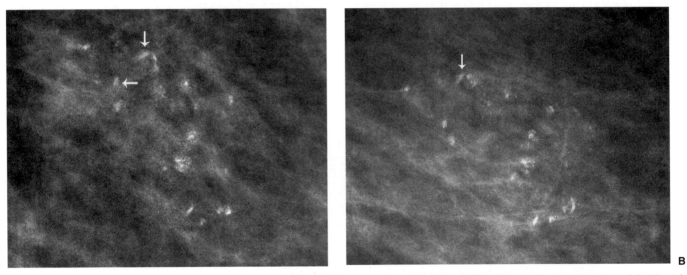

Figure 5.18 *Dystrophic calcifications in a nodular focus of hyalinized fibrosis.* Craniocaudal (*A*) and mediolateral oblique (*B*) spot compression magnification views show a cluster of linear calcifications with indistinct borders. On careful evaluation, a central lucency is seen in a few of the calcifications (*arrows*). Although the diagnosis was suspected based on the mammographic appearance, a biopsy is done. Category 4.

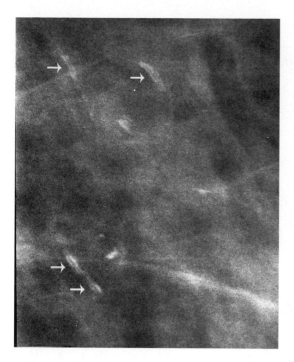

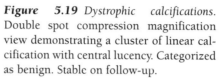

Figure 5.19 *Dystrophic calcifications.* Double spot compression magnification view demonstrating a cluster of linear calcification with central lucency. Categorized as benign. Stable on follow-up.

morphic clusters may be seen with or without an associated mass (Figure 5.21). Sequential mammograms demonstrate progressive deposition of calcium with coalescence and formation of larger calcifications (Figure 5.22). In some women, these calcified fibroadenomas are palpable. It is imperative that the benign nature of the palpable finding be described and that patient and referring physician be assured, so that the likelihood of biopsy is minimized.

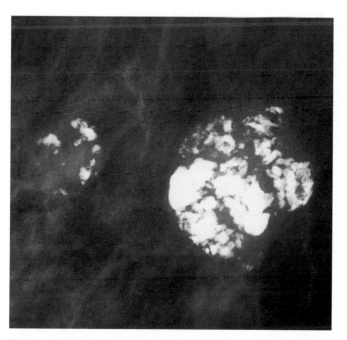

Figure 5.20 *Coarse, popcorn-like calcifications.* Hyalinized fibroadenomas. Category 2.

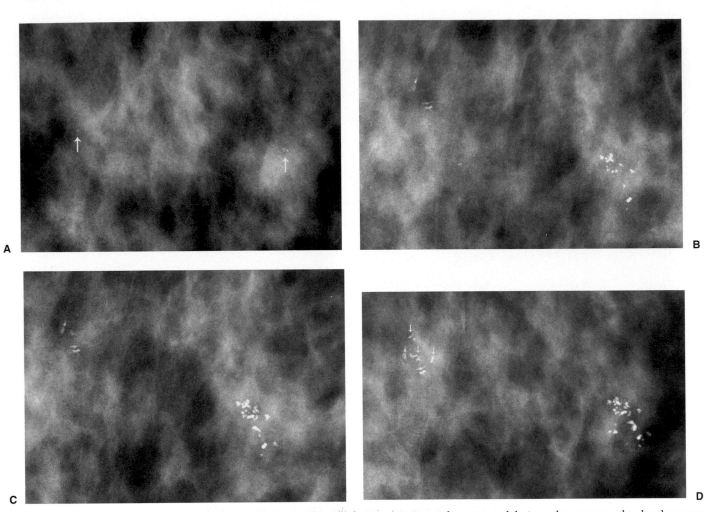

Figure 5.21 *Dystrophic calcifications.* Sequential craniocaudal views demonstrate the development of two clusters of calcifications. Other, similar clusters are present in the contralateral breast (not shown). *A.* Initial mammogram, showing foci of early calcification (*arrows*). *B.* One year later, additional calcifications have developed in each of the two clusters shown. *C.* Two years after the initial mammogram, additional calcifications have developed. *D.* Three years after the initial mammogram, some of the calcifications are coalescing and forming coarse calcifications. As fibroadenomas hyalinize, calcifications can develop in the stroma; as the calcifications coalesce, popcorn-like calcifications are formed. Notice the jagged edges or acute angles on some of the curvilinear calcifications (*arrows*). Category 2.

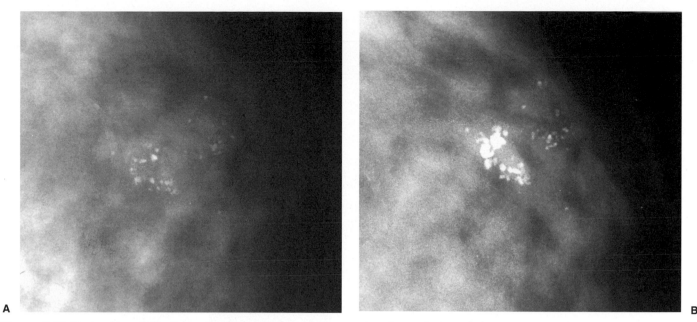

A   B

Figure 5.22 *Dystrophic calcifications.* Craniocaudal views demonstrating the evolution of dystrophic calcifications. *A.* Initial mammogram demonstrates a cluster of coarse, high-density calcifications with no linear forms or linear orientation. There is the suggestion of an associated bilobed nodule. Category 2. *B.* Craniocaudal view 2.5 years after the initial mammogram demonstrates progression of the calcification process. Large, coarse, high-density forms are present. Category 2.

DUCTAL CALCIFICATIONS

The precipitation of calcium salts in entrapped secretions in subsegmental ducts leads to the development of fusiform calcium casts of the dilated ducts (9,10). These calcifications (Figure 5.23) are:

- Rodlike or cigar shaped
- Coarse, high in density
- Smooth bordered
- Diffuse, bilateral, pointing toward the nipple
- Centrally lucency when periductal

They reflect the presence of duct ectasia, also called *periductal mastitis, secretory disease, comedo mastitis, plasma cell mastitis,* and *mastitis obliterans.* Histologically, the dilated ducts contain amorphous debris, foam cells, and less commonly, a crystalline-like lipid material. The epithelial cells normally lining the ducts are atrophic, appearing attenuated, deformed, and flattened or absent. The elastic tissue layer is disrupted and partially destroyed. In women with mastitis obliterans, fibrous tissue obliterates the epithelial lining and duct lumen. A chronic inflammatory process composed of plasma cells may be seen periductally.

This process is often bilateral and diffuse, less commonly unilateral, and rarely focal (Figure 5.24); branching of the calcifications can be seen. Because the epithelial lining of the ducts is flattened or denuded, the border of these calcifications is smooth (Figure 5.25). If the calcifications form periductally, a radiolucent center is seen. Coarse calcifications, associated with dense fibrotic breast tissue in the subareolar areas, reflect burned out plasma cell mastitis. These patients may describe a tender mass in one or both subareolar areas. A white, thick, cheeselike, and at times foul-smelling discharge may also be present, arising from multiple duct openings bilaterally.

Dense, coarse, cigar-shaped (linear) calcifications developing in large ducts are usually characterized by smooth borders reflecting an attenuated or denuded epithelial lining.

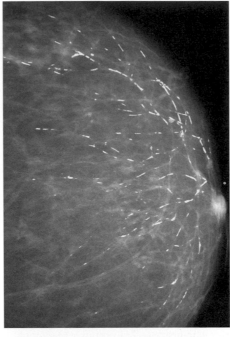

A

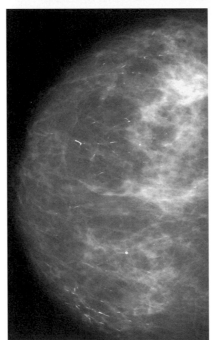

B

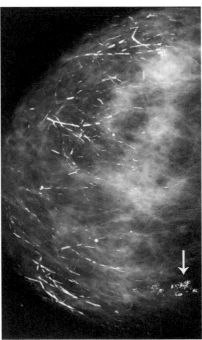

C

Figure 5.23 *Large, rodlike calcifications.* A. Craniocaudal view demonstrating large, rodlike calcifications diffusely involving the breast. The calcifications may have branch points and point toward the nipple. The process is usually diffuse and bilateral. B. Craniocaudal view in a different patient demonstrating scattered large, rodlike calcifications pointing toward the nipple. C. Two years later, many more large, rodlike calcifications have developed, and the preexisting calcifications are larger and more dense. A focus of dystrophic calcifications has also developed medially (*arrow*). Category 2.

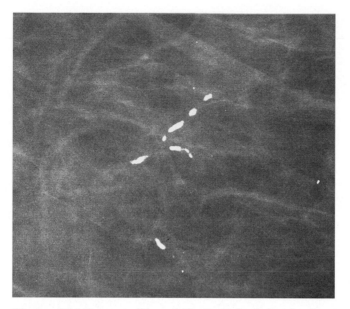

Figure 5.24 *Large, rodlike calcifications, focal.* Rarely, these types of calcifications can be focal. The calcifications are dense and smooth bordered. No pleomorphic calcifications of lower density are seen in the surrounding tissue. Category 2.

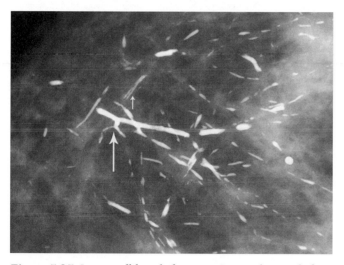

Figure 5.25 *Large, rodlike calcifications.* Coarse, dense calcifications with smooth borders reflecting a denuded or absent epithelial lining in the duct. Branch points may be seen (*long arrow*). A central lucency is noted when they form periductally (*short arrow*). Category 2.

LOBULAR CALCIFICATIONS

Lobules represent groupings of round glands called *acini*. It is in the acinar structures that milk is produced during late pregnancy and lactation. If the acini are not altered by proliferations of the surrounding fibrous perilobular tissue, as is seen in fibroadenomas and sclerosing adenosis, calcifications developing in acini are round, relatively high density, well defined or pearl-like, and smooth bordered. If the lumen of the glands is small, the calcifications may be punctate. In some patients they can occur in tight clusters (Figure

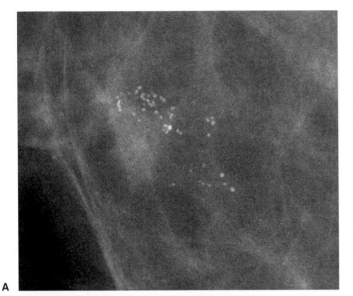

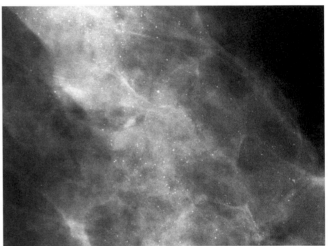

A

B

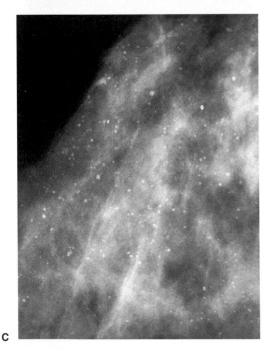

C

Figure 5.26 *Round and punctate calcifications.* A. A cluster of monomorphic, high-density, well-defined, round calcifications. *B.* Different patient. Monomorphic calcifications are scattered diffusely in the breast parenchyma. The calcifications are round, well defined, and high in density. *C.* Another patient with round and punctate calcifications diffusely scattered in dense tissue. All category 2.

5.26), reflecting sclerosing adenosis, or be diffusely scattered bilaterally (like "a thousand points of light").

When there is associated proliferation of perilobular stroma, as is seen with sclerosing adenosis and fibroadenomas, the acinar spaces may be deformed, compressed, and elongated, resulting in pleomorphic clusters of calcifications. These can be indistinguishable from those seen in some forms of DCIS, more commonly (but not exclusively) low- and intermediate-grade DCIS (11). A subgroup of calcifications occurring in fibroadenomas is fairly distinctive. These calcifications are high density, chunky, and "coral-like" with jagged edges, and some form acute angles (Figure 5.27). In our experience, these sometimes develop rapidly in patients with fibroadenomas during or after completion of chemotherapy for breast cancer.

If the acinar spaces are tiny and tightly apposed, we may not be able to resolve the individual calcification particles, but rather, see smudgy, ill-defined, or amorphous calcifications (Figure 5.28). When specimen radiography is done, using higher magnification factors than achievable in patients, these amorphous calcification clusters can sometimes be resolved into individual punctate calcifications reflecting tightly packed, adjacent acinar structures. Amorphous calcifications usually reflect the presence of sclerosing adenosis; they can be associated with DCIS, commonly low nuclear grade without central necrosis (Box 5.4). When the amorphous calcifications are diffuse and bilateral, in patients with dense tissue, our approach is careful follow-up. When they are unilateral and focal, particularly if new compared with prior studies, or if they are in an unusual location (e.g., lower inner quadrant), we recommend biopsy.

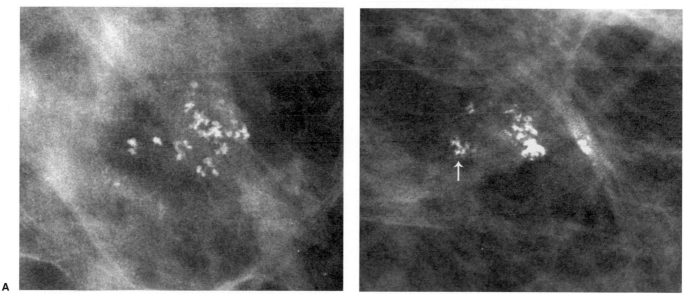

A **B**

Figure 5.27 *Fibroadenomas.* A. In fibroadenomas, the proliferating perilobular stroma can compress, deform, and elongate the acinar spaces. Calcifications developing in the epithelial elements and surrounding stroma can have a fairly distinctive appearance. The calcifications are high-density, chunky, and "coral-like" with jagged edges, and some form acute angles. Category 2. B. Different patient with "coral-like," high-density calcifications with jagged edges (*arrow*) and branches at acute angles. Category 2.

(*continued on next page*)

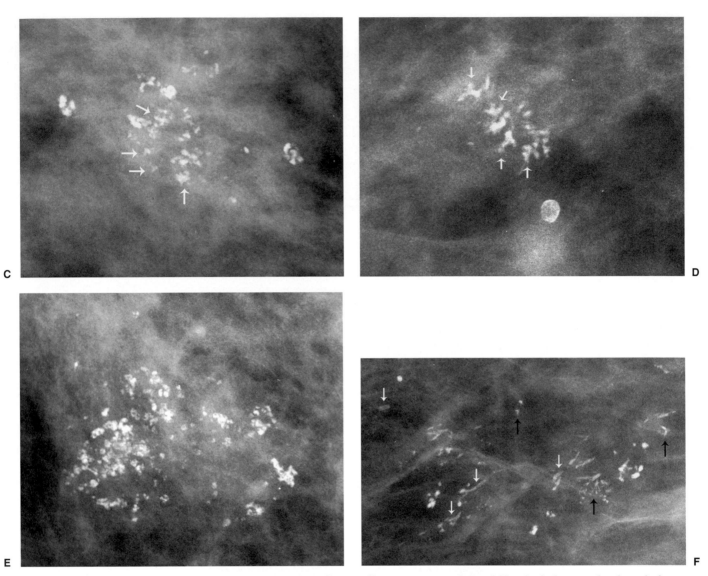

Figure 5.27 (continued) *C.* Different patient with coral-like, high-density, chunky calcifications with jagged edges (*arrows*). Category 2. *D.* Different patient with "coral-like," high-density calcifications with jagged edges and branches at acute angles (*arrows*). In a number of our patients, these types of calcifications have developed within a year of chemotherapy. It may be that the chemotherapy leads to hyalinization and calcification of preexisting fibroadenomas. Incidentally noted is a lucent-centered calcification. *E.* Dense calcifications, some with an associated central lucency ("bubbly"). Category 2. *F.* Linear calcifications, some with central lucencies (*white arrows*) mixed with coarse, "coral-like" calcifications having jagged edges and acute angles (*black arrows*). Although the diagnosis of a fibroadenoma was suspected based on the imaging findings, an imaging-guided biopsy is done, confirming the diagnosis.

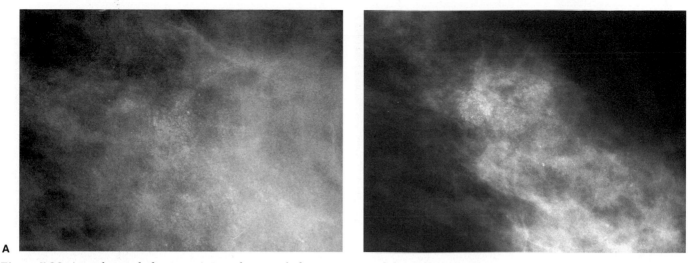

A   B

Figure 5.28 *Amorphous calcifications. A.* Low-density calcifications scattered throughout the dense parenchyma. The calcifications have a similar appearance on lateral views (e.g., no layering is noted). Although not all images are shown, this is a bilateral, diffuse process in this patient. *B.* No significant change is seen 5 years later. When this process is diffuse and bilateral, we follow patients at annual intervals. When focal, or if there are changes on follow-up studies, or if the cluster is in an unusual location, we recommend biopsy. These calcifications are tightly clustered, well-defined, tiny calcifications that appear amorphous because we are not able to resolve them into individual particles on routine images. When specimens are magnified at 3×, these amorphous calcifications can be resolved into individual, well-defined, tiny particles. Although assigned as category 3, our follow up for most of these patients is annual.

Box 5.4: Amorphous, "Smudgy" Calcifications

Milk of calcium (differential appearance between craniocaudal and lateral views)
Sclerosing adenosis
Ductal carcinoma *in situ* (more commonly low or intermediate grade without central necrosis)

CALCIFICATIONS ASSOCIATED WITH MASSES

Thin, well-defined, curvilinear calcifications can be seen when formed in the wall of cysts, oil cysts, and silicone granulomas. Some of these are lucent-centered calcifications or, when less than 1 mm thick, eggshell or rim-type calcifications (Figure 5.29).

Calcium can be present in suspension (Figure 5.30) or as discrete calcifications in microcysts or macrocysts (Figure 5.31). The hallmark of intracystic calcifications is their variation in appearance on orthogonal views (12–14). When viewed on the CC view, the calcium may appear as an amorphous, ill-defined, round smudge or as a cluster of high-density, tightly packed, round (polyhedral) calcifications. When viewed in the horizontal plane on a 90-degree lateral view (and often even on the MLO view), the calcium layers in the dependent portion of the cyst and is seen as sharp, high-density curvilinear calcifications or individual calcifications assuming a teacup or a meniscus-like configuration, enabling definitive diagnosis (Figure 5.32). Microcysts and milk of calcium can be multifocal and bilateral in women with dense tissue, or focal and unilateral. In some patients, the milk of calcium involves macrocysts.

Calcium in suspension (milk of calcium) is characterized by a differential appearance on orthogonal images: amorphous on the CC view and curvilinear and sharply defined on a 90-degree lateral view.

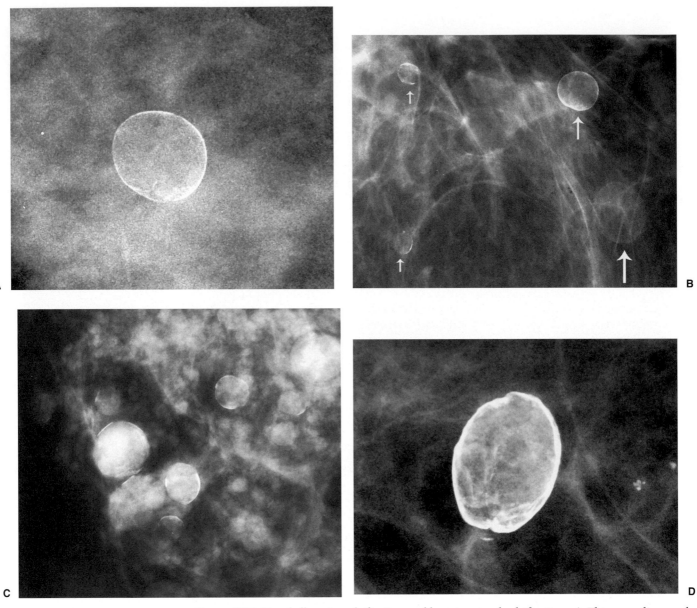

Figure 5.29 *Egg shell or rim calcifications and lucent-centered calcifications. A.* Thin, curvilinear calcification developing in the wall of cysts or oil cysts. *B.* Different patient. Multiple oil cysts with thin, rim calcification at various stages of development. Uncalcified oil cyst (*largest arrow*); complete rim calcification (*medium-sized arrow*); partially calcified oil cysts (*two small arrows*). *C.* Different patient. Rim calcifications developing around several silicone granulomas. *D.* Different patient. Lucent-centered calcifications are thicker and vary in size, from less than 1 mm to more than 1 cm.

(*continued on next page*)

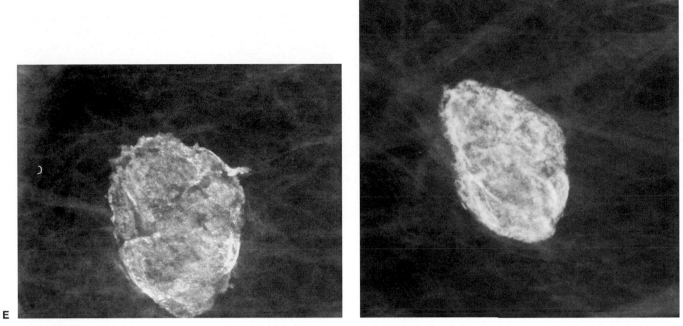

E   F

Figure 5.29 (continued) *E.* Different patient. Lucent-centered calcification can develop in areas of fat necrosis. *F.* On subsequent mammograms, these can stabilize or become denser and smaller in size or resolve completely. All are category 2.

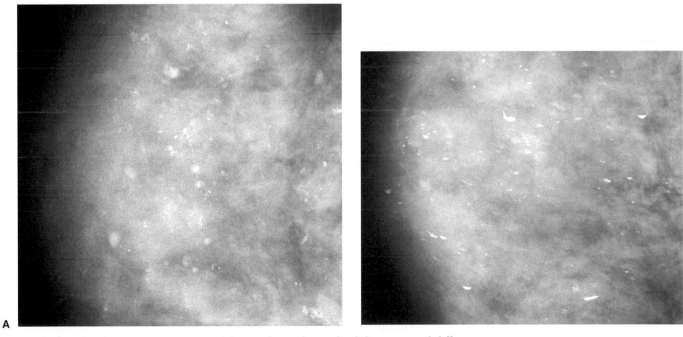

A   B

Figure 5.30 *Milk of calcium.* *A.* Craniocaudal view shows dense glandular tissue and diffuse, scattered, round, amorphous calcifications of varying sizes. *B.* The 90-degree lateral view demonstrates sharply defined, linear, and curvilinear calcifications ("teacups"). An appearance that changes between craniocaudal and mediolateral oblique (or 90-degree lateral) views is the hallmark of this type of calcification. Category 2.

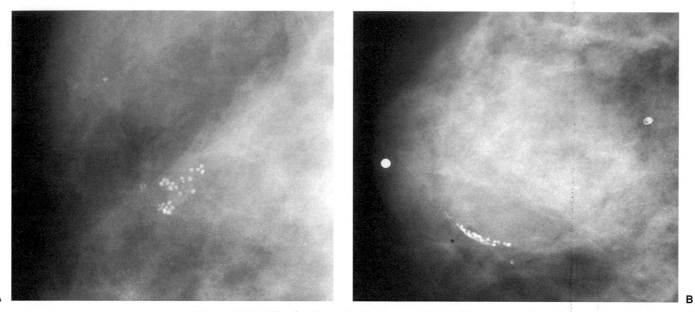

A   B

Figure 5.31 *Milk of calcium. A.* Craniocaudal view shows dense glandular tissue and a cluster of high-density, well-defined (possibly polyhedral) calcifications. *B.* The 90-degree lateral view demonstrates layering of the individual calcifications in what is now seen to be a macrocyst. With layering calcifications such as these, ultrasound is not absolutely necessary to evaluate the mass; the layering confirms that the mass is fluid filled. Category 2.

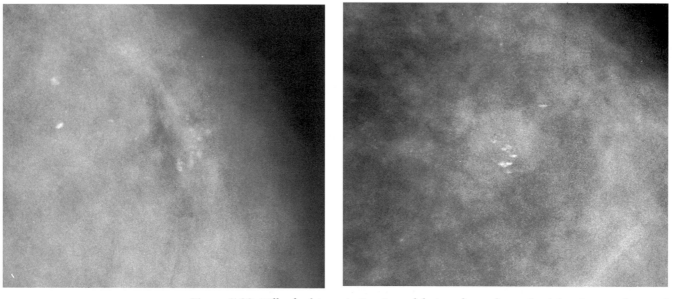

A   B

Figure 5.32 *Milk of calcium. A.* Craniocaudal view shows dense glandular tissue and amorphous calcifications. *B.* The 90-degree lateral view demonstrates better defined, now linear calcifications.

(*continued on next page*)

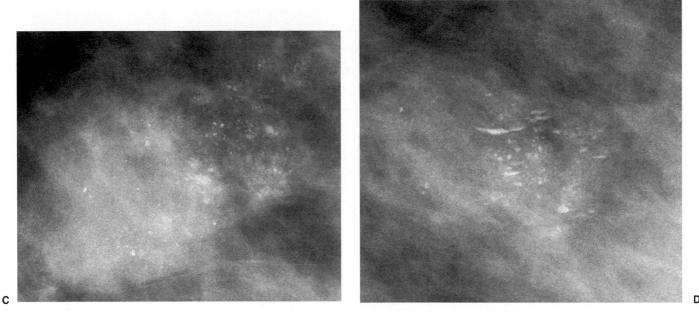

Figure 5.32 (continued) *C.* Craniocaudal view in a different patient shows dense glandular tissue and amorphous calcifications mixed with some round and punctate forms. *D.* The 90-degree lateral view demonstrates a significant change in the overall appearance of the calcifications. They are now better defined, and some are linear (teacups). Category 2.

SUTURE CALCIFICATIONS

Suture material in the breast can calcify (15,16). These calcifications may look like knots and be evenly spaced; they may be curvilinear, forming loops; or they may be linear calcifications with smooth borders limited to the biopsy site. These calcifications appear to be a rare occurrence in the nonirradiated breast. They occur with a higher frequency in women after lumpectomy and radiation therapy. It has been postulated that radiation-induced damage and alterations in tissue healing delay the reabsorption of catgut sutures, thereby providing a matrix for the depositing of calcium (15).

PARASITES

Sporadic case reports are available describing the imaging features of parasites localized to the breast. These include filariasis (*Wuchereria bancrofti* and *Brugia malayi*); onchocerciasis (*Onchocerca volvulus*) and loiasis (*Loa loa*), all of which tend to be localized to the subcutaneous tissues; cysticercosis; dracunculosis; and schistosomiasis (17,18). The deceased parasites calcify, leading to the development of linear, curvilinear, coiled, lacelike, beadlike, or serpiginous calcifications (Figure 5.33) in isolation or with an associated soft tissue component (as has been reported for cutaneous myasis—*Dermatobia hominis*) (19). Trichinosis (*Trichinella spiralis*) involves the pectoral muscles and spares breast tissue (20); fine, punctate, well-defined pearl-like calcifications, diffusely scattered bilaterally but limited to the pectoral muscles, are seen in these patients (Figure 5.34).

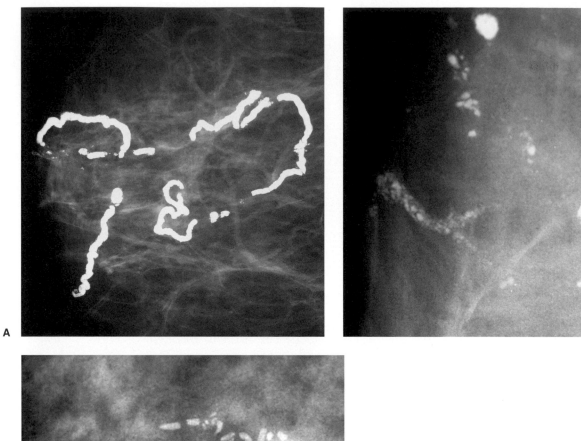

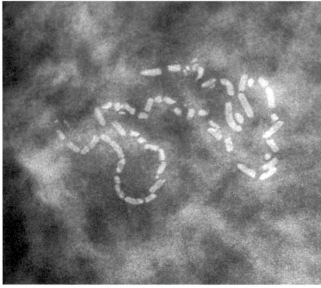

Figure 5.33 *Calcified parasites.* *A.* Parasites. Dense, coarse, linear, and serpiginous calcifications are seen. *B.* Photographic cone-down view, subareolar area demonstrating a slightly different appearance of the calcifications. *C.* Different patient. Linear, coiled, and serpiginous calcifications are seen.

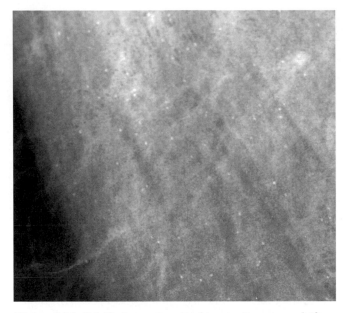

Figure 5.34 *Calcified parasites*. Trichinosis. Punctate calcifications diffusely involving the pectoral muscle are shown.

CALCIFICATIONS ASSOCIATED WITH MALIGNANCY

When considering calcifications associated with malignancy, we are primarily talking about proliferative cellular processes occurring in terminal ducts and DCIS. DCIS is cancer contained within these ducts; it is noninvasive or intraductal disease and should be distinguished from invasive (extraductal) breast cancer. The most common manifestation of DCIS is calcifications detected on screening mammograms in otherwise asymptomatic patients. Rarely, DCIS can present as a macrolobulated or spiculated mass, an area of distortion detected mammographically, a palpable mass, spontaneous nipple discharge (clear, serous, or bloody), or Paget's disease of the nipple (21,22).

> When associated with breast cancer, calcifications most commonly reflect the presence of intraductal cancer or DCIS.

Until the late 1980s, DCIS was considered a rare disease, being reported in 3% to 5% of all biopsies done for clinical findings (23). Rapid advances in mammographic technique and our ability to detect and characterize calcifications, coupled with increasing numbers of women undergoing screening mammography, have led to dramatic increases in the number of patients diagnosed with DCIS. In screening mammography programs, DCIS represents 22% to 45% of all detected breast cancers (22–25). An increase in the number of biopsies done for mammographically detected calcifications has driven the histologic descriptions of DCIS, classification schemes, and our overall appreciation for this disease. With the increases in DCIS detection has come significant controversy about the biologic significance of some of these lesions (25).

When discussing DCIS, it is critical to recognize that DCIS is a heterogeneous disease, that all cases should not be "lumped" into one basket. DCIS is heterogeneous in its mammographic, clinical, and histologic presentation and consequently its biologic behavior. Some forms of DCIS invariably progress to invasion and do so with a rapid time course, whereas others may remain stable in the duct for years, regress, or eventually progress to low-grade invasive ductal carcinomas. The daunting challenge we face is knowing how to manage patients with some forms of low-grade DCIS appropriately. These are the lesions that may never progress to invasion; consequently, some patients diagnosed with these lesions are overtreated (e.g., mastectomy or using radiation therapy after lumpectomy), whereas others are undertreated. This reflects our current inability to distinguish insignificant lesions from those that may recur, invade, and metastasize.

> DCIS is a heterogeneous disease process.

Proliferative cellular processes, occurring in the terminal ducts, are usually mammographically occult unless associated with calcifications. The duct wall is composed of loose connective tissue forming the basement membrane, a discontiguous layer of myoepithelial cells at the base of a contiguous layer of epithelial cells lining the lumen of the duct; normal ducts are therefore characterized by a two-cell layer. *Hyperplasia* refers to an increase in the number of epithelial or myoepithelial cells lining the ducts. It can be qualified by pathologists as mild, moderate, or severe. As the proliferating cells acquire atypical cytologic features, the term *atypical ductal hyperplasia* (ADH) may be used. It is important, however, to emphasize that the diagnosis of ADH is, to some extent, subjective and defined differently by pathologists (26). Given the importance of some of the decisions made when a patient is diagnosed with ADH, it behooves radiologists involved in imaging-guided procedures to work closely with the pathologists and to have some understanding of their approach to this diagnosis. In some patients, ADH may progress to the development of DCIS.

Based on three-dimensional studies of ducts (27) involved with DCIS, biologic markers, and associated invasive lesions, consider at least two large subgroups of DCIS: (a) those that appear to evolve over time from proliferative processes in the ducts, including ductal hyperplasia and ADH, eventually leading to low-nuclear-grade DCIS without central necrosis; and (b) those arising *de novo* in the duct, characterized by central necrosis and short intraductal phases. The proliferative processes associated with the first group are in a state of flux and multifocal in the involved ducts. That is, a normal segment of duct may be adjacent to an area of low-grade DCIS, next to an area of ductal hyperplasia, and next to an area of atypical ductal hyperplasia, abutting yet another focus of low-nuclear-grade DCIS. The calcifications we detect mammographically likely develop in secretions within the duct lumen in association with hyperplasia, ADH, or low-grade DCIS without central necrosis. Because the effects of the proliferative process on the duct lumen overlap, it is not surprising that the mammographic appearance of the calcifications in these different processes is indistinguishable (28). In some patients, low-grade DCIS without central necrosis may give rise to low-grade invasive carcinoma.

It is likely that the other major subgroup of DCIS arises *de novo* in the duct rather than evolving from a preexisting process (e.g., high-grade DCIS does not arise from low-grade DCIS, although they can coexist in a given lesion). These lesions are unifocal and contiguous in the duct and are often high nuclear grade with central necrosis. Areas of microinvasion may be apparent.

Histologically, ducts involved with DCIS are distended, compared with normal ducts. Low-nuclear-grade DCIS is characterized by monomorphic nuclei lacking nucleoli, low mitotic rates (low thymidine-labeling rates), cell polarization toward the duct lumen, no cell necrosis or autophagocytosis, and probably, long intraductal phases. The cells can form rigid cribriform spaces, roman bridges, or micropapillary projections. In some patients, a more solid growth pattern may be seen histologically.

High-grade DCIS is characterized by pleomorphic nuclei having multiple nucleoli, high mitotic rates (high thymidine-labeling rates), lack of cellular polarization, presence of cell necrosis and autophagocytosis, and a short intraductal phase. Most of these lesions are obligate invaders. The cells circumferentially encroach and narrow the lumen of the distended ducts. The lumen contains necrotic cellular debris within which the calcifications form. In some patients, there is an intense inflammatory reaction surrounding the involved ducts, making it difficult to identify areas of microinvasion. High-nuclear-grade DCIS lesions are likely to give rise to poorly differentiated, high-nuclear-grade invasive lesions. These are the types of lesions that we should be striving to diagnose mammographically. Without intervention, these types of DCIS lesions progress to invasion; their detection and excision may serve to reduce the likelihood of invasive disease in the future.

The calcifications we detect mammographically, in association with these cellular proliferative processes, develop in luminal secretions or in the necrotic cellular debris found in the lumen of the distended ducts (29). Calcifications, developing in secretions occurring in the cribriform spaces formed by the proliferating cells, are well-defined, punctate, oval, round (Figure 5.35), or amorphous (Figure 5.36) with variable densities within a

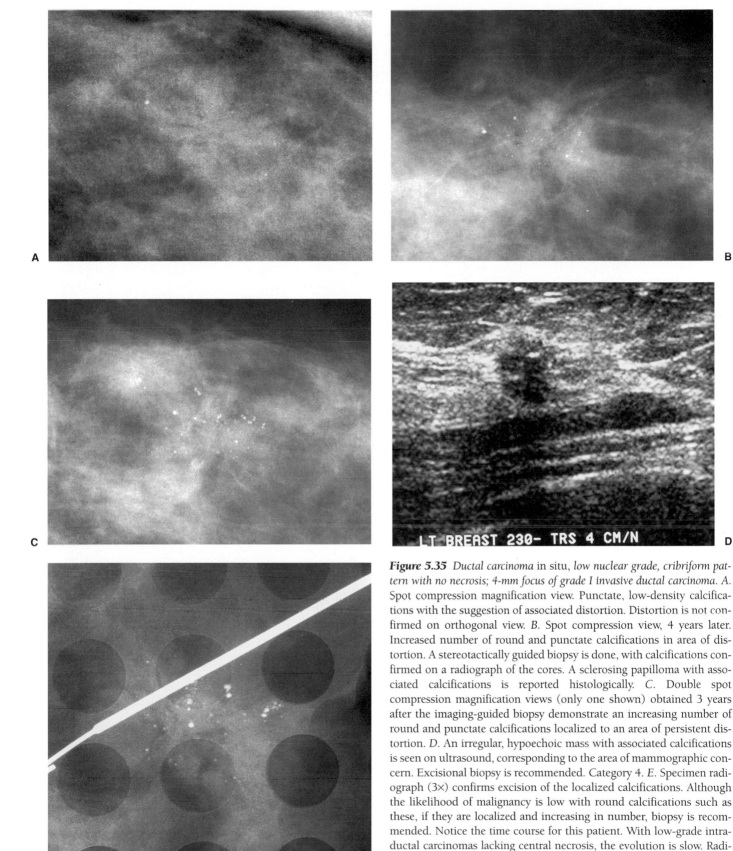

Figure 5.35 *Ductal carcinoma* in situ, *low nuclear grade, cribriform pattern with no necrosis; 4-mm focus of grade I invasive ductal carcinoma. A. Spot compression magnification view. Punctate, low-density calcifications with the suggestion of associated distortion. Distortion is not confirmed on orthogonal view. B. Spot compression view, 4 years later. Increased number of round and punctate calcifications in area of distortion. A stereotactically guided biopsy is done, with calcifications confirmed on a radiograph of the cores. A sclerosing papilloma with associated calcifications is reported histologically. C. Double spot compression magnification views (only one shown) obtained 3 years after the imaging-guided biopsy demonstrate an increasing number of round and punctate calcifications localized to an area of persistent distortion. D. An irregular, hypoechoic mass with associated calcifications is seen on ultrasound, corresponding to the area of mammographic concern. Excisional biopsy is recommended. Category 4. E. Specimen radiograph (3×) confirms excision of the localized calcifications. Although the likelihood of malignancy is low with round calcifications such as these, if they are localized and increasing in number, biopsy is recommended. Notice the time course for this patient. With low-grade intraductal carcinomas lacking central necrosis, the evolution is slow. Radiographic follow-up in 6 months is probably not very helpful in these patients. Changes, if they occur, often take years.*

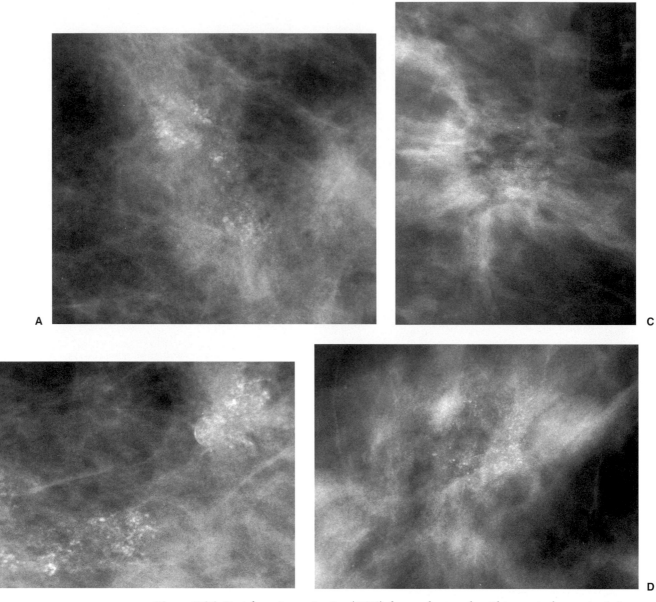

Figure 5.36 *Ductal carcinoma* in situ *(DCIS), low nuclear grade with no central necrosis. A.* Screening view demonstrates a developing cluster of amorphous calcifications. *B.* Spot compression magnification view confirming clusters of amorphous calcifications occupying a larger area than that suspected on the screening view. Category 4. *C.* In a different patient, the craniocaudal view demonstrates an area of distortion with central lucency and low-density calcifications. *D.* Double spot compression magnification view demonstrates a cluster of amorphous calcifications associated with an area of distortion. A 5-mm focus of grade I invasive ductal carcinoma associated with the DCIS is reported on the lumpectomy specimen in this patient.

cluster and among clusters. In some patients, linear orientation and segmental distribution of round and punctate calcifications can be seen (Figure 5.37). When associated with DCIS, it is more commonly low or intermediate-nuclear-grade DCIS; high nuclear grade is diagnosed in a small percentage of patients with these types of calcifications. Mammographically, we tend to underestimate the extent of these processes. In general, what we see may be the "tip of the iceberg" (30). It is also important to recognize that the calcifications we see may be in areas of hyperplasia (Figure 5.38) or atypical hyperplasia (Fig-

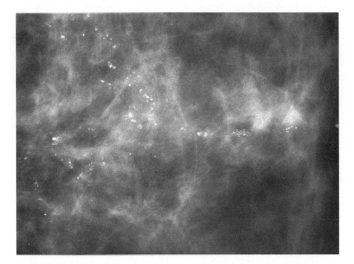

Figure 5.37 *Ductal carcinoma* in situ *(DCIS), micropapillary, cribriform pattern with no necrosis.* Double spot compression magnification view of the left subareolar area demonstrating round, punctate, and amorphous calcifications in a linear orientation. Although not shown, the patient's breast is diffusely involved with round and punctate calcifications, and a mass is palpated in the upper central portion of the breast. This 48-year-old patient had not had a mammogram in 9 years. A grade I invasive ductal carcinoma is reported histologically, with 8 of 19 axillary lymph nodes positive for metastatic disease. It has been suggested that low-grade DCIS is not a true cancer. Biologically, however, low-grade DCIS with associated low-grade invasive lesions can metastasize, particularly if neglected.

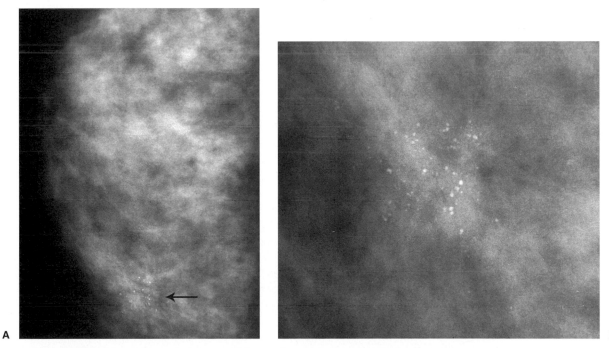

A   B

Figure 5.38 *Epithelial hyperplasia.* A. Craniocaudal view from a screening study demonstrating a new cluster of calcifications (mediolateral oblique view not shown) in the medial aspect of the right breast. Category 0. Magnification views are recommended. B. Double spot compression magnification views demonstrate round, punctate, and amorphous calcifications of variable density. Because these are new compared with prior studies, and in an unusual location, biopsy is recommended. Category 4.

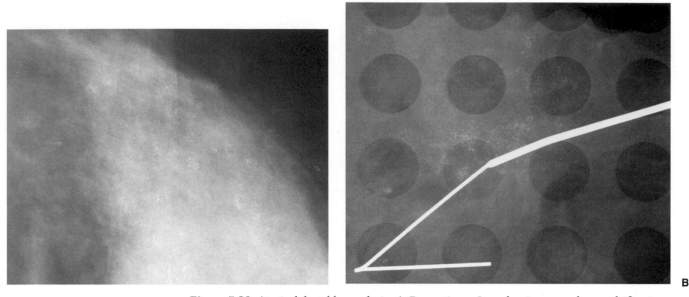

A   B

Figure 5.39 *Atypical ductal hyperplasia.* A. Dense tissue. Low-density, amorphous calcifications are seen. B. Higher magnification on a specimen radiograph (3×) demonstrates tightly packed punctate calcifications.

ure 5.39), that are next to an area of low-grade DCIS that has no associated calcifications. When targeting these types of calcifications during imaging-guided biopsies, we need to be aware that there may be an inherent sampling bias, so that increasing the numbers of cores obtained to include uncalcified tissue may be appropriate. Targeting the calcifications may yield a diagnosis of hyperplasia or atypical ductal hyperplasia (Chapter 10) adjacent to an area of noncalcified DCIS. Although controversial, excisional biopsy may be preferred to imaging-guided biopsy in some of these patients; this ensures adequate sampling to establish a diagnosis.

Calcifications developing in DCIS associated with central necrosis (regardless of nuclear grade) are commonly linear with irregular borders and clefts, variable in density with linear, segmental, or less commonly, regional distribution.

Calcifications developing in necrotic cellular debris have a fairly distinctive mammographic appearance. These calcifications are molded actively by the rapidly proliferating epithelial cells and develop in the dying cells. The calcifications are linear, with clefts and irregular borders reflecting the active cellular proliferative process (Figure 5.40). They are variable in density within a given lesion and among patients (Figure 5.41). Focally, segmentally, or regionally distributed, they may also have a linear orientation and extend to the nipple. Mammographically, we estimate the extent of the disease fairly accurately (30). Where we see calcifications is where the pathologist finds DCIS. Targeting this type of calcification with imaging-guided biopsies has a high diagnostic yield. The calcifications are molded and in intimate contact with the proliferating cells. Associated round and punctate calcifications may be seen among the linear calcifications.

Lesions characterized by central necrosis tend to be rapidly growing and the calcifications, as reflectors of an ongoing dynamic process, can change rapidly (Figures 5.42 to 5.46). In contrast, low-grade processes lacking central necrosis, evolve slowly and remain intraductal for longer periods of time. Slow mammographic changes usually characterize these processes. Careful comparison with prior mammographic images is helpful. Focal increases in round or punctate calcifications in a given cluster, particularly if the cluster is in an unusual location, may warrant a biopsy recommendation (Figure 5.35).

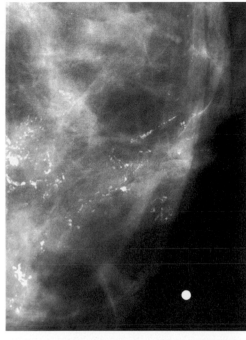

A

Figure 5.40 *Ductal carcinoma* in situ, *high nuclear grade with central necrosis. A.* Metallic BB placed on palpable area. Pleomorphic calcifications demonstrating irregular linear, round, and punctate forms. Linear orientation of some of the calcifications and a regional distribution are seen. *B.* A hypoechoic, macrolobulated mass with associated calcifications corresponding to palpable area. No invasion, however, is reported after excisional biopsy. With larger areas of calcification or tightly packed linear calcifications, ultrasonography may demonstrate an associated soft tissue component. If an abnormality is seen on ultrasound, imaging-guided biopsy can be done with ultrasound guidance. Category 5. *C.* In a different patient, the mediolateral oblique double spot compression magnification view demonstrates pleomorphic calcifications with linear forms and linear orientation. Category 4.

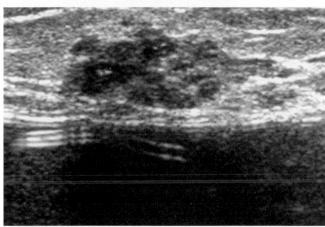

B

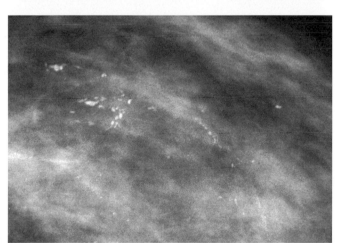

C

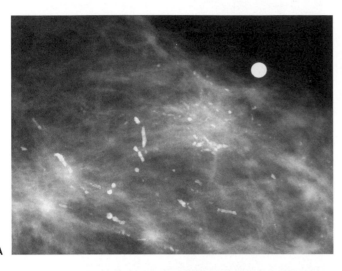

A

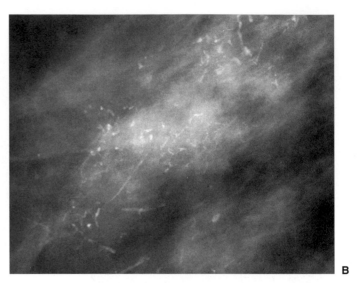

B

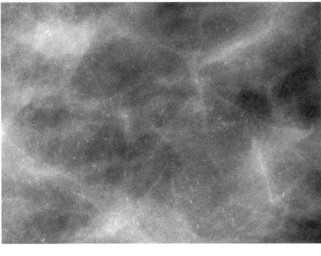

C

Figure 5.41 *Ductal carcinoma* in situ *(DCIS). A.* Mediolateral oblique view demonstrating a mixture of high- and low-density linear and round calcifications. Clefts can be seen in many of the linear calcifications. Although palpable, ultrasonographic evaluation is normal throughout this area. DCIS with a cribriform and solid growth pattern associated with necrosis and a 5.5-cm grade III invasive ductal carcinoma with extensive lymphovascular space involvement are reported histologically. *B.* Different patient, double spot compression magnification view in the craniocaudal projection demonstrating thin, linear calcifications. High-nuclear-grade DCIS with central necrosis and a 1-mm focus of grade II invasive carcinoma are reported histologically. *C.* In a different patient, double spot compression magnification view demonstrates many low-density linear calcifications regionally distributed. These patients help illustrate the variability that can be seen in the size and density of calcifications associated with DCIS within and among lesions.

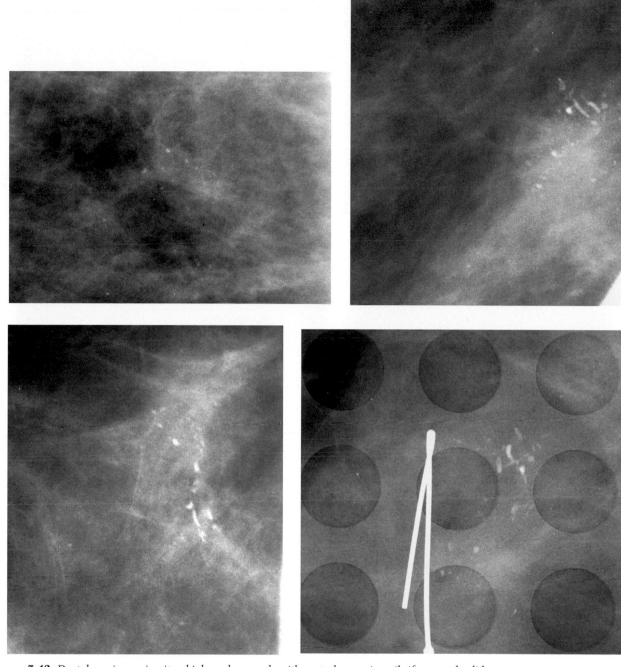

Figure 5.42 *Ductal carcinoma* in situ, *high nuclear grade with central necrosis, cribriform, and solid growth patterns. A.* Mediolateral oblique spot compression magnification view demonstrates punctate calcifications. Mediolateral oblique (*B*) and craniocaudal (*C*) double spot compression magnification views, 6 months later. There are now linear calcifications with linear orientation surrounded by lower-density round and punctate calcifications. Category 4. *D.* Specimen radiograph.

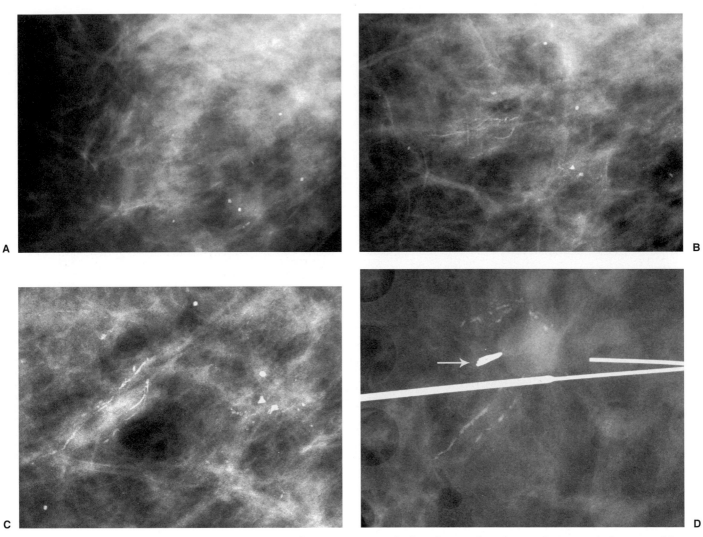

Figure 5.43 *Ductal carcinoma* in situ, *high nuclear grade with central necrosis. A.* Craniocaudal view demonstrating scattered, round calcifications. Follow-up in 6 months was recommended. *B.* Craniocaudal view 6 months later demonstrates development of linear calcifications with linear orientation. The round calcifications that prompted the follow-up are stable. *C.* Double spot compression magnification view in the craniocaudal projection. Stereotactically guided biopsy is done. *D.* Specimen radiograph. Metallic clip (*arrow*) deployed after 11-gauge vacuum-assisted biopsy is seen next to localization wire. The high-nuclear-grade lesions are characterized by a more rapid time course with a short intraductal phase.

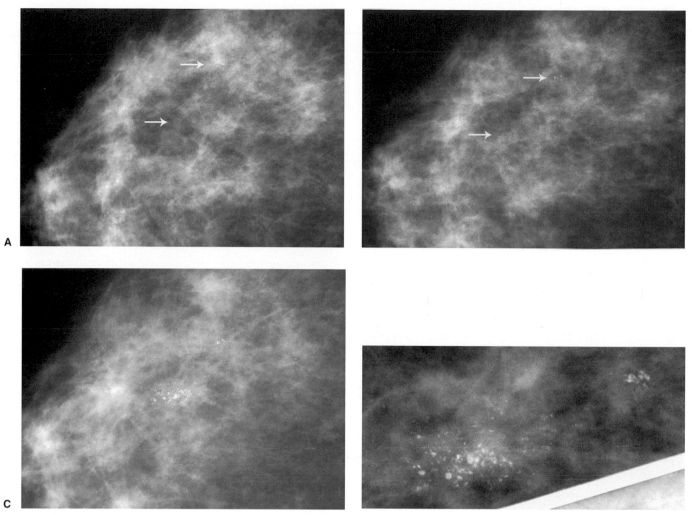

Figure 5.44 *Ductal carcinoma* in situ, *high nuclear grade with central necrosis. A.* Craniocaudal view showing scattered, tiny, low-density calcifications (*arrows*). *B.* One year later, a few more punctate calcifications (*arrows*) have developed. *C.* Two years later, many more calcifications are present. *D.* Double spot compression views are obtained in the mediolateral projection. The calcifications are pleomorphic, with variable densities and a few linear forms.

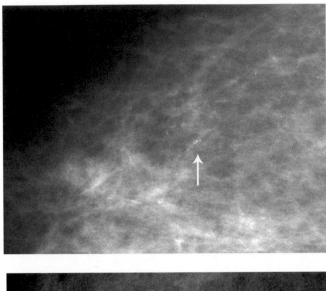

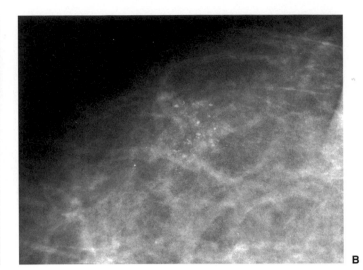

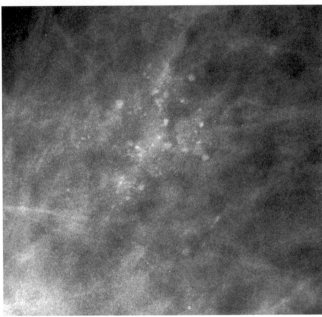

Figure 5.45 *Ductal carcinoma* in situ, *high nuclear grade with central necrosis. A.* Craniocaudal view demonstrating some low-density punctate calcifications (*arrow*). *B.* One year later, many more calcifications are seen at this site. *C.* Double spot compression magnification views are obtained in the craniocaudal projection. A cluster of pleomorphic round, punctate, and amorphous calcifications is shown. Given the rapid evolution and the focal nature of the findings, biopsy is done.

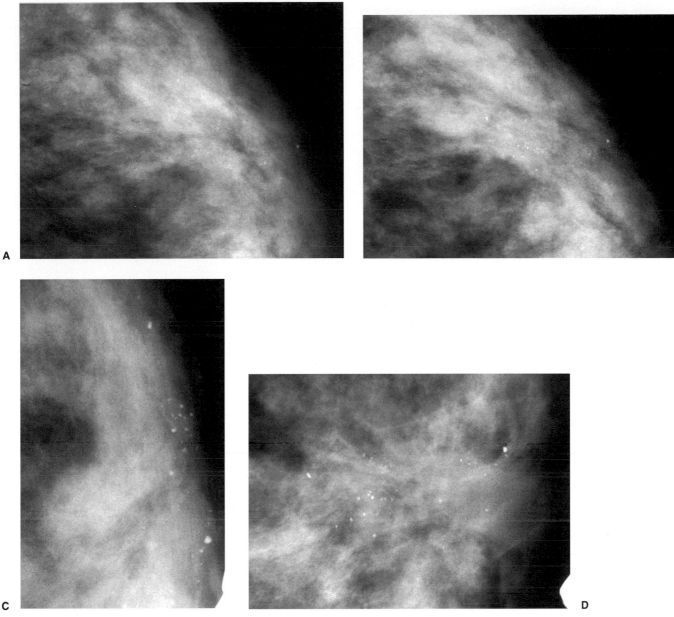

Figure 5.46 *Ductal carcinoma* in situ, *intermediate nuclear grade with scattered areas of necrosis. A.* Craniocaudal view demonstrating scattered punctate calcifications. *B.* Four years later, more calcifications have developed at this site. Double spot compression magnification views in craniocaudal (*C*) and mediolateral oblique (*D*) projections demonstrate a cluster of calcifications with pleomorphism and variable density. Biopsy is done.

VAN NUYS PROGNOSTIC INDEX

As mentioned previously, management of some women diagnosed with DCIS is controversial. Additional research is needed to help establish the biologic significance of some of these lesions so that appropriate treatment recommendations can be made. In 1995, Silverstein and colleagues (31) proposed the use of a prognostic index, the Van Nuys Prognostic Index (VNPI), to facilitate selection of a treatment option for patients with DCIS.

Incorporating pathologic classification, tumor size, margin width, and patient age, the VNPI was developed in an effort to provide a guideline in determining appropriate treatment and management recommendations for patients diagnosed with DCIS.

Table 5.2: Modified University of Southern California/Van Nuys Prognostic Index

Score	Tumor Size	Margins	Pathologic Classification	Age (Yr)
1	≤15 mm	≥10 mm	Non–high grade, no necrosis	>60
2	16–40 mm	1–9 mm	Non–high grade w/ necrosis	40–60
3	≥41 mm	<1 mm	High grade with or without necrosis	<40

Pathologic classification, tumor size, and width of margins were used to assess the risk for local recurrence. In 1997, this was modified to include the age of the patient in calculating the index. Each of these four prognostic features is assigned a score using a scale of 1 to 3 (worst) as outlined in Table 5.2. The scores are totaled to determine the overall modified University of Southern California/VNPI score that can range from 4 to 12 (32–33).

The size of the nuclei, as compared with the diameter of a red blood cell, along with the appearance of the chromatin and the presence of nucleoli, are used in determining the nuclear grade of lesions. Grade I nuclei have diameters comparable to that of one or one and one half red blood cells, diffuse chromatin, and unapparent nucleoli. Grade II nuclei have diameters equivalent to that of one or two red blood cells, coarse chromatin, and infrequent nucleoli. Grade III nuclei have a diameter greater than that of two red blood cells, vesicular chromatin, and one or more nucleoli. Necrosis is present, regardless of the cellular architectural pattern, when necrotic neoplastic cells of ductal origin are found in the lumen of the involved ducts (33).

To date, no statistically significant differences in mortality were reported when patients treated with mastectomy, lumpectomy and radiation therapy, or lumpectomy alone were compared. Significant differences are noted among these treatment options when local recurrence rates are considered. In many patients, recurrences simulate the primary lesion (Figure 5.47). However, about half of the local recurrences after conservative treatment of DCIS are invasive; hence, local recurrence is a particularly important consideration. In patients with DCIS treated with mastectomy, the likelihood of local recurrence is almost completely eliminated. In women treated conservatively for DCIS, Silverstein and colleagues (33) reported recurrence rates of 2%, 22%, and 52% in patients with VNPIs of 4, 5, or 6; 7, 8, or 9; and 10, 11, or 12, respectively. Recurrences were invasive in 0%, 46%, and 43% of patients with VNPIs of 4, 5, or 6; 7, 8, or 9; and 10, 11, or 12, respectively.

About 30% of patients diagnosed with DCIS have VNPIs of 4, 5, or 6. This subset of patients may not gain much benefit when radiation therapy is added to the lumpectomy. Patients with VNPIs of 10, 11, or 12 gain the most from postlumpectomy radiation therapy; however, local recurrence rates are high, and as such, these patients should be considered for mastectomy. As with most classification systems, the intermediate group, those with VNPIs, of 7, 8, or 9, present the greatest challenge. Depending on the overall score and some of the individual category scores, some of these patients are likely to benefit from radiation, whereas others are better served by undergoing a mastectomy (33).

Although there will undoubtedly be other classification systems, or modifications to the VNPI as results of ongoing randomized control trials are reported, it is clear that a system like this is helpful in selecting from available treatment options. It is presented here in its more basic form and should prompt additional, more detailed readings beyond the scope of this book.

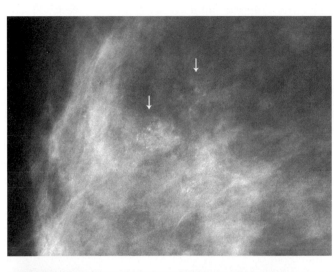

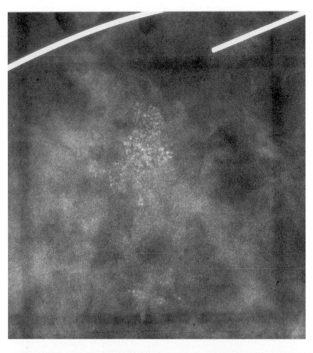

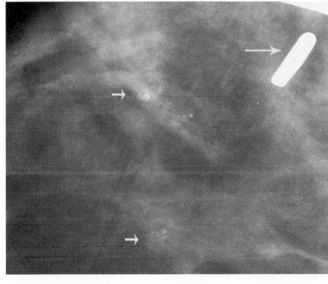

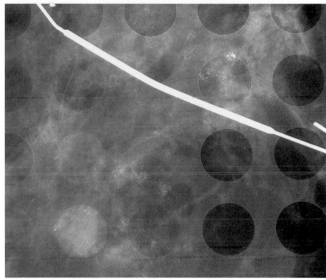

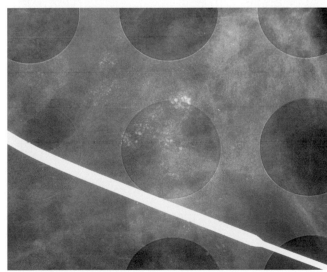

Figure 5.47 *Ductal carcinoma* in situ, *cribriform and solid pattern, low and intermediate grade with no necrosis. A.* Mediolateral spot compression magnification view. Amorphous calcifications (*arrows*). *B.* Specimen radiograph. Tightly packed punctate calcifications are present. *C.* Double spot compression magnification view of the lumpectomy site 5 years after surgery. Two clusters of amorphous calcifications have developed (*small arrows*). Metallic clip (*large arrow*) from the lumpectomy is seen. *D.* Specimen radiograph with photographic cone. *E.* Multiple clusters of tightly packed punctate calcifications. What is seen on the magnification view is the "tip of the iceberg"—many more calcification clusters are evident on the specimen. The appearance of the calcifications is similar to the initial presentation. Histologically, a recurrence is diagnosed.

ARTIFACTS, MIMICRY

High-density particles (gold) resembling calcifications can be seen in axillary lymph nodes of patients with rheumatoid arthritis treated with gold.

Artifacts can simulate calcifications and, although usually easy to identify, can sometimes present a challenge. Fingerprints, scratch marks, dust on the screen, deodorants, zinc oxide ointment, hair, and tattoos projecting on the breast parenchyma are some of the more common artifacts that may simulate breast calcifications (Figure 5.48). High-density particles reflecting shrapnel from gunshot wounds (Figure 5.49) or gold deposited bilaterally in lymph nodes after treatment of rheumatoid arthritis may also mimic the appearance of calcifications (34). Meticulous attention to detail, appropriate screen maintenance, and patient preparation can minimize the occurrence of artifacts. If questions persist about the presence of underlying calcifications or artifact simulating calcifications, repeat films can be obtained after the potential cause of the artifact has been addressed.

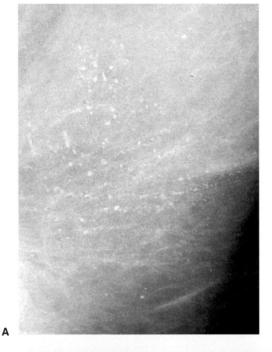

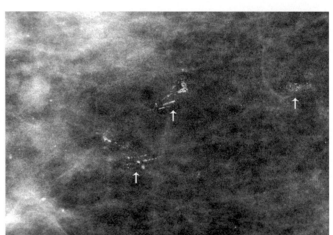

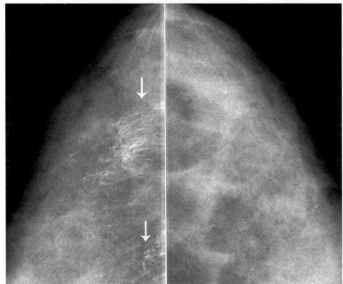

Figure 5.48 *Artifacts. A.* Deodorant. High-density linear material usually seen in the axillary area. *B.* Different patient; water droplets on the cassette (*arrows*). *C.* Different patient; hair (*arrows*).

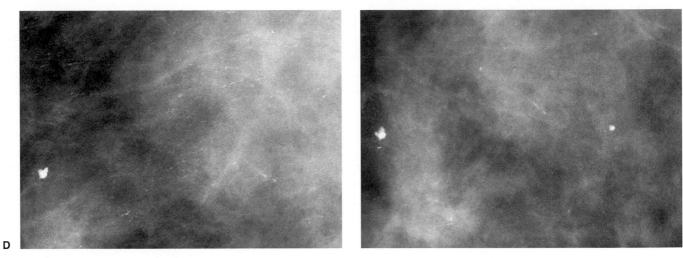

D   E

Figure 5.48 Continued *D.* Different patient; polymixin B sulfate (Neosporin) on skin. Low-density material, linear with curvilinear orientation, simulates calcifications. *E.* Follow-up image after skin is cleaned confirms skin artifact.

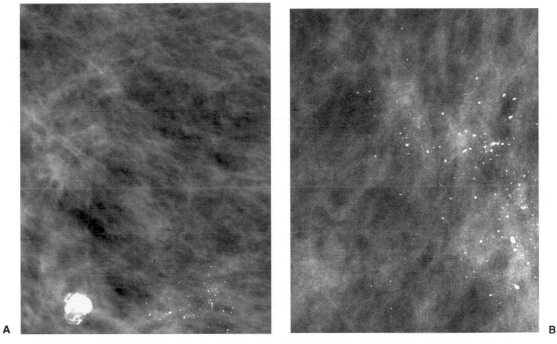

A   B

Figure 5.49 *Shrapnel. A.* High-density material describes bullet trajectory. *B.* Photographic cone on largest collection. The density of these particles is much higher than that seen with breast calcifications.

ULTRASTRUCTURE

Polarizing microscopy may be needed to see calcifications composed of calcium oxalate.

Chemically, breast calcifications are classified into two major types. Type I calcifications are composed of calcium oxalate (weddellite) and occur in association with benign secretory processes and cystic changes. They are colorless and may not be seen on hematoxylin and eosin–stained tissue viewed with routine microscopy. They are, however, visible as birefringent crystals with polarizing microscopy. Type II calcifications are composed of calcium phosphate crystals (hydroxyapatite) that have been identified in benign and malignant breast tissue and are thought to develop in conjunction with cell necrosis. Type II calcifications are readily seen using hematoxylin and eosin, with deeply basophilic staining. They are not birefringent when viewed with polarizing microscopy (35,36).

REFERENCES

1. American College of Radiology (ACR). *Breast imaging reporting and data system (BI-RADS)*, 3rd ed. Reston, VA: ACR, 1998.
2. Kopans DB, Meyer JE, Homer MJ, et al. Dermal deposits mistaken for breast calcifications. *Radiology* 1983;149:592–594.
3. Sickles EA. Breast calcifications: mammographic evaluation. *Radiology* 1986;160:289–293.
4. Bassett LW. Mammographic analysis of calcifications. *Radiol Clin North Am* 1992;30:93–105.
5. Moshyedi AC, Puthawala AH, Kurland RJ, et al. Breast arterial calcifications: association with coronary artery disease. *Radiology* 1995;194:181–183.
6. Doeger KM, Whaley DH, Berger PB, et al. Breast arterial calcification detected on mammography is a risk factor for coronary artery disease. *Radiology* 2002;225:553[abst].
7. Fuster M, Saez JJ, Orozco D, et al. Breast arterial calcification: a new cardiovascular risk marker. *Radiology* 2002;225:553–554[abst].
8. Bassett LW, Jackson VP, Jahan R, et al. *Diagnosis of diseases of the breast*. Philadelphia: WB Saunders, 1997:357–443.
9. Asch T, Frey C. Radiographic appearance of mammary duct ectasia with calcification. *N Engl J Med* 1962;266:86–87.
10. Dixon JM, Anderson TJ, Lumsden AB, et al. Mammary duct ectasia. *Br J Surg* 1983;70:601–603.
11. MacErlean DP, Nathna BE. Calcification in sclerosing adenosis simulating malignant breast calcification. *Br J Radiol* 1972;45:944–945.
12. Sickles EA, Abele JS. Milk of calcium within tiny benign breast cysts. *Radiology* 1981;141:655.
13. Linden SS, Sickles EA. Sedimented calcium in benign breast cysts: full spectrum of mammographic presentation. *AJR Am J Roentgenol* 1989;152:967–971.
14. Moy L, Slanetz PJ, Yeh DE, et al. The pendant view: an additional projection to confirm the diagnosis of milk of calcium. *AJR Am J Roentgenol* 2001;177:173–175.
15. Davis SP, Stomper PC, Weidner N, et al. Suture calcification mimicking recurrence in the irradiated breast: a potential pitfall in mammographic evaluation. *Radiology* 1989;172:247–248.
16. Stacey-Clear A, McCarthy KA, Hall DA, et al. Calcified suture material in the breast after radiation therapy. *Radiology* 1992;183:207–208.
17. Chow CK, McCarthy JS, Neafie R, et al. Mammography of lymphatic filariasis. *AJR Am J Roentgenol* 1996;167:1425–1426.
18. Friedman PD, Kalisher L. Case 43: filariasis. *Radiology* 2002;222:515–517.
19. de Barros N, D'Avila MS, Bauab SP, et al. Cutaneous myiasis of the breast: mammographic and US features—report of five cases. *Radiology* 2001;218:518–520.
20. Aspesteguia L, Murillo A, Biurrun J, et al. Calcified trichinosis of pectoral muscle: mammographic appearance. *Eur Radiol* 1995;5:414–416.
21. Stomper PC, Connolly JL, Meyer JE, et al. Clinically occult ductal carcinoma in situ detected with mammography: analysis of 100 cases with radio-pathologic correlation. *Radiology* 1989;172:235–241.
22. Poplack SP, Wells WA. Ductal carcinoma in situ of the breast: mammographic-pathologic correlation. *AJR Am J Roentgenol* 1998;170:1543–1549.
23. Haagansen CD, ed. *Disease of the breast*, 3rd ed. Philadelphia: WB Saunders, 1986.
24. Stomper PC, Connolly JL. Ductal carcinoma in situ of the breast: correlation between mammographic calcification and tumor subtype. *AJR Am J Roentgenol* 1992;159:483–485.

25. Ernster VL, Barclay J, Kerlilowske K, et al. Incidence of and treatment for ductal carcinoma in situ of the breast. *JAMA* 1996;275:913–918.

26. Rosai J. Borderline epithelial lesions of the breast. *Am J Surg Pathol* 1991;15:209–221.

27. Faverly DRG, Burgers L, Bult P, et al. Three dimensional imaging of mammary ductal carcinoma in situ: clinical implications. *Semin Diagn Pathol* 1994;11:193–198.

28. Dinkel HP, Gassel AM, Tschammler A. Is the appearance of microcalcifications on mammography useful in predicting histological grade of malignancy in ductal carcinoma in situ? *Br J of Radiol* 2000;73:938–944.

29. Holland R, Hendricks JHCL. Microcalcifications associated with ductal carcinoma in situ: mammographic-pathologic correlation. *Semin Diagn Pathol* 1994;11:181–192.

30. Holland R, Hendricks JHCL, Verbeek ALM, et al. Extent, distribution and mammographic/histologic correlations of breast ductal carcinoma in situ. *Lancet* 1990;336:519–522.

31. Silverstein MJ, Lagios MD, Craig PH, et al. A prognostic index for ductal carcinoma in situ of the breast. *Cancer* 1996;77:2267–2274.

32. Silverstein MJ. Current status of the Van Nuys Prognostic Index for patients with ductal carcinoma in situ of the breast. *Semin Breast Dis* 2000;3:220–228.

33. Silverstein MJ, Recht A, Lagios MD, eds. *Ductal carcinoma in situ of the breast*, 2nd ed. Philadelphia: Lippincott William & Wilkins, 2002:459–474.

34. Bruwer A, Nelson G, Spark R. Punctate intranodal gold deposits simulating microcalcifications on mammograms. *Radiology* 1987;163:87–88.

35. Frappart L, Boudeulle M, Boumendil J, et al. Structure and composition of microcalcifications in benign and malignant lesions of the breast. *Hum Pathol* 1984;15:880–889.

36. Ahmed A. Calcifications in human breast carcinomas: ultrastructural observations. *J Pathol* 1975;117:247–251.

BENIGN MASSES

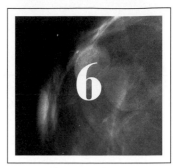

6

Although we place much emphasis on detecting microcalcifications and anguish over their characterization, we need to recognize that most invasive ductal carcinomas present as a mass. In contrast, when associated with malignancy, microcalcifications usually reflect intraductal, noninvasive breast cancer. Our primary goal with screening mammography is the recognition or perception of a possible mass or distortion related to an underlying mass. Our characterization of masses and management recommendations are predicated on spot compression, rolled or microfocus spot magnification views, and breast ultrasound. In some women, what appears to be a mass on screening images is shown to be superimposition of normal glandular tissue, and what appears as an innocuous asymmetry is identified as likely malignant with further workup. By integrating patient history; clinical, mammographic, and ultrasonographic findings; and an understanding of breast histopathology, it is possible to approximate a diagnosis and have significant confidence in the appropriate management recommendation.

Relevant history is reviewed in evaluating and managing women with a breast mass. Women with a personal history of breast cancer, or a history of breast cancer involving a first-degree relative (mother, father, daughter, sister), are at increased risk for developing breast cancer. This risk is increased if the relative developed breast cancer premenopausally or had bilateral breast cancer. The age and menopausal status of the patient, hormone replacement therapy, and physical findings should be known and factored in the formulation of a differential (Box 6.1).

In women older than 30 years of age presenting with a focal finding (e.g., lump, dimpling, focal tenderness), a metallic BB is used to mark the area of concern, and mediolateral oblique (MLO) and craniocaudal (CC) views are obtained bilaterally (1). A spot tangential view of the focal finding is also obtained. Correlative physical examination and ultrasound are done. Ultrasonography is not absolutely indicated if completely fatty tissue is imaged and it correlates to the site of concern to the patient.

Physical examination and ultrasonography are done in women who are pregnant, lactating, or younger than 30 years of age and present with a lump. If any concerns persist after this initial evaluation, an MLO may be done to exclude calcifications associated with an intraductal carcinoma that may not be apparent on ultrasound. If an underlying malignancy is suspected, mammographic images are obtained to evaluate the patient fully.

As defined by the American College of Radiology Breast Imaging and Reporting Data System (BI-RADS), a *mass* is a "space occupying lesion seen in two different projections." This is to be distinguished from *density*, a term used "if a potential mass is seen in only one projection . . . until it is three dimensionally confirmed" (2). Masses are three dimensional and have a bulging or convex contour and an abrupt density change at the margin. They may produce architectural distortion and have associated calcifications. Depending on location,

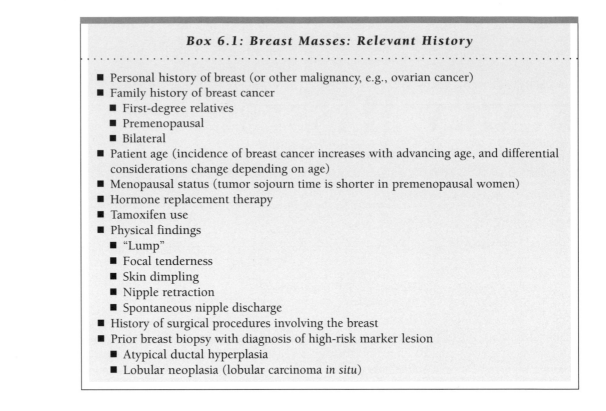

Box 6.1: Breast Masses: Relevant History

- Personal history of breast (or other malignancy, e.g., ovarian cancer)
- Family history of breast cancer
  - First-degree relatives
  - Premenopausal
  - Bilateral
- Patient age (incidence of breast cancer increases with advancing age, and differential considerations change depending on age)
- Menopausal status (tumor sojourn time is shorter in premenopausal women)
- Hormone replacement therapy
- Tamoxifen use
- Physical findings
  - "Lump"
  - Focal tenderness
  - Skin dimpling
  - Nipple retraction
  - Spontaneous nipple discharge
- History of surgical procedures involving the breast
- Prior breast biopsy with diagnosis of high-risk marker lesion
  - Atypical ductal hyperplasia
  - Lobular neoplasia (lobular carcinoma *in situ*)

size, internal matrix, and surrounding tissue, the mass may be palpable. Asymmetric tissue is planar, changing significantly between different projections; is scalloped; is inhomogeneous; and has a gradual density change at the margins. It is not palpable (3).

Compression, rolled, and magnification views done with the spot compression paddle are used to establish the shape, margins, and density of breast masses. *Round, oval, lobular*, and *irregular* (if "shape cannot be characterized") are the terms in BI-RADS to describe the shape of a mass. *Circumscribed, microlobulated, obscured* (margins "hidden by superimposed or adjacent normal tissue"), *indistinct*, and *spiculated* are the terms used to describe the margins of a mass. The x-ray attenuation or density of a mass is described as high, equal, low (but not fat containing), or fat containing (radiolucent) and is relative to an equal volume of fibroglandular tissue (2) (Table 6.1).

Additional features to consider when evaluating masses are listed in Box 6.2. Establishing the presence of associated calcifications and their morphology is helpful in assessing the etiology of a mass. Benign calcifications are usually associated with benign masses (Figure 6.1). If malignant-appearing calcifications are associated with a mass, then invasive ductal carcinoma with an associated intraductal component is the most likely diagnosis (Figure 6.2). Likewise, establishing the presence of satellite lesions is helpful (Figure 6.3). Although maligned, the halo sign is a good indicator of benignity (4–6). The *halo sign* is defined narrowly as a 1-mm sharp lucency surrounding or par-

Table 6.1: American College of Radiology, Lexicon Terms for Masses

Shape	Margins	Density (Water Density)
Round	Circumscribed	High
Oval	Microlobulated	Low (but not fat containing)
Lobulated	Obscured	Equal
Irregular	Indistinct	Fat containing
	Spiculated	

Adapted from American Collee of Radiology (ACR). Breast imaging reorting and data systems (BI-RADS), 3rd ed. Reston, VA, American College of Radiology, 1998, with permission.

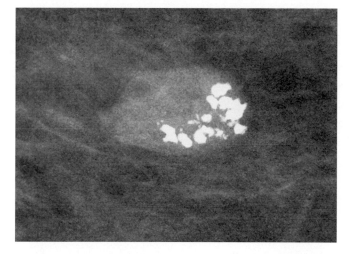

Figure 6.1 *Fibroadenoma, hyalinizing.* Oval mass with well-circumscribed margins and coarse, dystrophic calcifications consistent with a fibroadenoma undergoing hyalinization and calcification. Masses associated with benign calcifications are usually benign. Category 2.

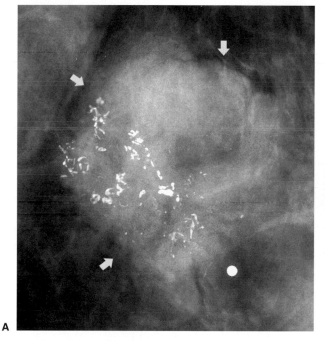

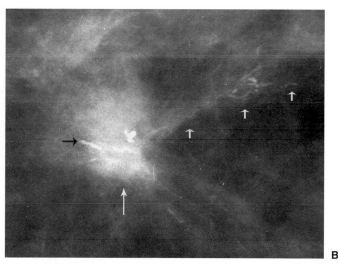

A

B

Figure 6.2 *Invasive ductal carcinoma,* not otherwise specified (NOS), with ductal carcinoma *in situ* (DCIS). *A.* A 62-year-old patient with a palpable mass (metallic BB), left breast. Mediolateral oblique view. Oval mass (*arrows*) with ill-defined margins and pleomorphic calcifications, including linear (casting) calcifications as well as round and punctate forms. The mass reflects the presence of an invasive ductal carcinoma (grade III), and the calcifications are found in an area of solid DCIS with central necrosis. Category 5. *B.* An 84-year-old patient with a screen-detected abnormality. Double spot compression magnification view demonstrates an ill-defined mass (*long white arrow*) with linear (casting) calcifications (*black arrow*). Linear calcifications with linear orientation can be seen extending for 1 cm posterior to the mass (*short white arrows*). This is consistent with an invasive ductal carcinoma having an associated intraductal component and central necrosis. Category 5. Clinically or mammographically detectable masses with casting-type calcifications most commonly reflect the presence of an invasive ductal carcinoma, NOS, with associated ductal carcinoma *in situ.*

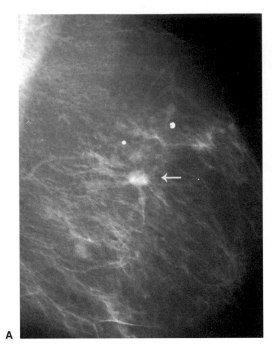

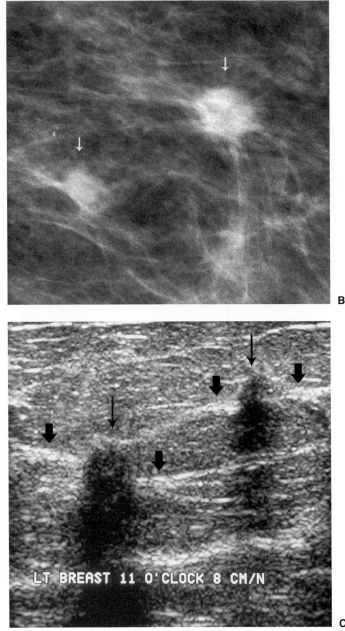

Figure 6.3 *Invasive ductal carcinoma*, not otherwise specified. *A.* A 60-year-old patient who underwent right mastectomy for breast cancer 11 years before this screening study, left breast. A new mass (*arrow*) is detected. Category 0. *B.* Spot compression views demonstrate two spiculated masses (*arrows*), one of which was not readily apparent on the screening study. Margin definition and unsuspected satellite lesion are defined best on spot compression views. *C.* On ultrasound, two adjacent irregular masses with shadowing are imaged (*long arrows*), corresponding to the masses seen mammographically. Both of these are taller than wide and are disrupting and crossing ligaments (*short arrows*). Category 5. Invasive ductal carcinoma is diagnosed at both sites. Three of 28 axillary lymph nodes are positive.

tially surrounding a mass (Figure 6.4). Not all masses with a true halo are benign, but many are (4,5). The halo sign is probably as good a sign of benignity as spiculation is a sign of malignancy. The halo sign may reflect active changes in the size of the mass.

The presence of multiple masses with similar mammographic features is suggestive of benignity. However, do not be lulled into a false sense of security by multiplicity. Women with multiple masses can develop breast cancer. It has been reported that since the frequency of cancer development among women not recalled for evaluation of multiple masses and the stage of the cancers diagnosed in these women are no different than those seen in the general screening population, evaluation of multiple masses appears not to be justified (7). Others advocate ultrasound evaluation in these patients (8). Although controversial, our approach to the patient presenting for the first time with multiple masses is to evaluate each mass as though it were a single finding. Our decisions are based on the mammographic and ultrasonographic features of the masses evaluated. On subsequent mammograms in these patients, we only evaluate new, developing masses.

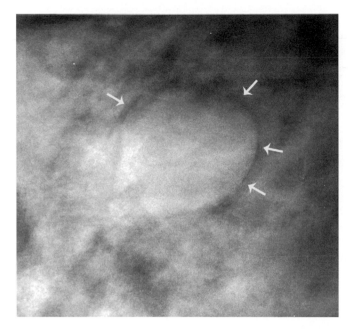

Figure 6.4 *Cyst: halo sign.* A 1-mm sharp radiolucency partially outlines this oval mass (*arrows*) with partially well-circumscribed margins. Although a halo sign can be seen with malignant masses, it is more common with benign masses that are changing actively in size. A cyst was imaged at this site ultrasonographically (not shown).

Previous films are useful in the evaluation of masses. Although stability is not an absolute sign of benignity, if a mass with benign features (e.g., well circumscribed) has been present for several years with no change, the likelihood of malignancy is low, and recommending follow-up in 6 months is not appropriate. If the mass has features of malignancy (e.g., spiculation, distortion) that are not explained easily (e.g., prior trauma or surgery at the site), it may represent a low-grade invasive lesion, and biopsy is indicated (Figure 6.5).

When reviewing prior films, use films from at least 2 or 3 years previously because subtle changes may not be apparent from one year to the next. Also, if available, review several years' worth of studies because benign lesions can fluctuate.

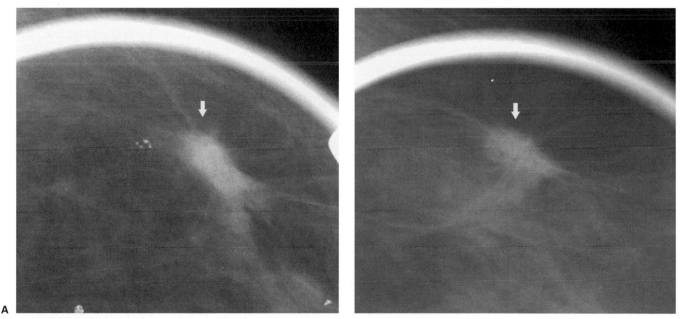

A

B

Figure 6.5 *Tubular carcinoma.* A. A 77-year-old patient who underwent right mastectomy for breast cancer 25 years before the current study. Spot compression view demonstrates a spiculated mass (*arrow*) in the left breast. B. Comparison spot compression view of this mass (*arrow*) 12 years previously. No definite change is noted; however, the patient has no history of surgery or trauma to this area. Tubular carcinoma or well-differentiated ductal carcinoma, not otherwise specified is prospectively considered. Category 4. Tubular carcinoma with associated low-nuclear-grade ductal carcinoma *in situ* with a cribriform pattern, is diagnosed histologically. The sentinel lymph node is negative. Stability of a lesion with malignant features (e.g., spiculation, distortion) that can not be explained does not ensure a benign etiology and warrants biopsy.

In selecting prior films for comparison, try to use films from at least 2 years previously, if available. Subtle changes may not be apparent from one year to the next but may be striking when comparison is made to studies from 2 or 3 years previously.

SKIN MASSES

Masses on the skin include moles, accessory nipples, skin tags, sebaceous cysts, and neurofibromas. They can often be distinguished from intraparenchymal lesions because they are partially or completely outlined by air, seen as a thin curvilinear lucency surrounding the margins of the mass that protrude beyond the skin (Figure 6.6); this lucency is lost where the lesion attaches to the skin (see later). In some women, talc, calcification, or air outlines the crevices of moles (Figure 6.7). We mark skin lesions with a metallic BB before taking any films so that we do not call a patient back unnecessarily for a skin lesion (Figure 6.8).

Sebaceous cysts are common, often palpable, sharply marginated intradermal masses that may develop calcifications (Figure 6.9) and undergo changes in size from one year to the next. On physical examination, these may be visible, causing a smooth skin bulge, and the orifice of the gland may be visible as a blackhead. If squeezed, a white, thick, cheesy material may be expressed. If inflamed, incision and drainage may be needed. Complete removal of the cyst wall is required; otherwise, they recur. Mammographically, these lesions can be well-circumscribed, or when inflamed, the margins may be indistinct (Figure 6.10) or spiculated (Figure 6.11A); associated calcifications may be present. On spot tangential views, they are localized to the skin (Figure 6.10B). Ultrasonographically, they are intradermal, anechoic, hypoechoic, or echogenic, often with posterior acoustic enhancement (Figure 6.10C). With manipulation of the transducer, the skin track can be identified in some patients (Figure 6.11B).

Multiple skin lesions, diffusely involving the skin bilaterally, are seen clinically in patients with neurofibromatosis. These lesions may increase in size and number as the patient ages. Mammographically, the skin lesions are well circumscribed and partially or completely outlined by air (Figure 6.12). Evaluation of the breast parenchyma may be difficult because of the skin lesions. Extra care should be used to disregard the obvious benign findings in search of a possible unsuspected malignancy in these patients.

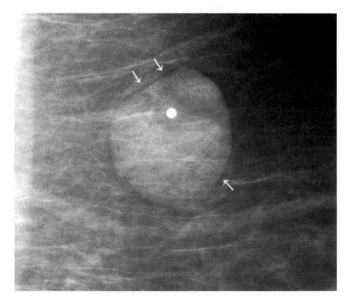

Figure 6.6 *Skin lesion.* Well-circumscribed, round mass with air outlining its contour (*arrows*). The sharp radiolucency, partially or completely surrounding a mass, is consistent with a dermal location. A metallic BB is use to mark skin lesions, and this is documented on the patient's history form by the technologist.

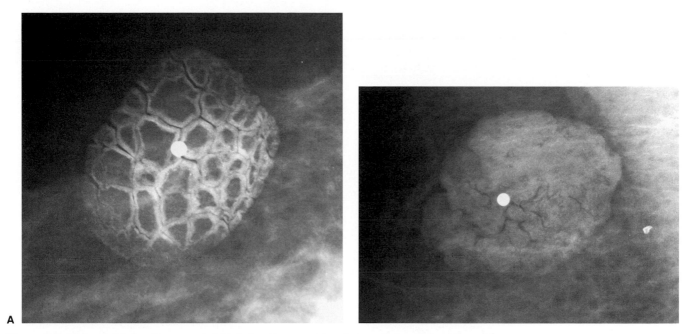

A   B

Figure 6.7 *Moles. A.* Mole with encrusted high-density material and air outlining the crevices of the lesion. *B.* Mole margin and crevices are well-defined because there is air outlining the contours. Although the appearance of these lesions is pathognomonic, we routinely use metallic BBs to mark skin lesions. This is documented on the patient's history form.

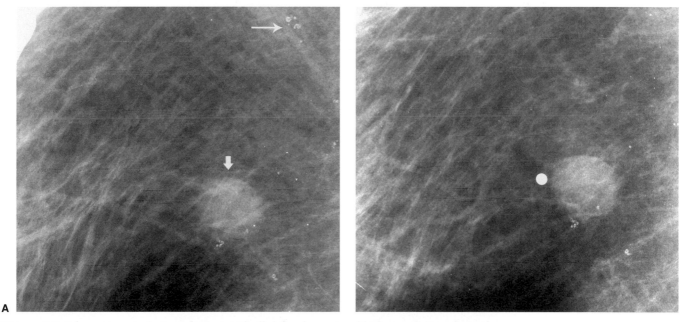

A   B

Figure 6.8 *Sebaceous cyst. A.* Round mass with ill-defined margins (*thick arrow*) just above the inframammary fold on this mediolateral oblique view. Additional views are indicated if the lesion is in the breast. The technologist should mark all obvious skin lesions so that callbacks for what turn out to be skin lesions are minimized. Incidentally noted are scattered skin calcifications (*thin arrow*). *B.* Metallic BB marking location of a sebaceous cyst. Category 2.

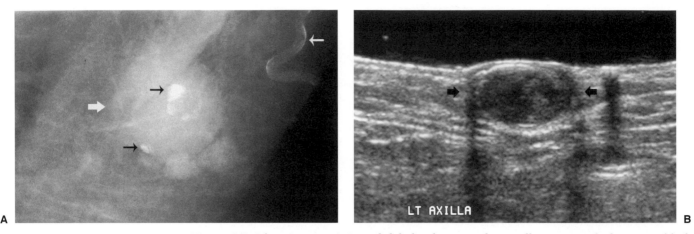

Figure 6.9 *Sebaceous cyst.* A. Round, lobulated mass with partially circumscribed margins (*thick white arrow*) and course calcifications (*thin black arrows*). Also noted are vascular calcifications (*thin white arrow*). B. Well-circumscribed, hypoechoic mass with a heterogenous echotexture and minimal posterior acoustic enhancement causing bulging of the skin surface (*arrows*). With pressure over the lesion, thick material is elicited, and follow-up films (not shown) demonstrate a decrease in the size of the lesion and a reduction in the calcifications. Radiography of the extruded material demonstrates calcifications.

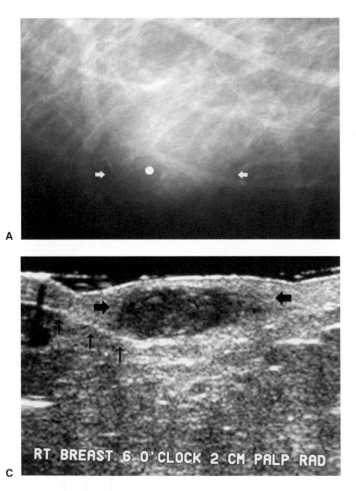

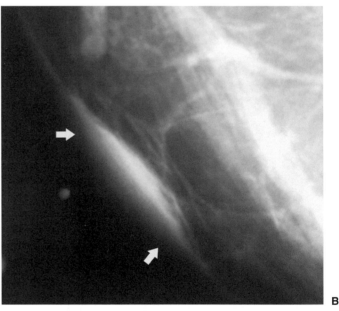

Figure 6.10 *Sebaceous cyst.* A. Patient presents with a tender, superficial mass. Metallic BB is used to mark the lesion. Increased density (*arrows*) is seen at the site without a definite mass. B. Spot compression tangential view places the lesion (*arrows*) tangent to the x-ray beam, thereby localizing it to the skin. C. A hypoechoic mass (*thick arrow*) is present in the dermis, consistent with a sebaceous cyst. The dermal layers are split by the developing mass; the deep dermal layer (*thin arrows*) is displaced inferiorly.

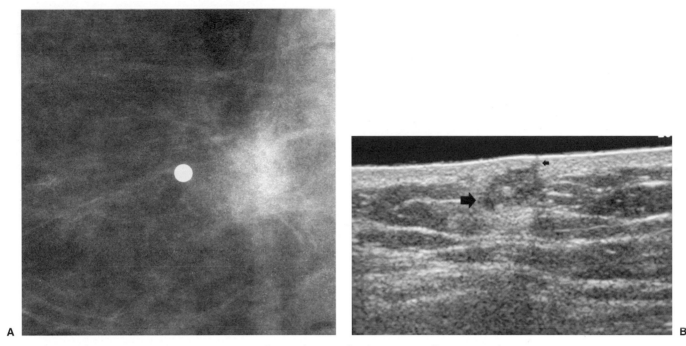

Figure 6.11 *Sebaceous cyst.* A. Patient presents with a tender superficial mass. Metallic BB is used to mark the lesion, which is seen as a round mass with spiculated margins. B. On ultrasound, an intradermal hypoechoic mass (*thick large arrow*) is imaged corresponding to the area of concern to the patient. The track to the skin surface is noted (*small arrow*).

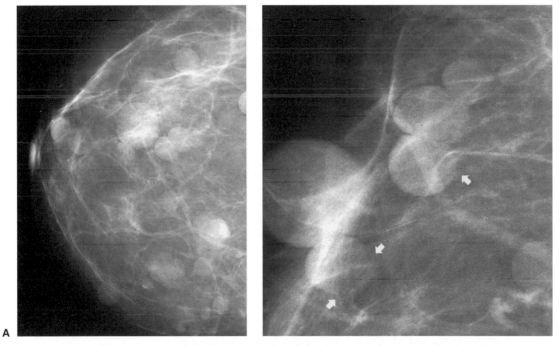

Figure 6.12 *Neurofibromatosis.* A. Multiple round and oval skin lesions with margins that are completely or partially outlined by air. B. Neurofibroma. The portion of the lesions that is surrounded by air is sharply delineated. This border definition, however, is lost where the lesion attaches to the skin. Transition points are marked for two of the lesion shown (*arrows*).

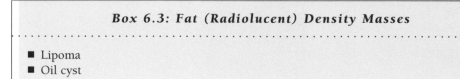

Box 6.3: Fat (Radiolucent) Density Masses

....

- Lipoma
- Oil cyst

Box 6.4: Mixed-Density Masses

....

- Intramammary lymph nodes
- Fibroadenolipomas (hamartomas)
- Fat necrosis, oil cysts
- Galactoceles
- Postoperative or posttraumatic fluid collections (hematomas, seromas)

FAT-CONTAINING LESIONS

Fat-containing lesions in the breast are benign (1,3). These masses can be completely fatty (Box 6.3) or mixed in density (Box 6.4). Although ultrasonographic findings are described, the diagnosis is reliably established when either completely lucent or mixed-density masses are seen mammographically.

LIPOMAS

Patients with lipomas can be asymptomatic or present with a hard or soft, mobile, palpable superficial mass. A well-circumscribed, radiolucent mass with a thin fibrous capsule is detected mammographically (Figure 6.13). Although the diagnosis is reliably made on

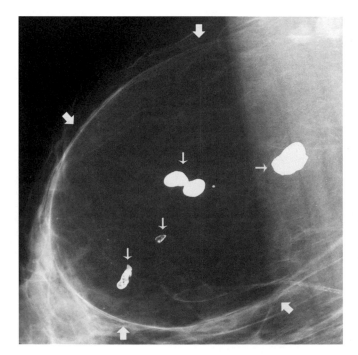

Figure 6.13 *Lipoma.* A radiolucent mass with a thin fibrous capsule (*thick arrows*) diagnostic of a lipoma. Category 2. Benign dystrophic calcifications are present (*thin arrows*).

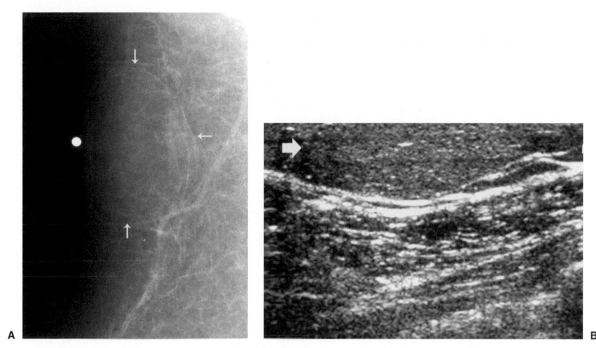

A   B

Figure 6.14 *Lipoma. A.* Patient presents with a soft palpable mass in the right breast; a metallic BB is used to mark the area. A radiolucent mass with a thin fibrous capsule (*arrows*) is imaged mammographically and is diagnostic of a lipoma. Category 2. *B.* On ultrasound, an oval homogeneously hypoechoic mass (*arrow*) is imaged corresponding to the palpable mass. Some mass effect on surrounding ligaments is noted.

mammographic findings, a well-circumscribed mass with a homogeneously hypoechoic to hyperechoic echotexture is imaged on ultrasound (9) (Figure 6.14). Histologically, these lesions are characterized by the presence of mature lipocytes surrounded by a thin capsule. If otherwise asymptomatic, no intervention or short-term follow-up is indicated (10,11).

OIL CYSTS

Oil cysts are radiolucent, solitary (Figure 6.15A) or multiple (Fig 6.16A), unilateral or bilateral masses. They vary, and can decrease, in size, resolving completely in some patients on subsequent mammograms. They are idiopathic or develop in areas of prior trauma or surgery and, in this setting, probably represent end-stage fat necrosis. Some women develop mural calcifications, resulting in lucent-centered (or eggshell) calcification (Figures 6.15B and 6.16B); whereas in others, the mural calcifications are seen *en phase* having a coarse, irregular, curvilinear appearance. In most women, oil cysts are asymptomatic, noted incidentally on screening mammography. Some patients may present describing a discrete, hard mass that is correlated to an oil cyst mammographically. In this situation, it is important to assure the patient and referring physician that the palpable finding is an oil cyst requiring no intervention or follow-up. Although the diagnosis is made mammographically and ultrasonography is not indicated, the ultrasonographic appearance of oil cysts is variable. They may be anechoic with through transmission indistinguishable from fluid-containing cysts (Figure 6.17); they may contain internal echoes; or intracystic, solid-appearing components may be seen (Figure 6.18). Sometimes, oil cysts appear solid.

In some women, oil cysts may be more appropriately characterized as mixed-density lesions because of thickened, ill-defined, or spiculated margins or the presence of a round

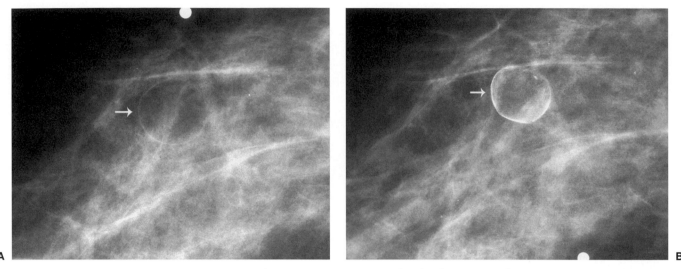

Figure 6.15 *Oil cyst*. Patient presents with a hard mass; metallic BB marks area. A well-circumscribed, round mass of fat density (*arrow*) is imaged corresponding to the palpable mass. This is pathognomonic of an oil cyst. No intervention or short-term follow-up is warranted. The report should specifically state that the palpable area of clinical concern corresponds to a benign finding requiring no surgical intervention. *B*. Four years later, calcification of the oil cyst wall is seen as a rim or eggshell-type calcification (*arrow*). Category 2.

or oval intracystic mass. With a history of trauma or surgery and if fat (radiolucency) is associated with these masses in two orthogonal projections, no intervention or short-term follow-up is warranted regardless of the spiculated margins or associated nodule (see Fat Necrosis).

Steatocystoma multiplex (12,13) is a rare condition with an autosomal dominant mode of inheritance associated with multiple intradermal oil cysts scattered over the body but with a predilection for the trunk and upper extremities. Although more commonly seen in men, women with this condition may be found to have multiple oil cysts in the breasts bilaterally.

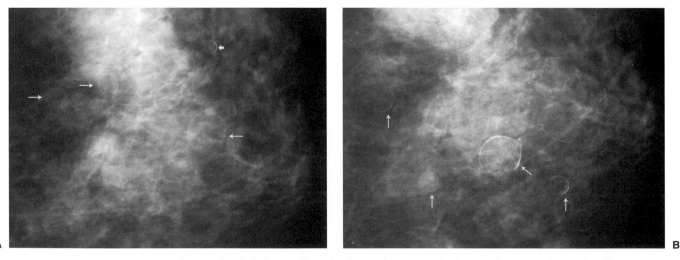

Figure 6.16 *Oil cysts*. A. Multiple, well-circumscribed, round masses of fatty density are present (*long arrows* mark some of these). One oil cyst has a partial calcification of rim or eggshell type (*short arrow*). B. Two years later, partial calcification involving the wall of several of the oil cysts is noted, resulting in rim or eggshell-type calcification (*arrows* mark some of these). Category 2.

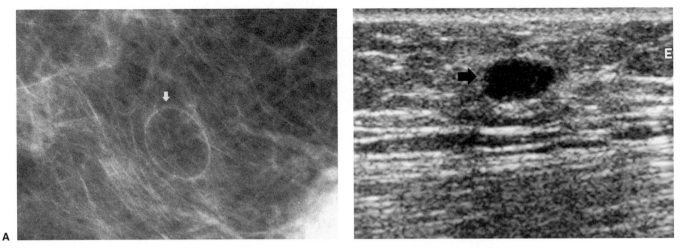

Figure 6.17 *Oil cyst.* A well-circumscribed, oval, radiolucent mass is identified mammographically (*arrow*). This is pathognomonic of an oil cyst. The diagnosis is made mammographically. Category 2. *B.* On ultrasound, a nearly anechoic mass (*arrow*) with some posterior acoustic enhancement is imaged corresponding to the oil cyst seen mammographically.

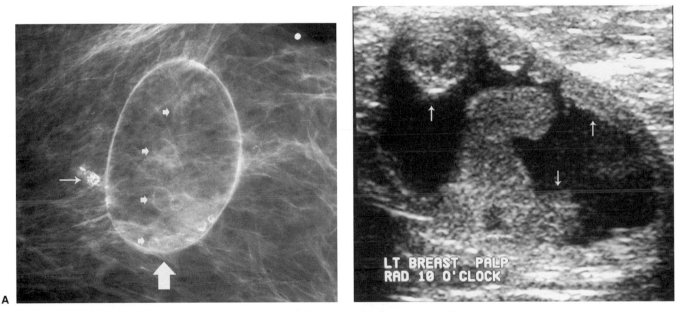

Figure 6.18 *Oil cyst. A.* Patient with a palpable mass; metallic BB marks the area. A well-circumscribed, oval, radiolucent mass (*large thick arrow*) with several internal small, round, radiolucent masses (*small thick arrows* mark some of these) is imaged mammographically. A dystrophic calcification is incidentally noted (*long thin arrow*). Category 2. *B.* On ultrasound, a complex cystic mass with mural nodules (*arrows*) is imaged corresponding to the palpable mass.

MIXED-DENSITY MASSES

LYMPH NODES

Intramammary and axillary lymph nodes are variable in number, size, density, shape, and location and are seen in as many as 5.4% of women undergoing screening mammography (14). Typically, they are round to oval, well-circumscribed, lobulated masses of mixed density located in the upper outer quadrants (Figure 6.19A, B); however, they can be found anywhere, including, rarely, the medial aspect of the breast. The presence of a variably sized fatty hilum either centrally or peripherally is required before assuming that a mass in the upper outer quadrant of the breast is a lymph node. Ultrasonographically, lymph nodes are well circumscribed, oval, hypoechoic masses with an area of hyperechogenicity either centrally or peripherally (Figures 6.19C and 6.20). In some patients, they can be strikingly hypoechoic with posterior acoustic enhancement simulating the appearance of cysts. They can fluctuate in size (Figure 6.21) and in some women can disappear only to reappear on subsequent studies.

Benign causes of intramammary and axillary lymphadenopathy (Figure 6.22) are listed in Box 6.5 (15).

Gold particles imaged as high-density, punctate particles mimicking microcalcifications can be seen bilaterally in the axillary and intramammary lymph nodes of women treated for rheumatoid arthritis with gold (16) (Figure 6.23). Coarse calcifications occurring in lymph nodes are often related to granulomatous disease and do not require intervention (Figure 6.24).

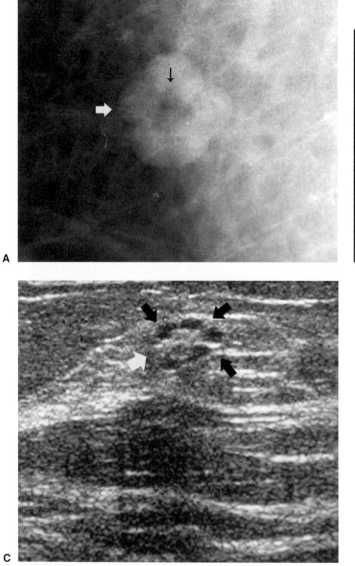

Figure 6.19 *Lymph node.* A. Well-circumscribed, macrolobulated mass (*white arrow*) with central radiolucency (*black arrow*) consistent with a lymph node. B. Different patient with a well-circumscribed, macrolobulated, mixed-density mass (*white arrow*) consistent with a lymph node. Central fatty hilum (*black arrow*) is seen. Mammogram is diagnostic. C. On ultrasound, a macrolobulated, well-circumscribed, hypoechoic mass (*black arrows*) is imaged with central hyperechogenicity (*white arrow*) diagnostic of a lymph node.

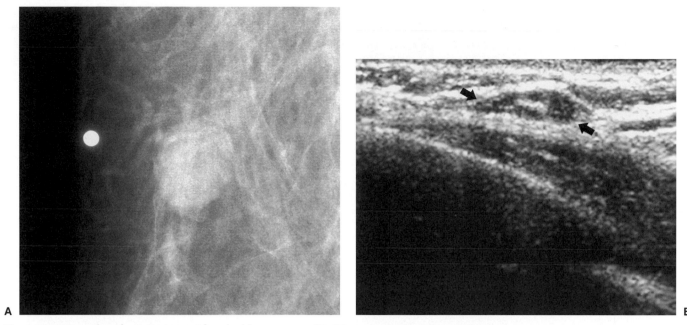

A   B

Figure 6.20 *Lymph node. A.* Patient with palpable mass; metallic BB marks the area. A round mass is imaged corresponding to the palpable area. No fatty hilum is imaged mammographically. *B.* A well-circumscribed, oval, hypoechoic mass (*arrows*) with central echogenicity consistent with an intramammary lymph node is imaged ultrasonographically corresponding to the palpable mass Category 2.

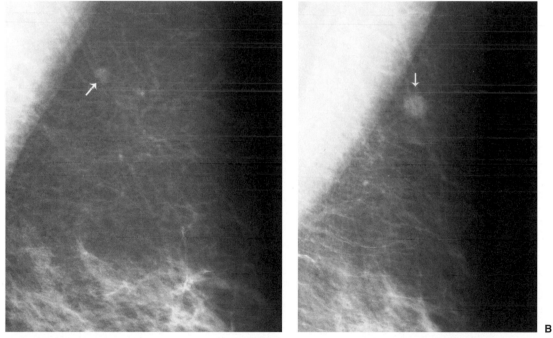

A   B

Figure 6.21 *Reactive lymph node. A.* A 76-year-old patient who underwent right mastectomy for breast cancer 1 year before this study. Mass in left axillary tail measures 4 mm, with the suggestion of a fatty notch (*arrow*) consistent with a lymph node. Category 2. *B.* Two years later, the mass measures 7 mm, and the notch is not apparent (*arrow*). Category 0.

(continued on next page)

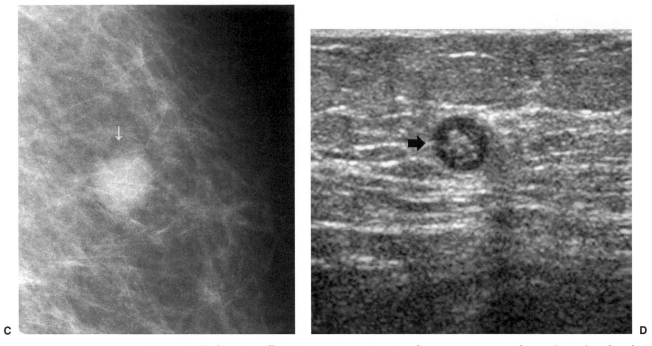

Figure 6.21 (continued) *C.* Spot compression view demonstrates a round mass (*arrow*) with indistinct margins. No fatty hilum is seen. *D.* Round, hypoechoic mass with hyperechogenic center consistent with intramammary lymph node (*arrow*); however, given the patient's personal history of contralateral breast cancer and the change in size, an ultrasound-guided needle biopsy is done. Category 4. A benign reactive lymph node is diagnosed histologically.

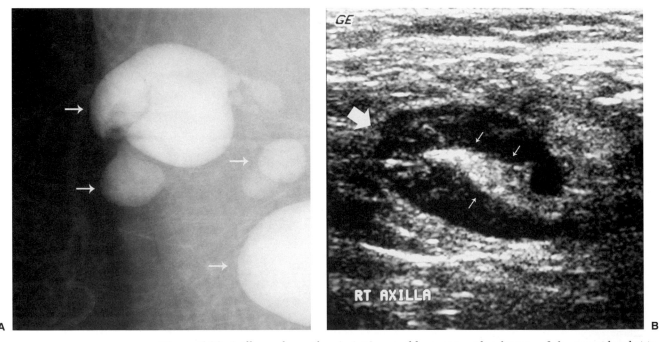

Figure 6.22 *Axillary adenopathy. A.* A 52-year-old woman with a history of rheumatoid arthritis. Well-circumscribed, dense, round masses (*arrows*) are seen bilaterally (left side is not shown). No fatty hila are identified mammographically. *B.* Hypoechoic mass (*thick arrow*) with central hyperechogenicity (*thin arrows*) consistent with a lymph node. Several other hypoechoic masses with central echogenicity are imaged bilaterally.

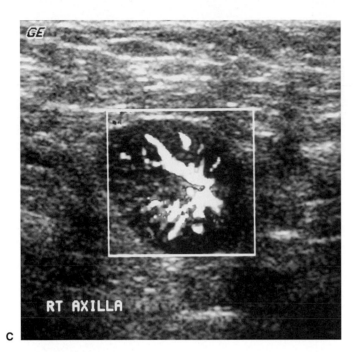

C

RT AXILLA

Figure 6.22 (continued)
C. Doppler demonstrates vascular structures entering through echogenic, hilar region.

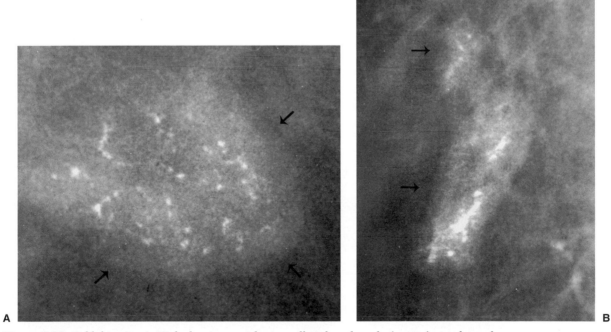

A   B

Figure 6.23 *Gold deposits. A.* High-density particles in axillary lymph node (*arrows*) simulate calcifications. This is gold in a patient with rheumatoid arthritis. *B.* Different patient; high-density particles in axillary lymph nodes (*arrows*). This is gold in a patient who received gold treatments for rheumatoid arthritis.

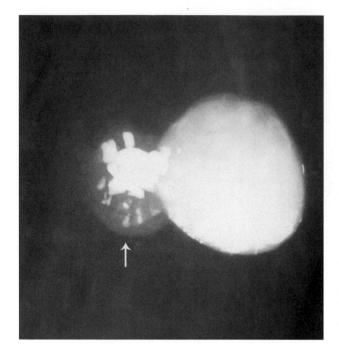

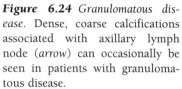

Figure 6.24 *Granulomatous disease*. Dense, coarse calcifications associated with axillary lymph node (*arrow*) can occasionally be seen in patients with granulomatous disease.

In a retrospective 5-year review, Lee and colleagues (17) reported unilateral enlargement of axillary or intramammary lymph nodes in 0.2% of their patients with otherwise normal mammograms. In their experience, biopsy is indicated in patients with a history of an underlying malignancy if the lymph node enlarges by more than 100% over baseline. If the woman does not have a history of a malignancy, the lymph node enlargement is small, the node is not palpable, and the node maintains a benign appearance, they suggest clinical and mammographic follow-up. In most of their patients, lymph node enlargement decreased on follow-up studies. Dershaw and associates (18) reported that spiculated adenopathy in patients with breast cancer is suggestive of extranodal extension of tumor into the perinodal fat and portends a poor prognosis. Walsh and co-workers (19) reported that although benign and malignant axillary adenopathy cannot be distinguished mammographically, biopsy should be recommended when nonfatty lymph nodes contain suspicious microcalcifications, are grossly enlarged (they suggest using 45 mm as the criteria for grossly enlarged), or have ill-defined or spiculated margins.

FIBROADENOLIPOMAS (HAMARTOMAS)

Because FALs contain normal breast tissue, breast cancer of any type can arise within them.

Fibroadenolipomas (FALs), or hamartomas, are characterized by the presence of a pseudocapsule within which fatty, glandular, and fibrous elements are admixed. This appearance has led some to describe them as a "breast within a breast" (Figure 6.25). The overall density of these lesions is variable depending on the proportions of fat and glandular tissue. In some women, a FAL may enlarge and present as a palpable mass (Figure 6.26). Because the lesions are made up of otherwise normal breast tissue, breast cancer of any type can arise in hamartomas (20). Development of pleomorphic calcifications and increasing density, particularly if ill defined or spiculated, in a FAL should prompt an imaging-guided biopsy (Figure 6.27). If the patient presents with a palpable mass in a FAL, imaging guidance is helpful in targeting areas of soft tissue in the FAL; otherwise, false-negative results may occur if fatty elements are sampled. On ultrasound, these lesions can be distinguished from the surrounding glandular tissue and have a heterogenous echotexture with admixed areas of hypoechogenicity and hyperechogenicity.

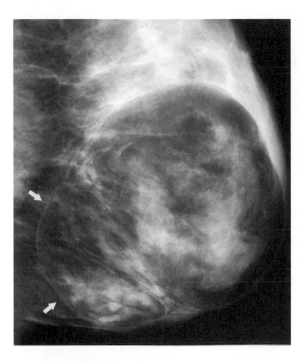

Figure 6.25 *Fibroadenolipoma.* A mixed-density mass. A thin pseudocapsule is seen (*arrows*) enclosing fatty and glandular elements. Some mass effect is seen superiorly. Category 2.

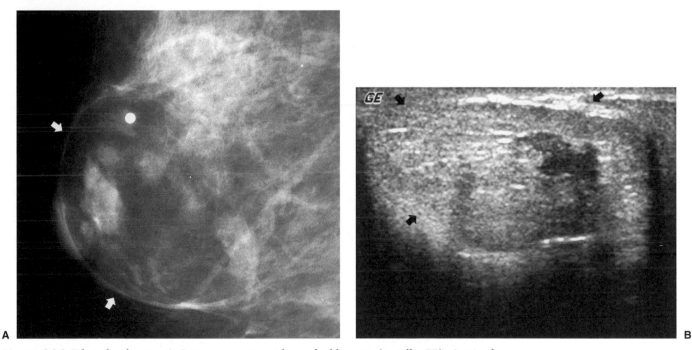

A   B

Figure 6.26 *Fibroadenolipoma.* *A.* Patient presents with a palpable mass (metallic BB). A mixed-density mass is imaged mammographically. Fatty and glandular tissue is admixed surrounded by fibrous pseudocapsule (*arrows*). Diagnosis is made based on mammographic finding. *B.* An oval mass (*arrows*) with a heterogenous echotexture is seen on ultrasound. Category 2.

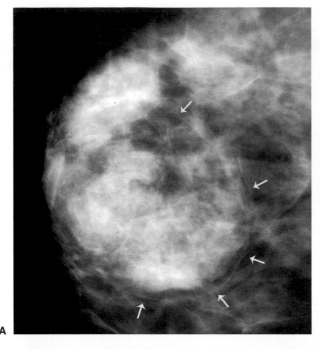

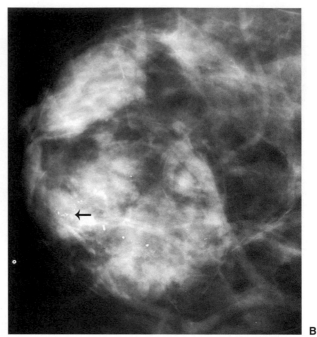

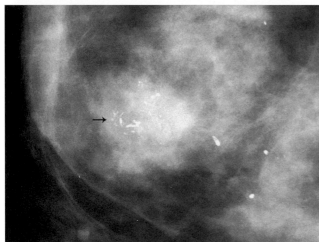

Figure 6.27 *Fibroadenolipoma and ductal carcinoma* in situ. *A.* A 64-year-old woman; screening mammogram. A mixed-density lesion (*arrows*) is identified consistent with a hamartoma or fibroadenolipoma (FAL). Category 2. *B.* Subsequent screening mammogram demonstrates developing calcifications (*arrow*) within the FAL. Category 0. Magnification views are indicated. *C.* Spot compression magnification view demonstrates a pleomorphic cluster of calcifications (*arrow*). Linear forms are present. Category 4. Ductal carcinoma *in situ*, high nuclear grade, with central necrosis developing in a FAL.

FAT NECROSIS

Trauma or surgery resulting in the release of fatty substances in the breast stroma can lead to an inflammatory response commonly characterized, in the acute setting, by a spiculated mass with architectural distortion (Figure 6.28); skin thickening and retraction may be present. Alternatively, a mixed-density mass with indistinct margins (Figure 6.29) or an irregular area of density (Figure 6.30) may be seen. As the inflammatory response subsides, the mammographic and ultrasonographic features of the lesion usually evolve. In some women, the spiculated or mixed-density mass becomes less dense, and a fatty center develops (Figure 6.31); as the ill-defined soft tissue component resolves, a smooth, thin-walled oil cyst may be all that remains. The progression from dense, spiculated mass to oil cyst is appreciated as films are viewed sequentially. In the intermediate stages, densities or nodules may be seen within the oil cyst. Calcifications developing in areas of fat necrosis can be dystrophic in appearance or, early in their formation, linear with irregular margins and pleomorphism indistinguishable from the microcalcifications associated with comedo necrosis in ductal carcinoma *in situ*. In other women, fat necrosis resolves com-

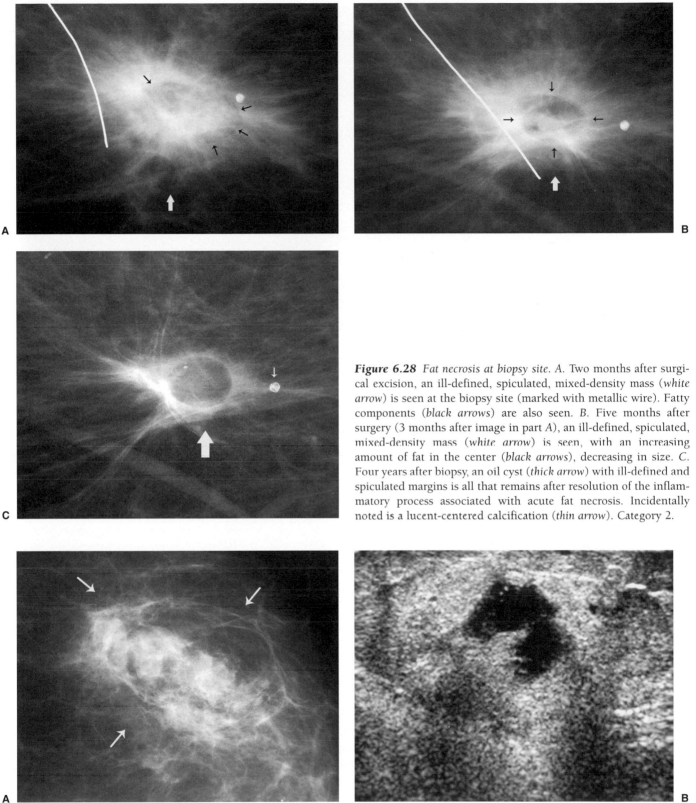

Figure 6.28 *Fat necrosis at biopsy site. A.* Two months after surgical excision, an ill-defined, spiculated, mixed-density mass (*white arrow*) is seen at the biopsy site (marked with metallic wire). Fatty components (*black arrows*) are also seen. *B.* Five months after surgery (3 months after image in part *A*), an ill-defined, spiculated, mixed-density mass (*white arrow*) is seen, with an increasing amount of fat in the center (*black arrows*), decreasing in size. *C.* Four years after biopsy, an oil cyst (*thick arrow*) with ill-defined and spiculated margins is all that remains after resolution of the inflammatory process associated with acute fat necrosis. Incidentally noted is a lucent-centered calcification (*thin arrow*). Category 2.

Figure 6.29 *Fat necrosis. A.* An ill-defined, oval, mixed-density mass (*arrows*) corresponding to trauma site. Category 2. *B.* Loss of normal tissue architecture with area of hyperechogenicity within which cystic changes are noted. In our experience, this is a common ultrasonographic appearance for acute fat necrosis. The 3-month follow-up shows complete resolution with no residual abnormality. When trauma or an inflammatory process is suspected (e.g., change is expected in a short period of time), a follow-up mammogram should be done in 3 months.

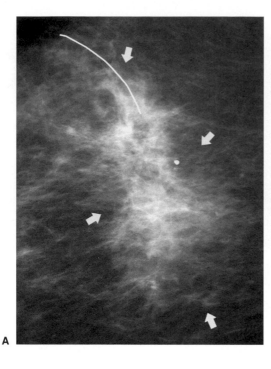
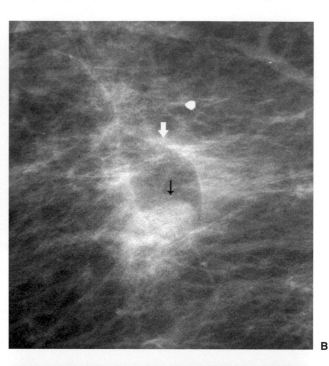
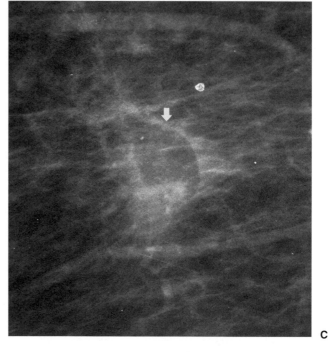

Figure 6.30 Fat necrosis. A. Ill-defined area of mixed density mass (*arrows*) at biopsy site. *B.* Three months later, much of the density has resolved. Oil cyst has formed with ill-defined margins (*white arrow*) and an intracystic nodule (*black arrow*). *C.* Four years later, the area has continued to decrease in size, and an oil cyst with only a small amount of residual surrounding ill-defined density (*arrow*) is seen. The intracystic nodule is almost completely resolved. Category 2.

pletely with no residual abnormality seen on subsequent studies (21). Less common appearances for fat necrosis include development of islands of parenchymal asymmetry (Figure 6.32) or trabecular thickening forming a fine reticular pattern (Figure 6.33).

Soo and colleagues (22) describe a wide range of ultrasound patterns for fat necrosis. In their experience, a complex mass with echogenic bands that may shift in position as the patient is moved is strongly suggestive of fat necrosis. They also found masses with echogenic mural nodules that evolve over time, solid-appearing masses, and anechoic masses with either posterior acoustic enhancement or shadowing as manifestations of fat necrosis on ultrasound. In our experience, one of the more common ultrasonographic fea-

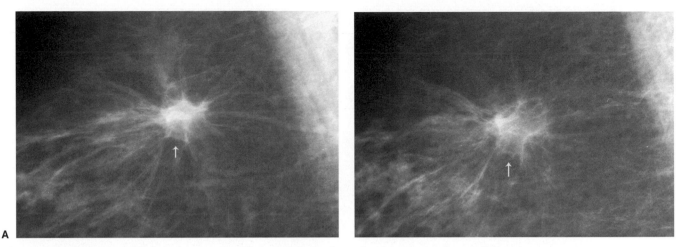

A   B

Figure 6.31 *Fat necrosis.* A. Spiculated mass with long spicules (*arrow*) at biopsy site, 1 year after surgery. B. Mixed-density spiculated mass (*arrow*) 2 years after biopsy. Increasing amounts of fat are seen in the center of the lesion, such that its overall density is decreasing. Progressive decreases in density and overall distortion (and associated soft tissue component) or stability in appearance after the first postbiopsy year is the expected evolution of fat necrosis. Increases in size, density, and distortion 1 year after the biopsy warrant biopsy.

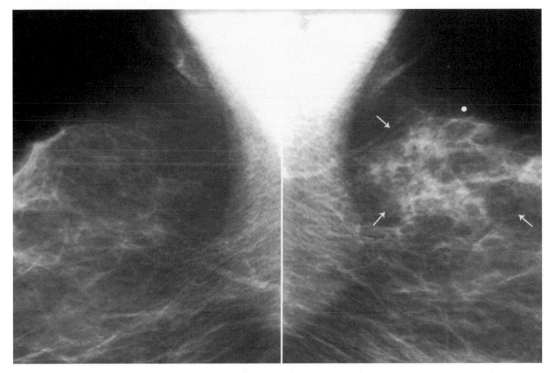

Figure 6.32 *Fat necrosis.* Palpable area (metallic BB) of parenchymal asymmetry (*arrows*) developing at site of chest wall trauma. Ultrasound (not shown) demonstrates disruption of the normal architecture with diffuse hyperechogenicity and associated small cystic spaces.

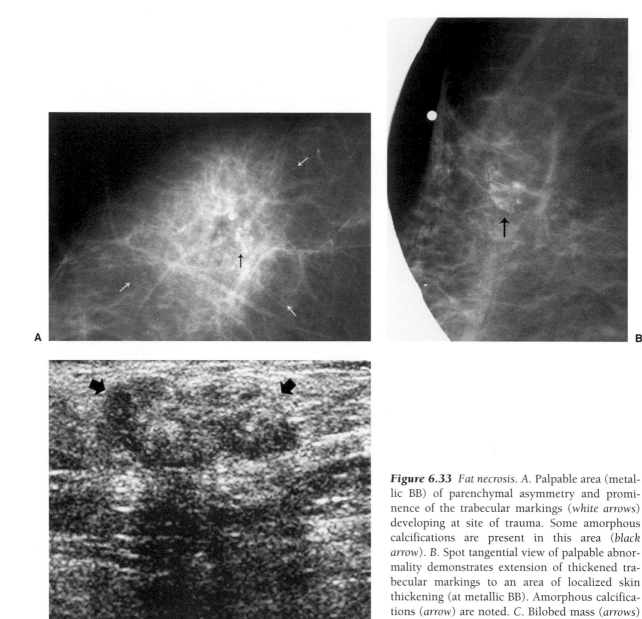

Figure 6.33 *Fat necrosis. A.* Palpable area (metallic BB) of parenchymal asymmetry and prominence of the trabecular markings (*white arrows*) developing at site of trauma. Some amorphous calcifications are present in this area (*black arrow*). *B.* Spot tangential view of palpable abnormality demonstrates extension of thickened trabecular markings to an area of localized skin thickening (at metallic BB). Amorphous calcifications (*arrow*) are noted. *C.* Bilobed mass (*arrows*) with heterogenous echotexture imaged at trauma (palpable) site.

tures of fat necrosis is an area of hyperechogenicity that may be well to ill defined and that is associated with cystic spaces or small, round or oval areas of hypoechogenicity (Figure 6.34).

A history of trauma or surgery and the appearance of the lesion on sequential mammograms provide the assurance needed to characterize these lesions as benign. Ultrasound is usually not needed for the diagnosis. It is critical to recognize that mammographic findings peak about 4 to 6 months after the biopsy or trauma, after which the findings stabilize or slowly resolve as described. If an area of spiculation and architectural distortion increases in size and density over time, it is unlikely to be fat necrosis. Fat necrosis can increase in size and density years after a biopsy; however, this is exceedingly rare and warrants a biopsy recommendation (Figure 6.35).

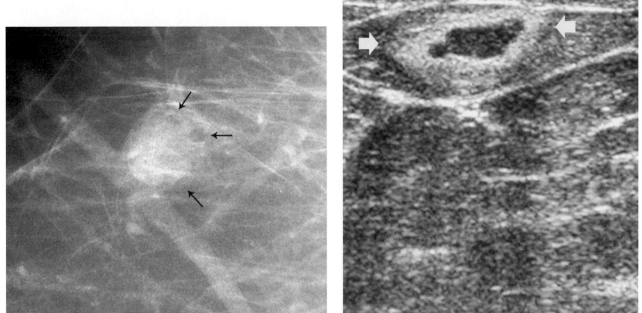

A   B

Figure 6.34 *Fat necrosis.* A. Round mass. Small locules of fat (*arrows*) can be seen associated with the mass in two projections (only one shown). B. A hyperechoic mass with central hypoechogenicity (*arrows*) is imaged ultrasonographically corresponding to the mass seen mammographically. In our experience, this is a common ultrasonographic appearance of fat necrosis.

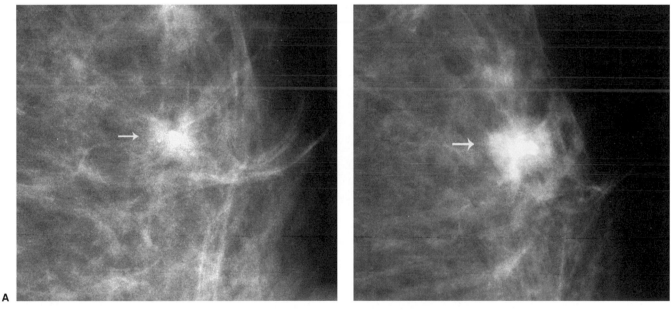

A   B

Figure 6.35 *Fat necrosis.* A. Ill-defined mass with coarse, dystrophic calcification (*arrow*) at biopsy site. B. One year later. Ill-defined mass with coarse dystrophic calcifications has increased in size and density (*arrow*).

(continued on next page)

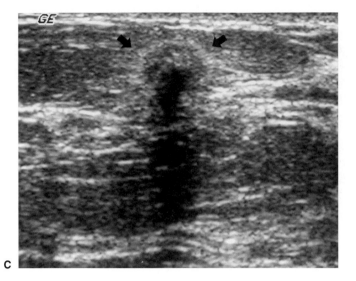

Figure 6.35 (continued) *C.* Mass with heterogenous echotexture and shadowing (*arrows*). Shadowing is related to dystrophic calcification. Fat necrosis is expected to stabilize or decrease in size, density, and associated distortion. In this patient, the mass at the biopsy site is increasing in size and density. Biopsy is indicated. Category 4. Fat necrosis is diagnosed histologically.

WATER-DENSITY MASSES

Some of the more common causes of benign and malignant round or oval masses are listed in Table 6.2, while some of the more common causes of benign and malignant spiculated masses are listed in Table 6.3.

Table 6.2: Water Density Round or Oval Masses

Benign	Malignant
Cyst	Infiltrating ductal carcinoma, NOS
Fibroadenoma (complex, tubular, and lactational adenomas)	Mucinous carcinoma
	Medullary carcinoma
Papilloma (solitary, multiple)	Papillary carcinoma
Fat necrosis	Lymphoma
Pseudoangiomatous stromal hyperplasia	Metastatic disease
Focal fibrosis	Ductal carcinoma *in situ*
Sclerosing adenosis	
Abscess	
Postoperative or posttraumatic fluid collections	
Vascular lesions	
Granular cell tumor	

Table 6.3: Water Density Spiculated Masses

Benign	Malignant
Fat necrosis (postoperative or posttraumatic)	Infiltrating ductal carcinoma, NOS
Mastitis	Tubular carcinoma
Focal fibrosis	Infiltrating lobular carcinoma
Sclerosing adenosis	Metastatic disease to lymph nodes
Complex sclerosing lesions	Ductal carcinoma *in situ*
Granulomatous disease	
Extraabdominal desmoid (fibromatosis)	

Cysts

Cysts are common breast lesions occurring in women of all ages. There is some predilection for the perimenopausal years, with a smaller peak of incidence in women in their late 70s and 80s. If women do not take hormone replacement therapy after menopause, cysts usually decrease in size, and most resolve spontaneously. Clinically, patients with cysts present with one or several lumps, focal tenderness, or rarely, nipple discharge. When the cyst is inflamed, erythema may be present at the site of the lump along with associated tenderness. In many women, cysts are asymptomatic, with a mass or multiple masses detected on screening mammography and characterized as a cyst on ultrasound.

Cyst fluid contains a variety of electrolytes, proteins, and hormones (23). Based on electrolyte content and cell lining, cysts can be separated into two primary groups. Epithelial-lined cysts are characterized by fluid high in sodium and low in potassium content, much like the composition of serum. It has been suggested that these cysts do not often recur after aspiration. Cysts lined with cells demonstrating apocrine metaplasia are characterized by fluid that is low in sodium and high in potassium content. This electrolyte content suggests a more active cellular process leading to the concentration of potassium. It may be that these cysts recur after aspiration more commonly than the epithelial-lined cysts (10,22,23).

Mammographically, cysts are variable in appearance. They can occur singularly (Figure 6.36A) or as multiple unilateral or bilateral masses (Figure 6.37) of varying sizes and densities. Although many are well circumscribed, some have obscured (Figure 6.36C) or ill-defined margins. Spiculation or distortion is rare. Calcifications can develop in the wall of cysts or within cysts (milk of calcium). Unless associated with milk of calcium, most cysts are indistinguishable from other water-density masses, including malignancies, and as such, ultrasonography is indicated for further evaluation.

On ultrasound, cysts are well circumscribed and anechoic, with posterior acoustic enhancement and thin edge shadows (Figure 6.36B). With small cysts deep in the breast, posterior acoustic enhancement may not be seen. Uncommon ultrasonographic features of

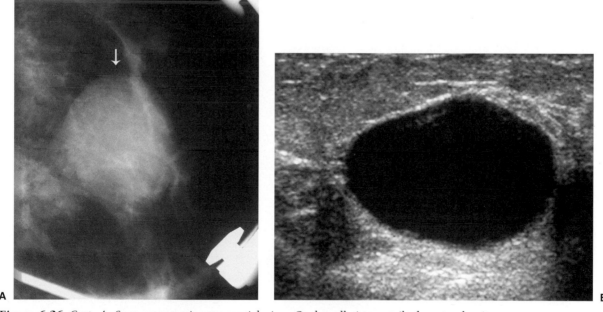

A   B

Figure 6.36 *Cyst. A.* Spot compression tangential view. Oval, well-circumscribed, water-density mass (*arrow*). *B.* Well-circumscribed, anechoic mass with posterior acoustic enhancement is seen on ultrasound. Category 2.

(continued on next page)

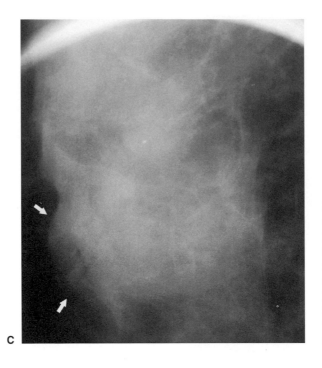

C

Figure 6.36 (continued) C. Spot compression view corresponding to palpable mass. Dense glandular tissue obscures visualization of the mass. A nodular contour is seen subcutaneously where the mass is partially surrounded by subcutaneous fat (*arrows*). A simple cyst is imaged ultrasonographically (not shown).

cysts include the presence of internal echoes that, if the transducer is left over the cyst, can be seen to be moving within the cyst (e.g., gurgling cysts) (Figure 6.38).

With optimal ultrasound equipment and meticulous technique, early cyst development, as acini within a lobule begin to distend, can be seen ultrasonographically as a cluster of small anechoic masses separated by thin echogenic septations (Figure 6.39). Posterior acoustic enhancement may also be seen. As the acini continue to distend, they fuse and give rise to larger cysts (Figure 6.39C). During real-time scanning, it is important to

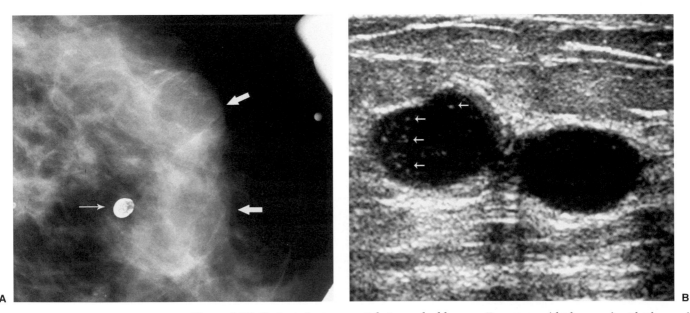

A   B

Figure 6.37 Cysts. A. Spot tangential view, palpable mass. Two masses (*thick arrows*) with obscured margins are imaged corresponding to the area of concern to the patient. A lucent-centered calcification is also noted (*thin arrow*). *B.* Two anechoic masses with posterior acoustic enhancement are imaged corresponding to the palpable mass. A few "floating" echoes are seen in one of the two cysts (*arrows*). Category 2.

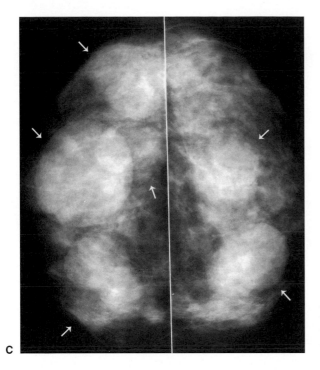

C

Figure 6.37 (continued) *C*. Multiple masses (*arrows*) of similar morphology bilaterally. On ultrasound, multiple cysts are present bilaterally.

evaluate the entire lesion and ensure that the septations are all thin. Now comfortable with these ultrasound findings, we are not routinely recommending short-interval follow-up or core biopsy of these areas. However, if there is any question about the correct diagnosis, core biopsy is appropriate. If a core biopsy is undertaken, these lesions decrease significantly in size and may disappear completely after the first or second pass through the lesion. Histologically, fragments of epithelial- and apocrine-lined cysts are reported after core biopsy of these areas.

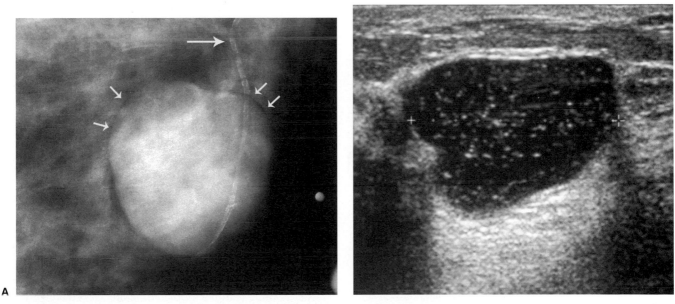

A   B

Figure 6.38 *Cyst.* *A*. Spot tangential view, palpable mass. Well-circumscribed, macrolobulated, oval mass with halo (*short arrows*) partially outlining contour. Incidentally noted is vascular calcification (*long arrow*). *B*. Well-circumscribed mass with internal echoes and posterior acoustic enhancement. During real-time scanning, the internal echoes swirl and shift in position consistent with a cyst ("gurgling"). We do not routinely aspirate this type of cyst unless the patient is symptomatic or another atypical feature is noted. Category 2.

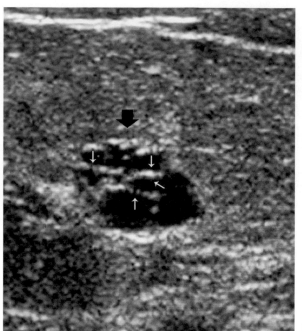

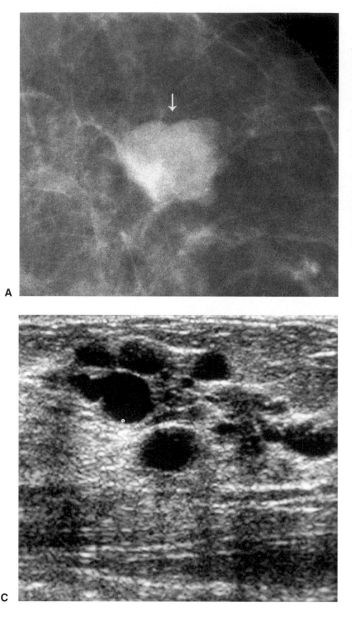

Figure 6.39 *Distending acini. A.* New, well-circumscribed macrolobulated mass (*arrow*). *B.* A cluster of small, anechoic, round masses (*black arrow*) is imaged ultrasonographically. Thin septations (*white arrows*) are seen separating the cysts. It is important that the septations be thin. Adjacent epithelial- and apocrine metaplasia-lined cysts are seen histologically. Given our own audit data and experience with the appearance of these lesions, we do not routinely recommend biopsy. If biopsy is undertaken, the lesion decreases or disappears after the first pass that goes through the lesion. *C.* Different patient. As the acini within a lobule continue to distend, the individual, small, clustered cysts can be imaged. Category 2.

Among our clinical colleagues, the traditional approach to women presenting with a palpable mass has been palpation-guided aspiration. If no fluid is obtained, a mammogram may or may not be ordered, and excisional biopsy may be recommended. With the availability of modern ultrasound units, we should challenge this approach. As a starting point, cysts are benign and often multiple and do not need to be aspirated unless the patient is tender or there are atypical ultrasonographic features. Some clinicians would suggest that patients with a palpable mass want it to go away. This is not the case with most of our patients. What women want is the reassurance that what they feel is not breast cancer. If this can be done with ultrasound (with the added benefit of evaluating the tissue surrounding the palpable area), aspiration is not needed, particularly because many cysts resolve spontaneously or fluctuate and some recur within days of an aspiration. Second, that fluid is not obtained during palpation-guided aspiration does not mean the lesion is not a cyst. A thick wall may preclude aspiration. Under ultrasound guidance, it is clear that some cysts are pushed away by the needle. The amount of pressure needed to puncture the cyst wall is best judged with imaging guidance. Finally, attempts to aspirate lesions may limit subsequent mammographic and ultrasonographic evaluations. It is recommended that mammographic and ultrasonographic studies be undertaken before any interventional procedures.

OTHER FLUID COLLECTIONS

Included in this group are galactoceles, postoperative (discussed at greater length in Chapter 10) or traumatic fluid collections (e.g., hematoma), and abscess. The mammographic appearance of these lesions is variable. Round and oval masses with indistinct margins are common. They can appear as cystic, complex cystic, or solid masses on ultrasound. Galactoceles develop in women who are pregnant, are lactating, or have stopped lactation within the last 2 to 3 years. A mixed-density mass or water-density mass can be seen mammographically. A fluid–fluid level may be present mammographically or ultrasonographically. Complex cystic masses, solid-appearing masses, or cysts are seen ultrasonographically (Figure 6.40).

Hematomas resulting from trauma may appear initially as water-density masses. As they liquefy and resolve, a mixed-density mass may be seen. They can appear as cystic or complex cystic masses; in some patients, a hyperechogenic mass may be seen (Figure 6.41). Postoperative fluid collections developing at lumpectomy sites are discussed in more detail in Chapter 10.

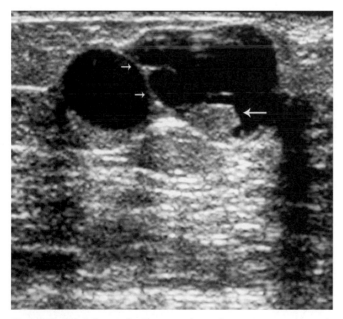

Figure 6.40 *Galactocele.* Patient who is lactating presents with a palpable mass. A complex cystic mass with posterior acoustic enhancement, septations (*small arrows*) and a seemingly solid component (*large arrow*) is seen on ultrasound. Thick, milky fluid aspirated with no residual abnormality after aspiration.

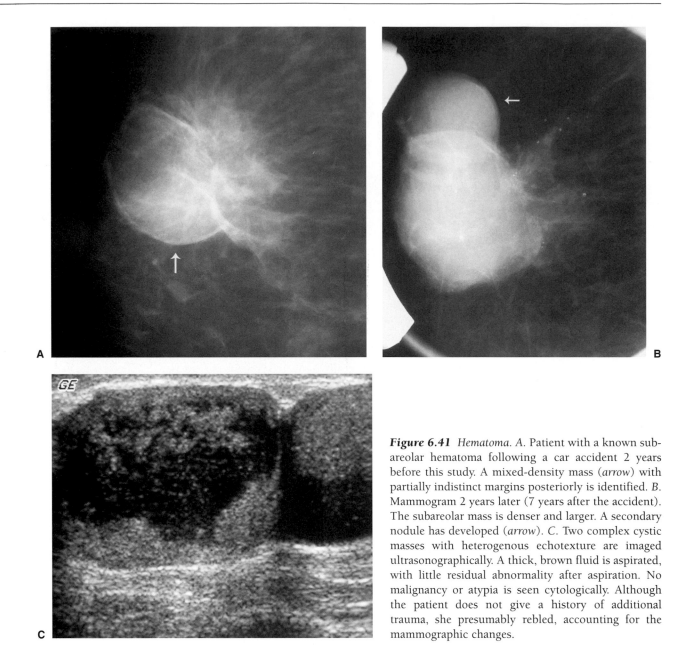

Figure 6.41 *Hematoma. A.* Patient with a known sub-areolar hematoma following a car accident 2 years before this study. A mixed-density mass (*arrow*) with partially indistinct margins posteriorly is identified. *B.* Mammogram 2 years later (7 years after the accident). The subareolar mass is denser and larger. A secondary nodule has developed (*arrow*). *C.* Two complex cystic masses with heterogenous echotexture are imaged ultrasonographically. A thick, brown fluid is aspirated, with little residual abnormality after aspiration. No malignancy or atypia is seen cytologically. Although the patient does not give a history of additional trauma, she presumably rebled, accounting for the mammographic changes.

Mastitis and abscesses are commonly seen during the first 6 weeks of lactation or weaning; however, they can involve women of all ages with no necessary antecedent. In the lactating patient, these are often associated with a crack or break in the skin, with *Staphylococcus aureus* being a common causative organism. These patients are treated with oral antibiotics. If symptoms do not improve, the development of an abscess should be considered, and percutaneous drainage may be indicated. Patients do not need to stop breast-feeding during treatment and probably should be encouraged to continue. With abscess formation, a mass with ill-defined or spiculated margins and associated distortion may be seen mammographically. A complex cystic mass is seen ultrasonographically (Figure 6.42). See Chapter 8 for an additional discussion of mastitis.

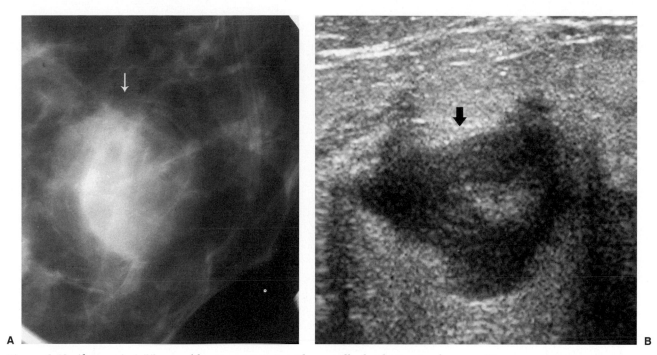

Figure 6.42 *Abscess. A.* A 39-year-old patient presents with a rapidly developing, tender mass. No recent pregnancy. An oval mass with obscured margins is seen mammographically (*arrow*). *B.* An irregular mass with a heterogenous echotexture is seen ultrasonographically (*arrow*). An aspiration is undertaken, yielding several milliliters of purulent fluid. Rapid improvement is attained with oral antibiotics.

ADENOMAS

FIBROADENOMAS

Fibroadenomas are common lesions, particularly in women in their 20s and 30s. In postmenopausal women, fibroadenomas decrease in size and increase in density as a result of hyalinization, and some develop calcifications. With estrogen replacement therapy, these changes may not develop, and preexisting fibroadenomas can enlarge or, rarely, develop in women postmenopausally (21). Clinically, women present with a mobile, rubbery, palpable mass. Some patients describe cyclical fluctuation in the size of the mass and associated tenderness.

Well-circumscribed, round (Figure 6.43), macrolobulated (Figure 6.44), or oval (Figure 6.45) masses are common. Fibroadenomas may have obscured or ill-defined margins; spiculation is rare. On ultrasound, a well-circumscribed, oval, homogenous hypoechoic mass is the most common finding (24); posterior acoustic enhancement may be seen, as may shadowing, particularly with hyalinization of the fibroadenoma. It is important, however, to emphasize that the mammographic and ultrasonographic appearance of fibroadenomas is highly variable (Figure 6.46). Clustered microcalcifications, with or without an associated mass, can be seen as can coarse popcorn-like calcifications. Fibroadenomas are variable in size and can enlarge; however, most stop growing after reaching 2 to 3 cm in diameter. Multiple fibroadenomas are reported in about 20% of women (21). On ultrasound, a well-circumscribed, oval mass (longer than it is wide) with a homogeneously hypoechoic echotexture is the most common presentation. One or two gentle macrolobu-

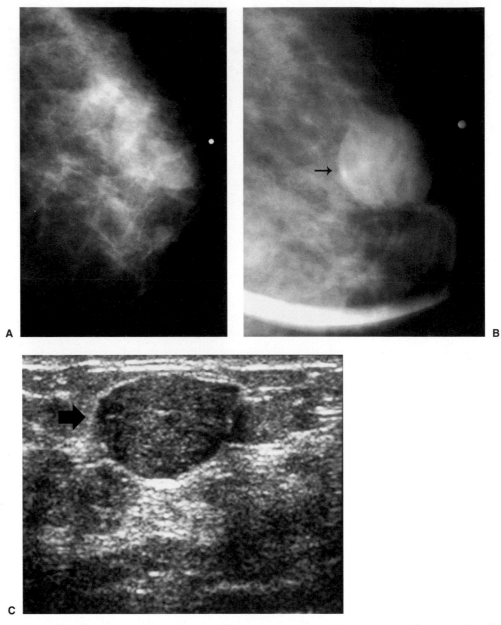

Figure 6.43 *Fibroadenoma. A.* A 39-year-old woman presents with a mass. Metallic BB marks the area. Glandular tissue obscures the lesion. *B.* Spot tangential view demonstrates well-circumscribed, round lesion (*arrow*) corresponding to the mass. *C.* Oval, hypoechoic mass with gentle lobulation and posterior acoustic enhancement (*arrow*).

lations may be present, as may posterior acoustic enhancement. With hyalinization, posterior acoustic shadowing may also be seen.

If a fibroadenoma is diagnosed on core biopsy, we do not routinely recommend post-biopsy follow-up in 6 months. Nor do we routinely recommend excisional biopsy when small increases in the size of core biopsy–proven fibroadenomas are noted on subsequent mammograms.

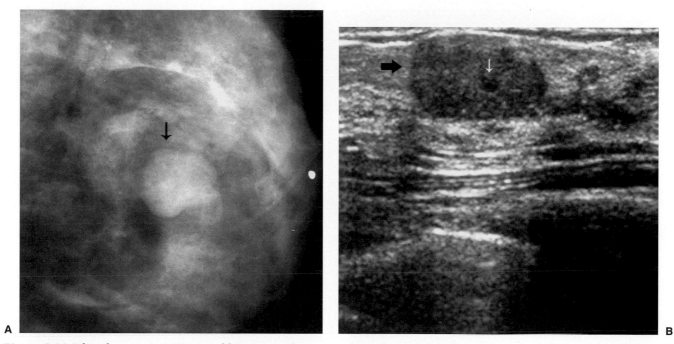

A   B

Figure 6.44 *Fibroadenoma.* A. A 43-year-old woman with a screen-detected mass. A well-circumscribed, macrolobulated mass (*arrow*) is identified. B. Oval, hypoechoic mass (*black arrow*) with posterior acoustic enhancement. A small cystic space is noted (*white arrow*) in the mass.

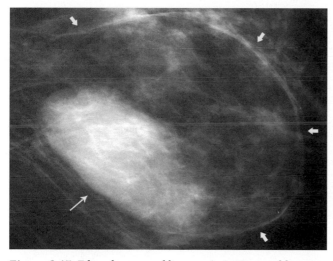

Figure 6.45 *Fibroadenoma and lipoma.* A. A 40-year-old woman with an oval, well-circumscribed mass with gentle lobulations (*thin arrow*). Also noted is a radiolucent mass with a thin, fibrous capsule (*thick arrows*). Diagnosis established following excisional biopsy done at the request of the patient. Included in the differential would be a fibroadenolipoma.

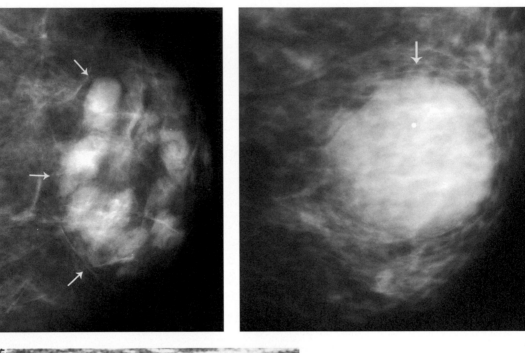

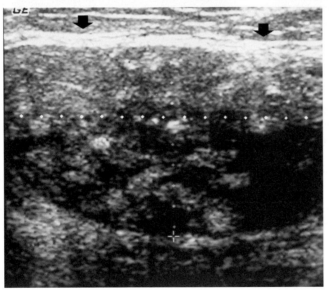

Figure 6.46 *Fibroadenomas. A.* A 41-year-old woman with a round mass of mixed density in the left subareolar area (*arrows*). A fibroadenolipoma would be the primary consideration, however, histologically, this proved to be a fibroadenoma with an atypical mammographic appearance. *B.* Different patient. A 37-year-old woman with a palpable mass. Metallic BB marks the area. A well-circumscribed, round mass (*arrow*) is seen corresponding to area of clinical concern. *C.* Oval mass with heterogenous echotexture (*arrows*). Given the ultrasound appearance, biopsy is undertaken.

COMPLEX FIBROADENOMAS

A term coined by Dupont and co-workers (25), *complex fibroadenomas* (CFAs), are fibroadenomas with superimposed fibrocystic changes, specifically the following:

- Cysts greater than 3 mm (Figure 6.47)
- Sclerosing adenosis (Figure 6.48)
- Epithelial calcifications (Figure 6.49)
- Papillary apocrine changes

In Dupont's study, about 33% of the fibroadenomas could be classified as complex. These lesions may be associated with an increased risk for the subsequent development of breast cancer. Reportedly, the risk is increased 3.88 times if proliferative changes are present in the stroma surrounding a CFA (25).

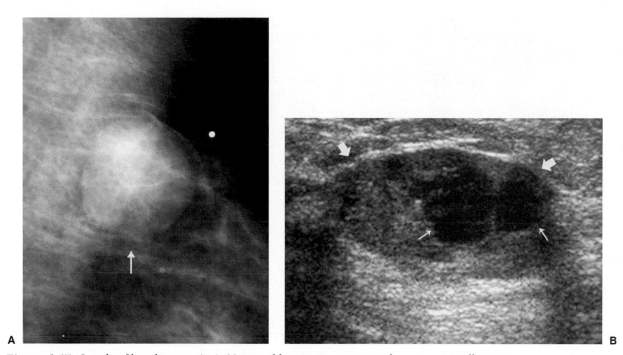

Figure 6.47 *Complex fibroadenoma.* A. A 32-year-old woman presents with a mass. Metallic BB marks the area. A round, well-circumscribed mass (*arrow*) is imaged. B. Complex mass (*thick arrows*) with cystic spaces (*thin arrows*) and posterior acoustic enhancement. Category 4. A complex fibroadenoma with cystic changes and epithelial hyperplasia is diagnosed histologically on imaging guided core biopsy.

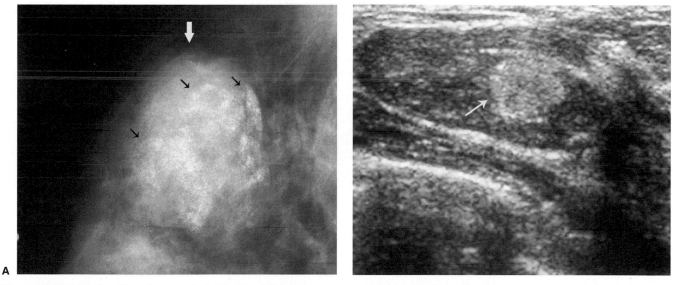

Figure 6.48 *Complex fibroadenoma.* A. A 35-year-old woman presents with a mass. An oval mass with partially indistinct borders (*white arrow*) and amorphous ("smudgy") calcifications (*black arrows*) is imaged at the site of clinical concern. B. Oval hypoechoic mass with a focal area of hyperechogenicity (*arrow*). Category 4. A complex fibroadenoma with superimposed sclerosing adenosis is diagnosed histologically on imaging guided core biopsy.

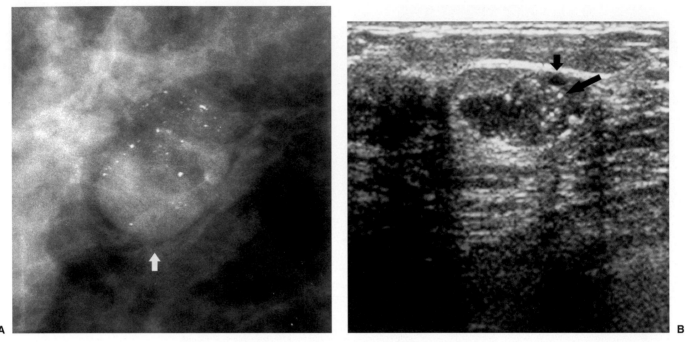

A   B

Figure 6.49 *Complex fibroadenoma.* A. A 45-year-old woman with screen-detected calcifications. Spot compression magnification view demonstrates an oval mass (*arrow*) with partially indistinct margins and associated pleomorphic calcifications. B. An oval mass with heterogenous echotexture and some posterior acoustic enhancement and a small cystic area (*short arrow*) superiorly is imaged ultrasonographically. High specular echoes (*long arrow*) in the mass are consistent with calcifications seen mammographically. Category 4. A complex fibroadenoma is diagnosed histologically on imaging guided core biopsy. The calcifications are identified in areas of epithelial hyperplasia.

The imaging features of CFAs are usually indistinguishable from those of fibroadenomas. In some patients, however, mammographic and ultrasonographic findings may suggest the diagnosis of a CFA. Epithelial calcifications may be seen mammographically as pleomorphic calcifications, including round, punctate, and less commonly, linear forms (Figure 6.49A). An associated mass may or may not be seen. Amorphous calcifications (Figure 6.48A) associated with a mass may reflect the presence of sclerosing adenosis within the fibroadenoma. Finally, a complex mass with cystic spaces (Figure 6.47B) may be seen on ultrasound, when the fibroadenoma is associated with cysts greater than 3 mm in size. Because, at most, this is a marker lesion for increased risk, we do not routinely recommend excision when diagnosed on core biopsy. Patients are imaged annually.

TUBULAR ADENOMAS

Women with tubular adenomas present in their 20s and 30s with palpable, movable masses. The imaging findings are indistinguishable from those described for typical fibroadenomas. A well-circumscribed, round (Figure 6.50) or oval mass is seen mammographically, and an oval, homogeneously hypoechoic mass is seen ultrasonographically (26). Pleomorphic clusters of calcifications may also be seen. With a diagnosis of tubular adenoma on needle biopsy of a well-circumscribed mass, we do not recommend excision. The patient is asked to return for annual mammography.

Grossly tubular adenomas lack a true capsule yet are well circumscribed and separable from the adjacent tissue. Histologically, these tumors are composed of uniformly small, closely packed tubular structures with scant surrounding stroma. Like normal breast ducts, the proliferating tubules are lined by a contiguous layer of epithelial cells and a discontinuous layer of basilar myoepithelial cells (10,11,23).

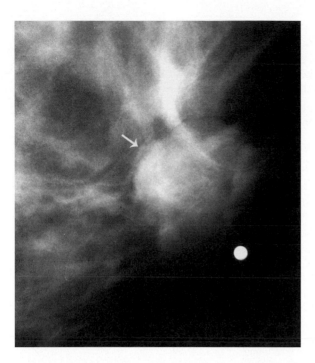

Figure 6.50 *Tubular adenoma.* A 58-year-old woman presents with a mass. Metallic BB marks the area. A round, well-circumscribed mass (*arrow*) is imaged at the site of clinical concern. On ultrasound, an oval mass with heterogenous echotexture is imaged (not shown). Category 4.

LACTATIONAL ADENOMAS

Patients with lactational adenomas typically present during pregnancy with a palpable, mobile mass; rapid growth may be noted by the patient. Because of the age of the patients, and their presentation during pregnancy or lactation, mammograms are not usually done. Macrolobulated, well-circumscribed, hypoechoic masses with posterior acoustic enhancement are among the ultrasound characteristics of lactating adenomas (27). Fibrous bands traversing the lesion and cystic spaces may also be seen (Figure 6.51).

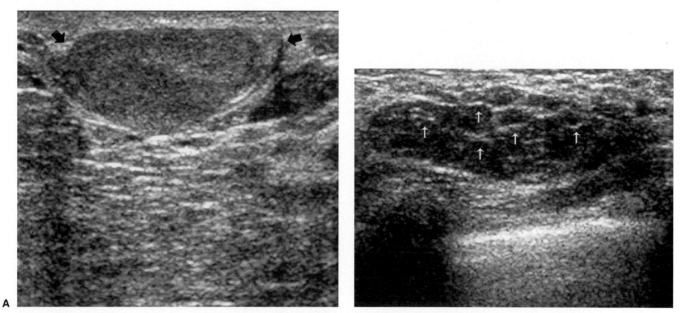

Figure 6.51 *Lactational adenomas.* A. A 46-year-old woman in third trimester of pregnancy presenting with a mass in the left subareolar area. A well-circumscribed, homogeneously hypoechoic mass (*arrows*) with minimal posterior acoustic enhancement is imaged ultrasonographically. Although a lactational adenoma was suspected, the patient requested core biopsy. B. A 33-year-old woman in the second trimester of pregnancy presents with a mass in the right breast. A hypoechoic mass with hyperechoic fibrous bands (*arrows*) is identified coursing through lesion. Lesion resolved after cessation of lactation.

The histologic appearance varies depending on the stage of pregnancy at the time of diagnosis. In women less than 6 months pregnant, the tubular structures, unlike those of tubular adenomas, vary significantly in size. The epithelial cells contain cytoplasmic vacuoles, and mitotic figures are common. Lesions diagnosed after the second trimester of pregnancy are characterized by large alveolar spaces filled with foamy material, variegated shape, and cytoplasmic vacuoles. These lesions may grow rapidly, and infarction with necrosis may occur (10,11,23). Most resolve, or decrease in size, following cessation of lactation

PHYLLODES

Phyllodes tumors are fibroepithelial tumors accounting for less than 1% of all breast neoplasms (23,28,29). Most are benign; however, metastases have been reported in 6% to 22% of patients (23). The mean age of patients with phyllodes is 45 years; however, they can occur in patients of all ages. As many as 80% of patients present with a palpable mass, whereas 20% are detected on screening mammography in asymptomatic women (28). A

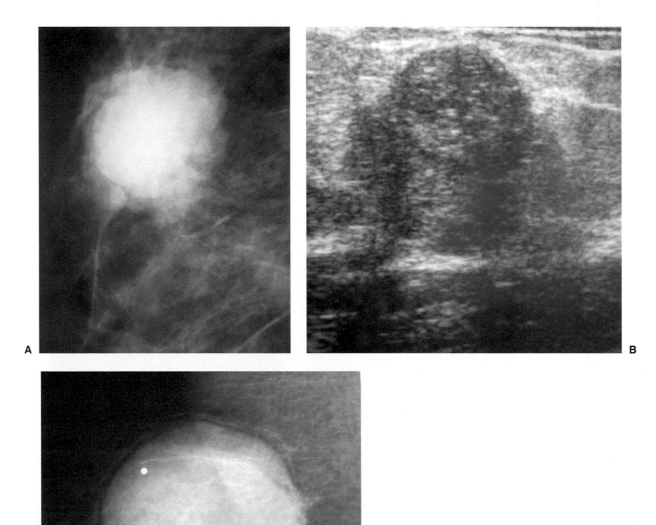

Figure 6.52 Phyllodes tumor. A. Macrolobulated mass with indistinct margins and some spiculation. *B.* Irregular hypoechoic mass. Cystic spaces can sometimes be seen within the mass on ultrasound. *C.* Different patient. A well-circumscribed mass (minimally indistinct margin posteriorly) is imaged corresponding to palpable mass metallic BB.

well-circumscribed mass that may be lobulated is the most common mammographic manifestation of phyllodes (Figure 6.52). Tumors that are larger than 3 cm in size are more likely to have histologic features suggestive of malignancy (28). On ultrasound, phyllodes are well-circumscribed, oval masses. Cystic changes may be seen and are more common in malignant tumors; however, this cannot be used to distinguish benign from malignant. Calcifications are uncommon (8%) and not useful in distinguishing benign from malignant tumors (28).

Histologically, the proliferation and appearance of the epithelial elements in phyllodes tumors and fibroadenomas are similar; the epithelial component in phyllodes is polyclonal. It is the cellularity of the stroma that distinguishes phyllodes from fibroadenomas; the stromal component in phyllodes is monoclonal. Increased cellularity of the stroma and projection of stromal elements into cystic spaces to create a leaflike (phyllodes) pattern characterize phyllodes tumors (10,11,23). The criteria used in the classification of phyllodes tumors as benign or malignant have varied. Border characteristics (infiltrative versus expansile), cellular atypism, mitotic activity, and stromal cellularity and overgrowth are used currently. Well-defined margins, no cytologic atypia, and fewer than five mitoses per high-power field characterize benign tumors. Features suggestive of malignancy include microscopically invasive margins, areas of stromal overgrowth, stromal hypercellularity with atypism, and prominent mitotic activity (more than five mitoses per high-power field) (10,11,23,28,29).

Management of these lesions requires complete surgical excision. Mastectomy may be indicated in women with malignant phyllodes. When metastases occur, they are hematogenous, and as such, axillary nodal dissections are not done. Local recurrences, reported in as many as 20% of patients, are usually related to incomplete surgical excisions.

SOLITARY PAPILLOMAS

Solitary papillomas develop in subsegmental ducts. Women with solitary papillomas commonly present with spontaneous nipple discharge. In these patients, ductography is helpful in establishing the presence, number, and location of lesions (30). Mammographic findings (31) include the following:

- Dilated subareolar duct
- Well-circumscribed, round or oval mass (Figure 6.53A)

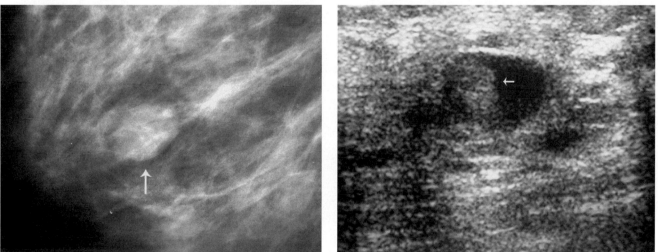

A   B

Figure 6.53 *Papilloma. A. Oval mass (arrow) detected on screening mammogram. B. Complex cystic mass seen on ultrasound; intracystic mass is present, suggesting a papilloma (arrow).*

(continued on next page)

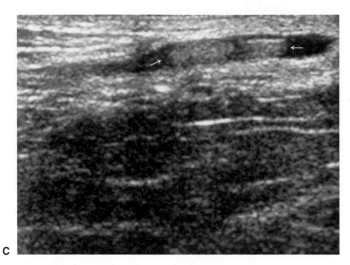

C

Figure 6.53 (continued) *C.* Different patient with spontaneous nipple discharge and an intraductal mass (*arrows*). Ultrasound is particularly helpful if the papilloma is subareolar in location, as in this patient.

- Spiculated mass (Figure 6.54)
- Cluster of punctate calcifications
- Coarse, curvilinear calcifications

On ultrasound of patients presenting with nipple discharge, intraductal lesions may be imaged, particularly if the lesion is close to the nipple and if the duct is dilated (Figure 6.53C). Intracystic papillomas are seen as solid mural nodules within cysts (Figure 6.53B).

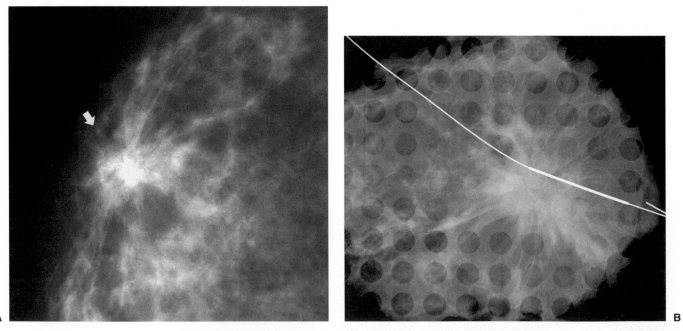

A   **B**

Figure 6.54 *Papilloma. A.* Spiculated mass (*arrow*). Category 4. Sclerosing intraductal papilloma with florid hyperplasia reported on core biopsy. Given a spiculated mass, however, this pathology is thought not to be congruent; excisional biopsy is recommended. *B.* Specimen radiograph. Spiculated mass excised. A sclerosing papilloma with focal areas of atypical ductal hyperplasia is diagnosed on the excisional biopsy.

If a pneumocystogram is done after aspiration, the lesion can be outlined by air. A homogeneously hypoechoic mass, indistinguishable from other solid masses, may also be seen.

Papillomas are small friable tumors with an epithelial lining contiguous with that of the duct and, therefore, characterized by the presence of a contiguous layer of epithelial cells and a discontinuous basilar layer of myoepithelial cells. The presence of a central fibrovascular core distinguishes these lesions from epithelial hyperplasia with papillary changes (papillomatosis).

MULTIPLE PAPILLOMAS

Multiple papillomas develop in the terminal ducts. Histologically, these lesions are identical to solitary papillomas. About 20% of women with multiple peripheral papillomas present with spontaneous nipple discharge (31). The other patients are usually asymptomatic with findings detected on screening mammography. A lobulated mass, multiple peripheral masses of varying sizes, or clusters of punctate calcifications unilaterally or bilaterally are the mammographic findings in women with peripheral papillomas (31) (Figures 6.55A and 6.56A). On ultrasound, multiple solid masses or a combination of intracystic, intraductal, and solid masses may be seen (Figures 6.55B and 6.56B, C). These patients may be at increased risk for breast cancer development; however, this has not been quantified.

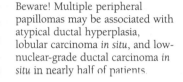

Beware! Multiple peripheral papillomas may be associated with atypical ductal hyperplasia, lobular carcinoma *in situ*, and low-nuclear-grade ductal carcinoma *in situ* in nearly half of patients.

FOCAL FIBROSIS

Clinically, focal fibrosis is usually diagnosed in premenopausal women presenting with a hard, discrete mass on physical examination. Various terms have been used to describe this entity, including focal breast fibrosis, breast fibrosis, breast sclerosis, fibrous mastopathy, and fibrous tumor. Theories on pathogenesis include selective hormonal stimulation of the fibroelastic tissue of the breast, a normal involutional change, or the end result of an inflammatory process (11).

The reported incidence of focal fibrosis on imaging-guided biopsy ranges from 2.1% to 15% (29–33). Mammographically, an oval or round mass with well-circumscribed (Fig-

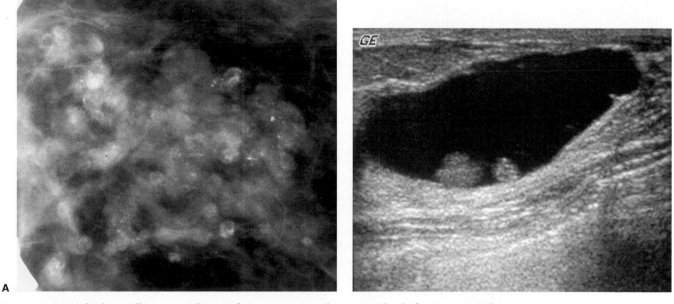

A **B**

Figure 6.55 *Multiple papillomas. A.* Cluster of masses some with associated calcifications. *B.* Different patient. Predominantly cystic mass with two solid intracystic masses.

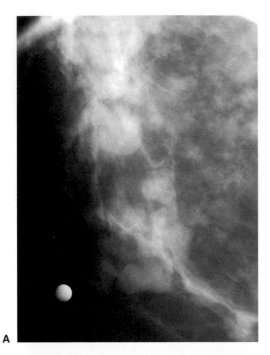

A

Figure 6.56 *Multiple papillomas. A.* Metallic BB marks location of palpable area. Spot tangential view demonstrates a cluster of masses. *B.* In some portions of this lesion, complex cystic masses with mural nodules (*arrows*) are imaged. *C.* In other portions of this lesion, intraductal lesions (*arrows*) are seen on ultrasound. Surgical exasion is indicated.

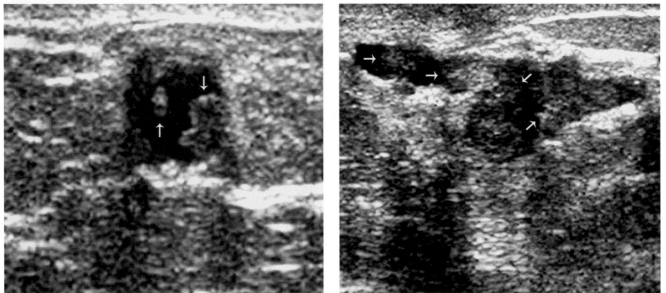

B

C

ure 6.57) to partially obscured to ill-defined margins (Figures 6.58 and 6.59) is the most common finding reported in as many as 72% of women diagnosed with this entity. A developing area of asymmetric density, architectural distortion, and a spiculated mass are less common imaging findings (32–36).

On ultrasound, a hypoechoic mass with well-circumscribed, lobulated, or ill-defined margins is the most common finding (Figures 6.57B). In some patients, the mass is isoechoic or centrally echogenic with a hypoechoic rim (Figure 6.58B). Posterior acoustic enhancement and shadowing have been reported in 17% to 21% and 14% to 40% of lesions, respectively; 44% to 68% of lesions demonstrate neither of these two features (29–33).

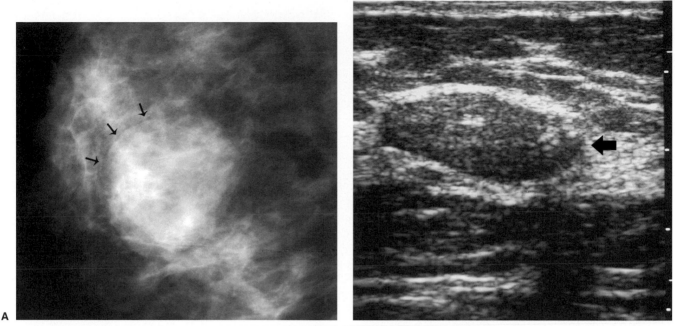

A B

Figure 6.57 *Focal fibrosis.* *A.* Round mass detected on screening mammogram. A halo sign is partially visualized (*arrows*). *B.* Oval, well-circumscribed hypoechoic mass (*arrow*) with some round areas of hyperechogenicity. Appearance simulates that of fibroadenomas. The assessment category depends on what prior studies show. If this mass is new or has increased in size, biopsy is indicated. If this mass is stable, no intervention is warranted. If no prior studies are available, and in consultation with the patient, this could be classified as category 3, with follow-up in 6 months recommended to establish stability.

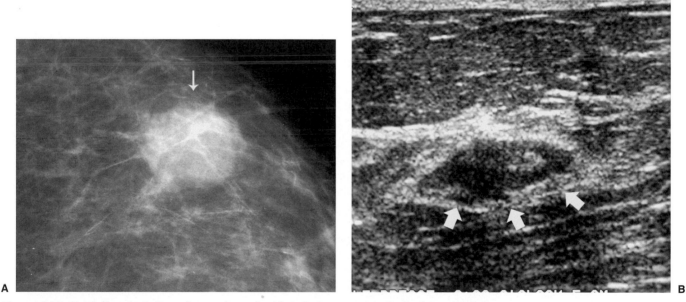

A B

Figure 6.58 *Focal fibrosis.* *A.* Round mass (*arrow*) with indistinct margins. *B.* Oval mass seen on ultrasound with associated areas of hyperechogenicity. Margins are irregular and possibly spiculated (*arrows*). Category 4.

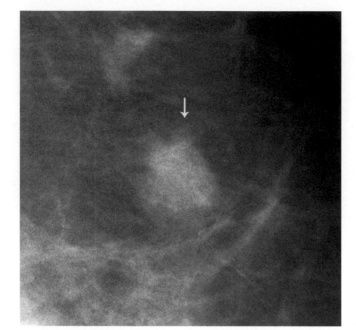

Figure 6.59 *Focal fibrosis. Round mass with indistinct margins (arrow). Category 4.*

The diagnosis of focal fibrosis after an imaging-guided biopsy can be considered congruent with the imaging findings provided targeting of the lesion is accurate and the lesion under question does not have features highly suggestive of malignancy (e.g., spiculation). Repeat core biopsy or excisional biopsy is appropriate for lesions with imaging features highly suggestive of malignancy.

Histologically, there is proliferation of the fibrous stroma with a decrease or obliteration of ductal and lobular elements. This process may be localized to the perilobular or interlobular stroma, or it may involve both. Vascular structures and nerves are sparse, and no perivascular or perilobular inflammatory infiltrate is seen (10). Review of pathology in some patients with an initial diagnosis of stromal fibrosis or fibrous tumors, may demonstrate that pseudoangiomatous stromal hyperplasia is a more appropriate diagnosis (37).

DIABETIC MASTOPATHY

Diabetic mastopathy is an uncommon entity usually reported in premenopausal women (38); however, it can also be seen in men (39). Significantly, these patients have a history of long-standing, juvenile-onset insulin-dependent diabetes; at the time of presentation with breast symptoms, many of these patients have other diabetes-related complications, including retinopathy, nephropathy, and neuropathy. Patients present with ill-defined, firm, nontender, mobile breast masses of varying sizes. Synchronous or metachronous breast lesions are not uncommon. This is a self-limited condition that may regress spontaneously.

Reported imaging findings include dense tissue mammographically and intense posterior acoustic shadowing ultrasonographically (Figure 6.60). Although many of these patients are young, vascular calcifications maybe present (38). In the appropriate clinical and histologic context, core biopsy can reliable establish the diagnosis.

Dense fibrosis, characterized by thick bundles of collagen with keloidal features and periductal, lobular, and vascular inflammatory infiltrates, are the histologic hallmarks of diabetic mastopathy. An autoimmune etiology has been proposed for this condition. It has been suggested that glycosylation and abnormal cross-linking of collagen somehow impede degradation (10).

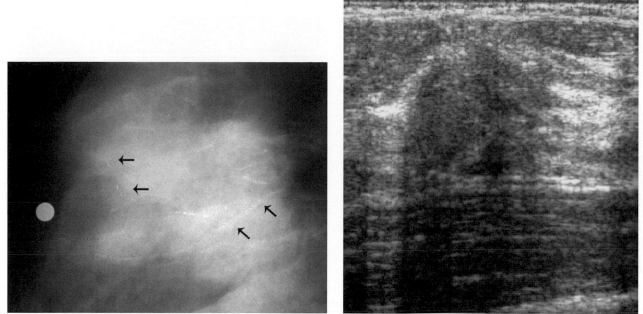

Figure 6.60 *Diabetic fibrous mastopathy. A.* A 40-year-old, long-standing insulin-dependent diabetic woman with a hard palpable mass. Metallic BB marks the area. Dense glandular tissue with arterial calcification corresponds to palpable area (*arrows*). *B.* Dense shadowing mass corresponding to palpable area. Diagnosis established on imaging guided core biopsy.

PSEUDOANGIOMATOUS STROMAL HYPERPLASIA

The clinicopathologic spectrum of pseudoangiomatous stromal hyperplasia (PASH) ranges from an incidental microscopic change reported as a focal lesion, in as many as 23% of breast biopsy specimens, to a less common mammographically or clinically apparent mass (40). Multifocality has been reported in as many as 60% of patients. Symptomatic patients presenting with a firm, mobile, nontender mass are typically premenopausal or postmenopausal women on hormone replacement therapy. In men, PASH has been reported as an incidental component of gynecomastia in nearly half of patients. These lesions are typically progesterone receptor positive and estrogen receptor negative. A hormonal etiology for this lesion has been suggested.

A noncalcified mass with well- to ill-defined margins (Figure 6.61) and rarely spiculation is the typical mammographic presentation of PASH. A well-circumscribed hypoechoic mass is seen ultrasonographically (41,42). Cystic spaces may be seen in the lesion (Figure 6.62), as may acoustic enhancement or shadowing. These lesions can enlarge over time (Figure 6.62) and may recur after excision (Figure 6.63). A diagnosis of PASH after imaging-guided biopsy is considered congruent with the imaging findings, provided targeting of the lesion is accurate and the lesion under question does not have features highly suggestive of malignancy (e.g., spiculation). Repeat core biopsy or excisional biopsy is appropriate for lesions with imaging features highly suggestive of malignancy.

Histologically, PASH may be mistaken for a low-grade angiosarcoma. In PASH, disruption and separation of collagen fibers in the intralobular stroma create a pattern of anastomosing slitlike (capillary-like) spaces that are incompletely lined by spindle myofibroblasts lacking a basement membrane. Mucopolysaccharides occupy the pseudovascular spaces. In angiosarcomas, the lumina are open, are lined by endothelial cells, and contain red blood cells. The pleomorphism, mitotic activity, and necrosis

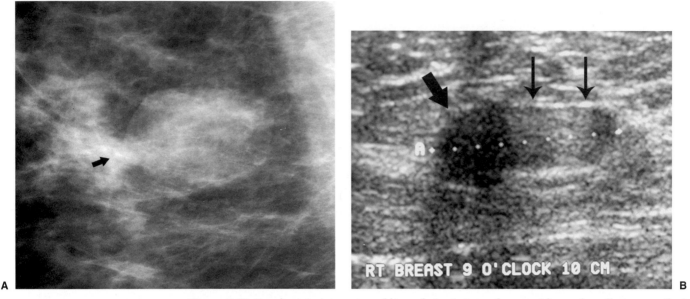

Figure 6.61 *Pseudoangiomatous stromal hyperplasia. A.* An oval mass with mostly well-circumscribed margins except anteriorly, where they are partially obscured (*arrow*). *B.* An oval mass with heterogenous echotexture. Posterior acoustic shadowing is noted with more hypoechoic area (*thick arrow*) and minimal enhancement in portion of mass that is hypoechoic to slightly hyperechoic (*thin arrows*). Diagnosis established on imaging guided core biopsy.

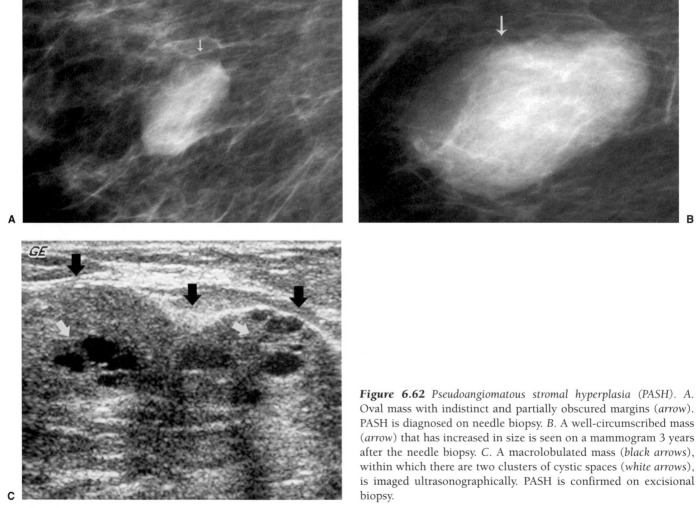

Figure 6.62 *Pseudoangiomatous stromal hyperplasia (PASH). A.* Oval mass with indistinct and partially obscured margins (*arrow*). PASH is diagnosed on needle biopsy. *B.* A well-circumscribed mass (*arrow*) that has increased in size is seen on a mammogram 3 years after the needle biopsy. *C.* A macrolobulated mass (*black arrows*), within which there are two clusters of cystic spaces (*white arrows*), is imaged ultrasonographically. PASH is confirmed on excisional biopsy.

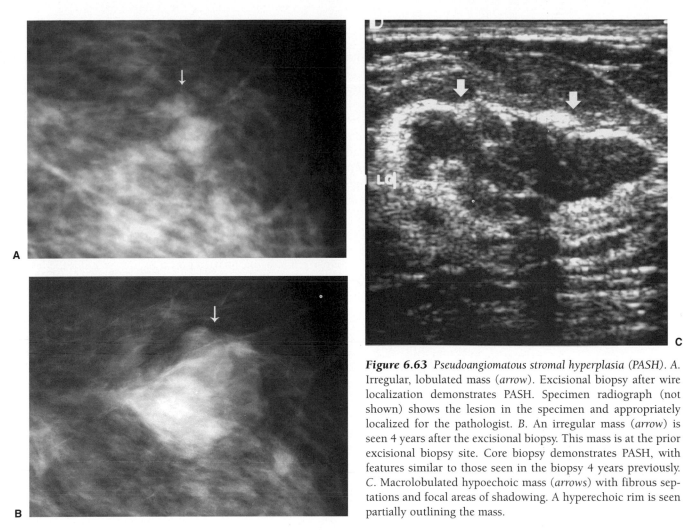

Figure 6.63 *Pseudoangiomatous stromal hyperplasia (PASH). A. Irregular, lobulated mass (arrow). Excisional biopsy after wire localization demonstrates PASH. Specimen radiograph (not shown) shows the lesion in the specimen and appropriately localized for the pathologist. B. An irregular mass (arrow) is seen 4 years after the excisional biopsy. This mass is at the prior excisional biopsy site. Core biopsy demonstrates PASH, with features similar to those seen in the biopsy 4 years previously. C. Macrolobulated hypoechoic mass (arrows) with fibrous septations and focal areas of shadowing. A hyperechoic rim is seen partially outlining the mass.*

reported in angiosarcomas are not seen in PASH. Also, factor VIII, an endothelial-specific marker, is not identified in PASH; however, reactivity for CD34 and muscle actin is seen (10,11,23).

COMPLEX SCLEROSING LESIONS (RADIAL SCARS)

The etiology of complex sclerosing lesions (CSLs) and radial scars is unknown. They are not, however, related to prior trauma or surgery. It has been suggested that radial scars may be related to an inflammatory process or to ischemia and infarction occurring in areas of proliferative change (43). Radial scars are distinctive histologic lesions seen commonly by pathologists as an incidental finding in breast tissue. By definition, these lesions measure less than 1 cm and are therefore not usually identified mammographically. CSLs have histologic features similar to those of radial scars; however, these lesions measure more than 1 cm in size. These lesions are not as common. Most of the lesions detected mammographically are larger than 1 cm and as such represent CSLs.

When clinical and imaging findings are considered, the presence of a CSL can sometimes be suggested prospectively. Mammographically, architectural distortion with fat in the center of the lesion and minimal (if any) central mass formation, long curving spicules, and a differential appearance of the lesion on orthogonal views (e.g., lesion is

Radial scars and CSLs are similar histologically; when less than 1 cm in size, they are designated as radial scars; when greater than 1 cm in size, they are considered CSLs.

more evident in one projection compared with the orthogonal view) are the hallmarks (44–54) (Figures 6.64, 6.65, and 6.66). Calcifications may be seen in as many as 37% of patients with CSLs (46). Although these lesions are often 1.5 to 3 cm in size, the physical examination in these patients is usually normal. Invasive ductal carcinomas that measure 1.5 to 3 cm in size are typically palpable, and the palpable abnormality feels larger than the lesion seen mammographically.

Cohen and Sferlazza (49) reported that radial scars are often seen on ultrasound and have greater conspicuity ultrasonographically than mammographically. Our own experience with ultrasonography in these patients is that it is not as helpful. In our hands, many of lesions are subtle on ultrasound; when imaged, they are hypoechoic, with variable amounts of shadowing (Figure 6.66C). They may only be seen in one orientation of the transducer and not easily confirmed as the transducer is rotated over the area of concern.

The management of these lesions remains controversial. Some advocate excisional biopsy when a CSL is suspected prospectively, based on imaging findings, and excisional biopsy following a diagnosis of a CSL on an imaging-guided core biopsy. Others advocate routine imaging-guided core biopsy of these lesions with no excision required if the lesion is not associated with atypical ductal hyperplasia, the biopsy included at least 12 specimens, and the mammographic findings are reconciled with the histologic findings (54). There are three related issues to consider (53,54):

1. Is the pathologist able to distinguish CSL reliably from tubular carcinoma? (It is also sometimes difficult to distinguish CSL from sclerosing adenosis, although because this is a benign lesion, this potential misdiagnosis can be viewed as not significant.)
2. In a woman with a spiculated mass and distortion, can we accept the diagnosis of radial scar or CSL after core biopsy?
3. Are these lesions associated with other lesions, such as atypical ductal hyperplasia, lobular neoplasia, low-nuclear-grade ductal carcinoma *in situ*, and tubular carcinomas, often enough to warrant excision in all patients?

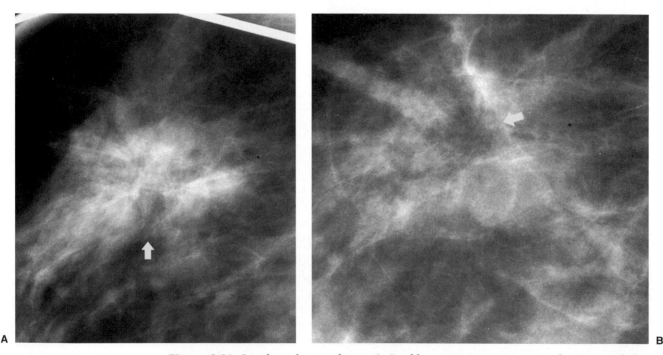

Figure 6.64 Complex sclerosing lesion. A. Double spot compression magnification. Mediolateral oblique (MLO) view demonstrating an area of distortion and spiculation (*arrow*). B. Double spot compression magnification, craniocaudal projection. Distortion with central fat (*arrow*). The appearance is less striking than that seen on the MLO view. Not palpable on physical examination. An invasive ductal carcinoma of this size, and with the close proximity to the skin, should be readily palpable.

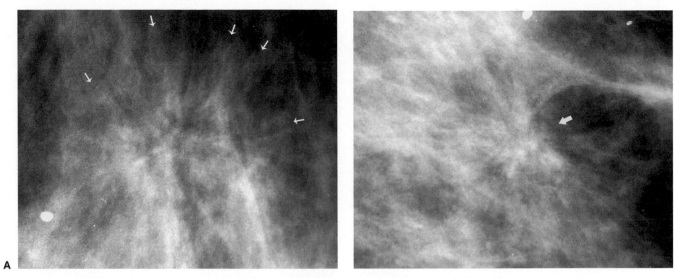

A
B

Figure 6.65 *Complex sclerosing lesion.* A. Double spot compression magnification. Mediolateral oblique view shows distortion with radiolucency centrally and fatty tissue outlining long spicules (*arrows*). B. Double spot compression magnification. Craniocaudal projection shows distortion that is less conspicuous but still visible (*arrow*), with central radiolucency and long spicules.

We continue to take a cautious and conservative approach to women with a CSL detected mammographically with findings as described earlier and distinguish these patients from those with incidentally noted radial scars on biopsies done for unrelated findings. If a CSL is suspected based on imaging findings, we still recommend excisional biopsy; and if core biopsy of a lesion is done and the diagnosis is CSL, we recommend excisional biopsy.

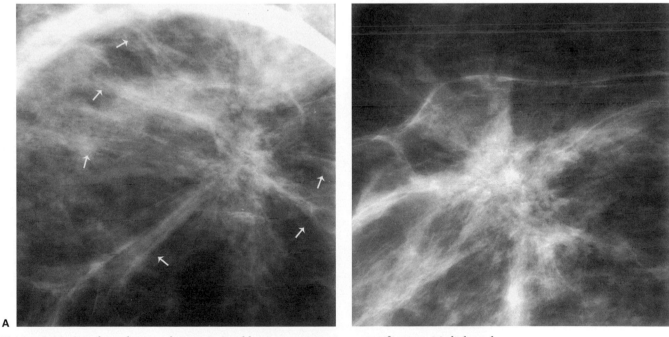

A
B

Figure 6.66 *Complex sclerosing lesion.* A. Double spot compression magnification. Mediolateral oblique (MLO) view shows central radiolucency and long spicules (*arrows*). B. Double spot compression magnification. Craniocaudal projection shows central radiolucency and long spicules.

(continued on next page)

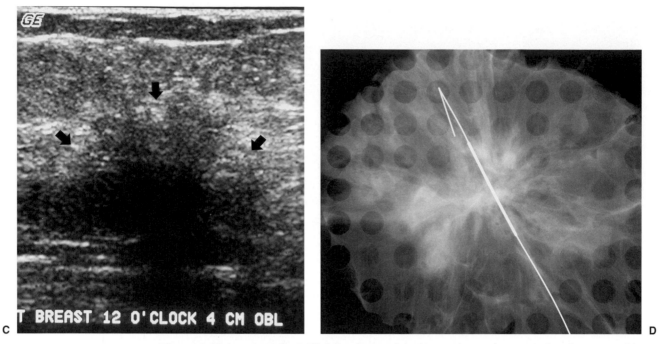

C   D

Figure 6.66 (continued) *C.* Ill-defined area of shadowing (*arrows*) is imaged at the expected location of the lesion. No palpable abnormality is appreciated as the lesion is imaged. *D.* Specimen radiograph demonstrating distortion and long spicules.

SCLEROSING ADENOSIS

Most women with sclerosing adenosis are asymptomatic with a cluster of either round and punctate or amorphous calcifications detected on a screening mammogram. Rarely, sclerosing adenosis can present with a clinically or mammographically detected mass (Figure 6.67). Mammographically, these masses can be either round or spiculated; associated distortion or calcifications may be seen.

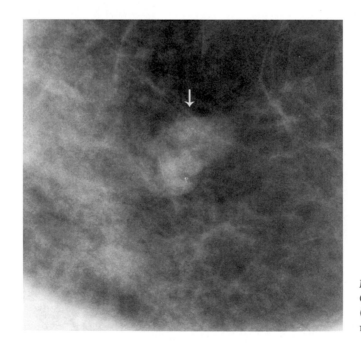

Figure 6.67 *Sclerosing adenosis. Oval, well-circumscribed mass (arrow) is detected on screening mammogram.*

This is a lobulocentric lesion characterized by the proliferation of acini and surrounding intralobular stroma. The acinar spaces can be compressed and elongated by the proliferating stroma. These lesions can sometimes be mistaken for tubular carcinomas. In sclerosing adenosis, the lumina of the glands are flattened or elongated, and there is a two-cell layer (epithelium and myoepithelium) lining the acini. In contrast, the glands in tubular carcinomas are round, uniform and angulated with no myoepithelial cells seen lining the proliferating glands.

EXTRAABDOMINAL DESMOIDS (FIBROMATOSIS)

Extraabdominal desmoids are rare lesions that may be associated with Gardner's syndrome. They are locally aggressive and require wide local excision. In about 20% of patients, they recur locally within the first 5 years. A spiculated mass that may be close to the pectoral muscle is seen mammographically. A hypoechoic mass with variable amounts of shadowing is seen ultrasonographically (Figure 6.68).

BENIGN VASCULAR LESIONS

A variety of benign vascular lesions may be seen arising in breast tissue. These include hemangiomas (perilobular, cavernous, capillary), angiomas, and venous hemangiomas. A round or oval mass is the most common finding mammographically; in some patients, punctate calcifications in isolation of a mass may be seen (Figures 6.69 and 6.70). On ultrasound, the masses may be hyperechoic or contain hyperechoic foci within them. The histologic differentiation of these lesions from angiosarcomas is critical.

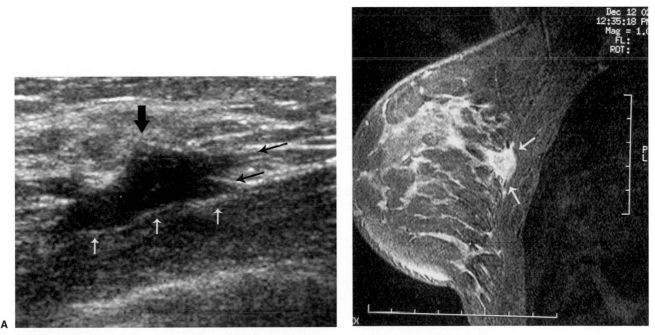

Figure 6.68 *Extraabdominal desmoid. A.* A 23-year-old woman presents with a palpable, tender mass. Mammogram (not shown) demonstrates dense glandular tissue with no discrete lesion seen on spot tangential view. Ultrasonographically, an irregular mass (*thick black arrow*) with apparent spiculation (*thin black arrows*) abuts the deep pectoral fascia (*white arrows*). *B.* Magnetic resonance imaging after gadolinium. An irregular enhancing mass abuts the pectoral (*arrows*). Wide local excisions are critical in reducing the likelihood of local recurrences in these patients.

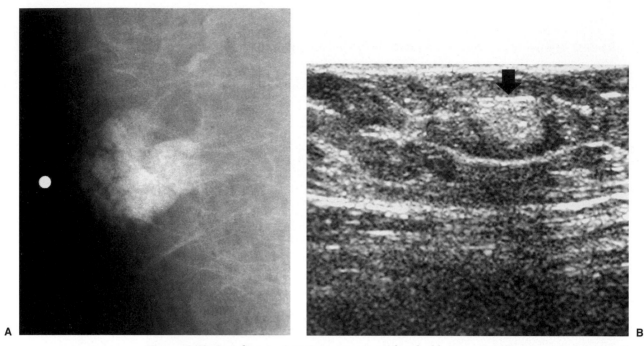

Figure 6.69 *Angiolipoma. A.* Patient presents with palpable mass. Metallic BB marks location. Spot compression tangential view demonstrates an irregular ("cloudlike") mass. *B.* Oval mass with heterogenous echotexture and focal areas of hyperechogenicity (*arrow*). Category 4.

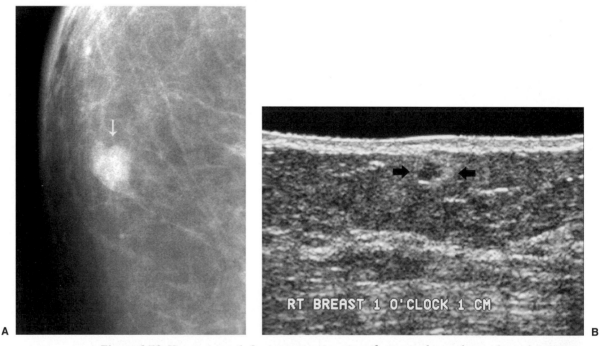

Figure 6.70 *Hemangioma. A.* Spot compression view of a screen-detected mass (*arrow*) in a 71-year-old woman. *B.* Ultrasonographically, a mass with a heterogenous echotexture is imaged corresponding to the area of mammographic concern. A central area of hypoechogenicity is almost completely surrounded by a thick rim of hyperechogenicity (*arrows*).

REFERENCES

1. Evans WP. Breast masses: appropriate evaluation. *Radiol Clin North Am* 1995;33:1085–1108.
2. American College of Radiology (ACR). *Breast imaging reporting and data system (BI-RADS)*, 3rd ed. Reston, VA, American College of Radiology, 1998.
3. Feig SA. Breast masses: mammographic and sonographic evaluation. *Radiol Clin North Am* 1992;30:67.
4. Cupples TE, Eklund GW, Cardenosa G. Mammographic halo sign revisited. *Radiology* 1996; 199:105.
5. Tabar L, Dean PB. Signs of primary importance in diagnosing circumscribed tumors. In: *Teaching atlas of mammography*. New York, Thieme, 1985:18.
6. Swann CA, Kopans DB, Koerner FC, et al. The halo sign and malignant breast lesions. *AJR Am J Roentgenol* 1987;149:1145.
7. Leung JWT, Sickles EA. Multiple bilateral masses detected on screening mammography: assessment of need for recall imaging. *AJR Am J Roentgenol* 2000;175:23–29.
8. Mendelson EB, Tobin CE. Critical pathways in using breast US. *Radiographics* 1995;15: 935–945.
9. Fornage BD, Tassin GB. Sonographic appearance of superficial soft tissue lipomas. *J Clin Ultrasound* 1991;19:215–220.
10. Tavassoli FA. *Pathology of the breast*, 2nd ed. New York: McGraw-Hill, 1999.
11. Rosen PP. *Rosen's breast pathology*, 2nd ed. Philadelphia: Lippincott Williams & Wilkins, 2001.
12. Pollack AH, Kuerer HM. Steatocystoma multiplex: appearance at mammography. *Radiology* 1991;180:836–838.
13. Mester J, Darwish M, Deshmukh SM. Steatocystoma multiplex of the breast: mammographic and sonography findings. *AJR Am J Roentgenol* 1998;170:115–116.
14. Murphy TJ, Mowad CM, Feig SA, et al. Breast imaging case of the day. *Radiographics* 1998;18: 536.
15. Leibman AJ, Wong R. Findings on mammography in the axilla. *AJR Am J Roentgenol* 1997;169: 1385–1390.
16. Bruwer A, Nelson G, Spark R. Punctate intranodal gold deposits simulating microcalcifications on mammograms. *Radiology* 1987,163:87–88.
17. Lee CH, Giurescu ME, Philpotts LE, et al. Clinical importance of unilaterally enlarging lymph nodes on otherwise normal mammograms. *Radiology* 1997;203:329–334.
18. Dershaw DD, Selland D, Tan LK, et al. Spiculated axillary adenopathy. *Radiology* 1996;201: 439–442.
19. Walsh R, Kornguth PJ, Scott Soo M, et al. Axillary lymph nodes: Mammographic, pathologic and clinical correlation. *AJR Am J Roentgenol* 1997;168:33–38.
20. Mester J, Simmons RM, Vazquez MF, et al. In situ and infiltrating ductal carcinoma arising in a breast hamartoma. *AJR Am J Roentgenol* 2000;175:64–66.
21. Hogge JP, Robinson RE, Magnant CM, et al. The mammographic spectrum of fat necrosis in the breast. *Radiographics* 1995;15:1347–1356.
22. Scott Soo M, Kornguth PJ, Hertzberg BS. Fat necrosis in the breast: sonographic features. *Radiology* 1998;206:261–269.
23. Elston CW, Ellis IO, eds. *The breast*, 3rd ed. Edinburgh: Churchill Livingstone, 1998.
24. Fornage BD, Lorigan JG, Andrey E. Fibroadenomas of the breast: sonographic appearance. *Radiology* 1989;172:671–675.
25. Dupont WD, Page DL, Parl FF, et al. Long-term risk of breast cancer in women with fibroadenoma. *N Engl J Med* 1994;331:10–15.
26. Scott Soo M, Dash M, Bentley R, et al. Tubular adenomas of the breast: imaging findings with histologic correlation. *AJR Am J Radiol* 2000;174:757–761.
27. Sumkin JH, Perrone AM, Harris KM, et al. Lactating adenoma: US features and literature review. *Radiology* 1998;206:271.
28. Liberman L, Bonaccio E, Hamele-Bena D, et al. Benign and malignant phyllodes tumors: mammographic and sonographic findings. *Radiology* 1996;198:121–124.
29. Czumm JM, Sanders LM, Titus JM, et al. Breast imaging case of the day (phyllodes). *Radiographics* 1997;17:448.
30. Cardenosa G, Doudna C, Eklund GW. Ductography of the breast: technique and findings. *AJR Am J Roentgenol* 1994;162:1081.
31. Cardenosa G, Eklund GW. Benign papillary neoplasms of the breast: mammographic findings. *Radiology* 1991;181:751.

32. Venta LA, Wiley EL, Gabriel H, et al. Imaging features of focal breast fibrosis: mammographic-pathologic correlation of noncalcified breast lesions. *AJR Am J Roentgenol* 1999;173:309–316.
33. Rosen EL, Soo MS, Bentley RC. Focal fibrosis: a common breast lesion diagnosed at imaging-guided core biopsy. *AJR Am J Roentgenol* 1999;173:1657–1662.
34. Harvey SC, Denison CM, Lester SC, et al. Fibrous nodules found at large-core needle biopsy of the breast: imaging features. *Radiology* 1999;211:535–540.
35. Revelon G, Sherman ME, Gatewood OMB, et al. Focal fibrosis of the breast: imaging characteristics and histopathological correlation. *Radiology* 2000;216:255–259.
36. Sklair-Levy M, Samuels TH, Catzavelos C, et al. Stromal fibrosis of the breast. *AJR Am J Roentgenol* 2001;177:573–577.
37. Piccoli CW, Feig SA, Palazzo JP. Developing asymmetric density. *Radiology* 1999;211:111–117.
38. Westinghouse Logan W, Hoffman Y. Diabetic fibrous breast disease. *Radiology* 1989;172:667–670.
39. Weinstein SP, Conant EF, Orel SG, et al. Diabetic mastopathy in men: imaging findings in two patients. *Radiology* 2001;219:797–799.
40. Ibrahim RE, Sciotto CG, Weidner N. Pseudoangiomatous hyperplasia of mammary stroma: some observations regarding its clinicopathologic spectrum. *Cancer* 1989;63:1154.
41. Cohen MA, Morris EA, Rosen PP, et al. Pseudoangiomatous stromal hyperplasia: mammographic, sonographic and clinical patterns. *Radiology* 1996;198:117–120.
42. Polger MR, Denison CM, Lester S, et al. Pseudoangiomatous stromal hyperplasia: mammographic and sonographic appearances. *AJR Am J Roentgenol* 1996;166:349–352.
43. Sewell CW. Pathology of benign and malignant breast disorders. *Radiol Clin North Am* 1995;33:1067–1080.
44. Tabar L, Dean PB. *Teaching atlas of mammography.* Stuttgart, Germany: Thieme-Verlag, 1985:88–89.
45. Mitnick JS, Vasquez MF, Harris MN, et al. Differentiation of radial scar from scirrhous carcinoma of the breast: mammographic-pathologic correlation. *Radiology* 1989;173:697–700.
46. Greenstein-Orel S, Evers K, Yeh IT, et al. Radial scar with microcalcification: radiologic-pathologic correlation. *Radiology* 1992;183:479–482.
47. Adler DD, Helvie MA, Oberman HA, et al. Radial sclerosing lesion of the breast: mammographic features. *Radiology* 1990;176:737–740.
48. Ciatto S, Morrone D, Catarzi S, et al. Radial scar of the breast: review of 38 consecutive mammographic diagnoses. *Radiology* 1985;187:757–760.
49. Cohen MA, Sferlazza SJ. Role of sonography in evaluation of radial scars of the breast. *AJR Am J Roentgenol* 2000;174:1075–1078.
50. Frouge C, Tristant H, Guinebretiere JM, et al. Mammographic lesions suggestive of radial scars: microscopic findings in 40 cases. *Radiology* 1995;195:623.
51. Nielsen M, Christesen L, Andersen J. Radial scars in women with breast cancer. *Cancer* 1987;59:1019.
52. Linnell F, Ljungberg O, Andersen I. Breast carcinoma: aspects of early stages, progression and related problems. *Acta Pathol Microbiol Scand* 1980;272[Suppl]:1.
53. Jacobs TW, Byrne E, Colditz G, et al. Radial scars in benign breast biopsy specimens and the risk of breast cancer. *N Engl J Med* 1999;340:430–436.
54. Brenner RJ, Jackman RJ, Parker SH, et al. Percutaneous core needle biopsy of radial scars of the breast: when is excision necessary? *AJR Am J Roentgenol* 2002;179:1179–1184.

MALIGNANT LESIONS

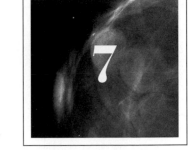

INVASIVE DUCTAL CARCINOMA

Invasive ductal carcinoma not otherwise specified (NOS), or no special type, is the most common type of breast cancer, representing 65% to 75% of mammary carcinomas (1,2). Patients may present with a hard, fixed, palpable mass that may cause skin thickening and retraction (Figure 7.1). When more advanced, breast cancer can deform the breast with a protruding, fungating (Figure 7.2), or ulcerating (Figure 7.3) mass. If the cancer develops close to the subareolar area, patients may describe progressive nipple inversion or retraction (Figure 7.4). Rarely, patients present with spontaneous nipple discharge, and less than 1% of patients present with metastatic disease to the axilla but no clinically or mammographically apparent primary lesion in the ipsilateral breast. In these patients, magnetic resonance imaging (MRI) may prove to be helpful in identifying the primary lesion (3).

With the increasing use of screening mammography, patients with invasive ductal carcinomas are diagnosed before signs of cancer are detected or symptoms have developed. A spiculated mass (Figure 7.5) is the most common mammographic finding in asymptomatic women. The mass may cause architectural distortion and have associated malignant-type calcifications indicating an associated intraductal component. Less commonly, invasive ductal carcinoma presents as a round or oval mass with well-circumscribed to ill-defined or indistinct margins (Figure 7.6A), focal parenchymal asymmetry (Figure 7.7), distortion (Figure 7.8), or diffuse changes (Figure 7.9). The density of the lesions is variable, and these masses can be low density (Figure 7.10).

In many women, the mammographic features of a mass (e.g., spiculated with linear, casting-type calcifications) are such that an ultrasound does not add significant information. In these patients, ultrasound is done primarily to help direct the imaging-guided biopsy. In other patients, however, ultrasonography is helpful and compliments mammography in characterizing lesions. As discussed in Chapter 4, when a patient presents with a palpable mass and dense tissue is seen mammographically at the site of clinical concern, ultrasonography is critical in the characterization of the palpable abnormality (Figure 7.11). On ultrasound, an irregular, ill-defined hypoechoic mass is often imaged corresponding to the mass seen mammographically or palpated clinically. Spiculation, microlobulation, vertical orientation, angular margins, calcifications, extension of tumor into ducts pointing toward the nipple, and branching of tumor away from the nipple with variable amounts of shadowing are additional findings associated with malignancy (4). In patients with predominantly fatty tissue, and less commonly glan-

Invasive ductal carcinomas, not otherwise specified, represent 65% to 75% of all diagnosed breast cancers.

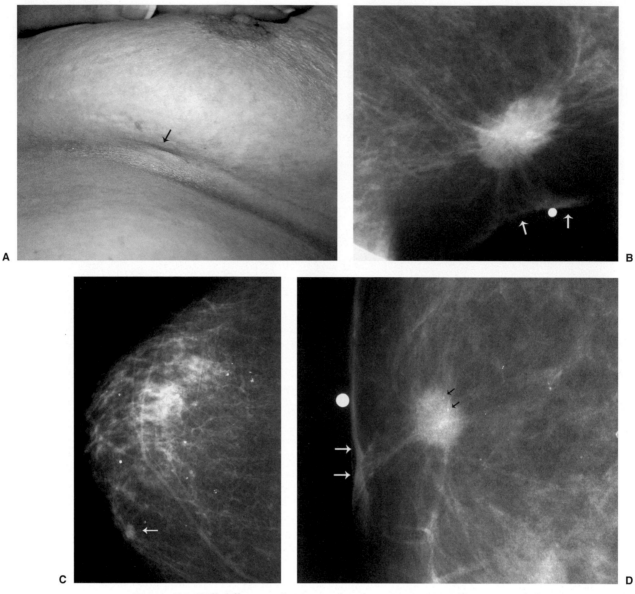

Figure 7.1 *Well-differentiated, invasive ductal carcinoma, not otherwise specified. A.* A 77-year-old patient presenting with dimpling (*arrow*) just above the inframammary fold on the left. In some patients, dimpling becomes apparent during compression. *B.* Spot tangential view taken at site of the dimpling. Spiculated mass with skin retraction and thickening (*arrows*). *C.* In an 84-year-old patient, the craniocaudal view identifies a mass (*arrow*) on the medial aspect of the right breast. *D.* Spot compression view demonstrates spiculated mass with associated calcifications (*black arrows*), skin thickening, and retraction (*white arrows*).

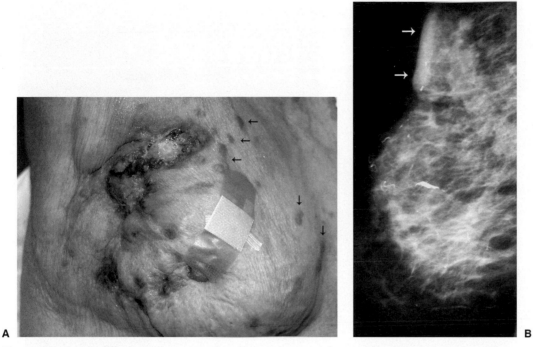

A   B

Figure 7.2 *Poorly differentiated, invasive ductal carcinoma, not otherwise specified. A.* A 97-year-old patient with advanced breast cancer. Marked deformity of the right breast is seen with ulceration. Small erythematous nodules (*black arrows*) represent skin metastases. *B.* Diffusely abnormal mammogram with decreased compressibility of the breast as well as skin and trabecular thickening. Prominent skin changes are noted at the site of ulceration (*arrows*). Some of the mammographic findings may be attributable to ipsilateral axillary adenopathy with resultant lymphatic obstruction.

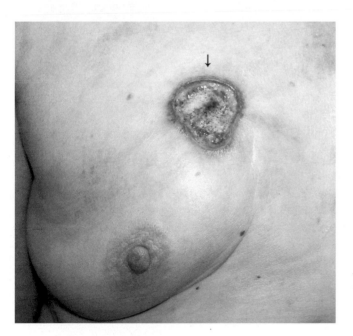

Figure 7.3 *Moderately differentiated invasive ductal carcinoma, not otherwise specified.* A 78-year-old patient with ulceration (*arrow*) secondary to underlying advanced breast cancer.

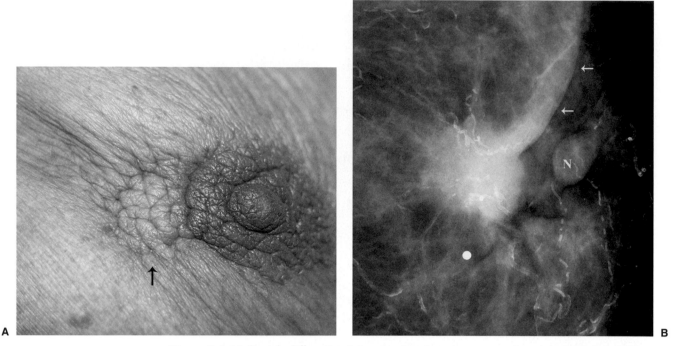

Figure 7.4 *Moderately differentiated, invasive ductal carcinoma, not otherwise specified. A. A 90-year-old patient presenting with retraction and dimpling (arrow), left periareolar region. B. Spot compression view demonstrates ill-defined mass (metallic BB) with associated skin thickening and retraction (arrows) adjacent to the left nipple (N). Extensive arterial calcification is present.*

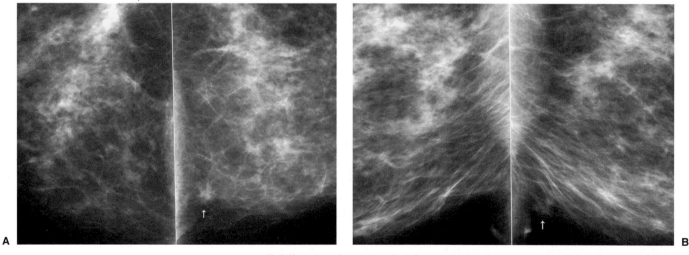

Figure 7.5 *Well-differentiated, invasive ductal carcinoma, not otherwise specified. Craniocaudal (CC) (A) and mediolateral oblique (MLO) (B) views in a 53-year-old patient. Screening mammogram. A possible mass (arrow) is detected medially on the left CC view. It is not definitely seen on the MLO view, however, it is suspected to be in the area just above the inframammary fold (arrow). Category 0: additional imaging evaluation is indicated.*

(continued on next page)

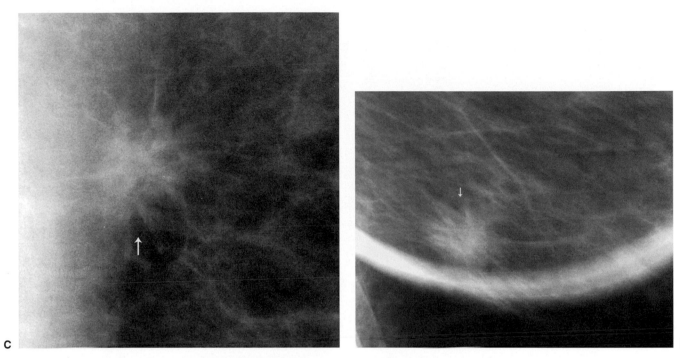

C   D

Figure 7.5 (continued) *C.* Spot compression view in the CC projection confirms the presence of a spiculated mass (*arrow*). *D.* Spot compression view in the MLO projection just above the inframammary fold demonstrates spiculated mass (infiltrative margins) in second projection (*arrow*). Category 4. Imaging-guided biopsy is undertaken using ultrasound (not shown) guidance.

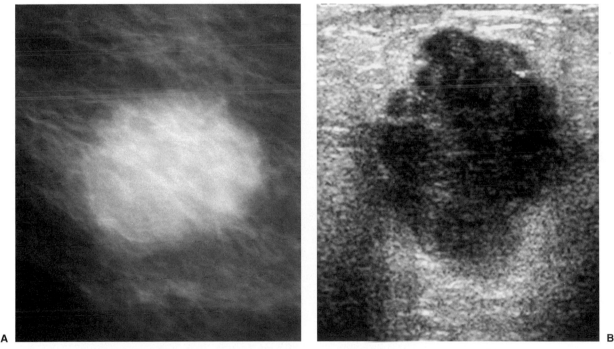

A   B

Figure 7.6 *Poorly differentiated, invasive ductal carcinoma, not otherwise specified. A.* A 45-year-old patient. Round mass with indistinct margins (expansile margins). *B.* Mass with heterogeneous echotexture; lobulated, angulated, ill-defined margins; and posterior acoustic enhancement. In our experience, many patients presenting with a round or oval mass (expansile margins) having posterior acoustic enhancement and marked hypoechogenicity are diagnosed with poorly differentiated, rapidly growing invasive ductal carcinoma.

(continued on next page)

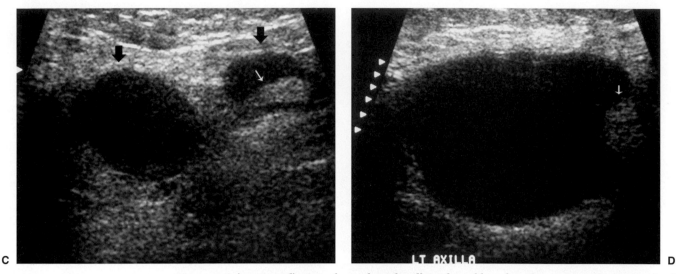

C

D

Figure 7.6 (continued) *C.* In the ipsilateral axilla, enlarged lymph nodes are imaged, characterized by a bulging cortex (*black arrows*), marked hypoechogenicity, complete loss or attenuation (mass effect) of the central fatty hilum (*white arrow*), and posterior acoustic enhancement. *D.* Third node in axilla: enlarged, nearly anechoic with posterior acoustic enhancement (simulates a cyst) and marked attenuation of the fatty hilum (*arrow*). Breast primary and metastatic disease to axillary lymph node diagnosed on imaging-guided core biopsies. Patient treated with neoadjuvant therapy followed by surgery.

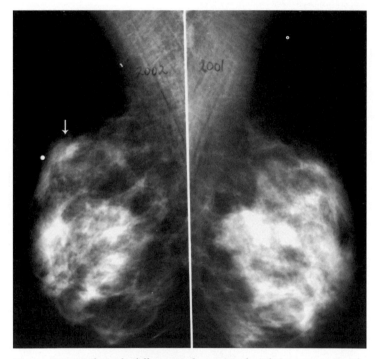

Figure 7.7 *Moderately differentiated, invasive ductal carcinoma, not otherwise specified. A.* Right mediolateral oblique views from 2002 and 2001 back to back. Patient presents with a lump in the right breast (metallic BB marks area). Focal parenchyma asymmetry (*arrow*) is developing compared with previous study and corresponds to area of clinical concern. Palpable areas of focal parenchymal asymmetry require spot compression views, correlative physical examination, and ultrasound evaluation.

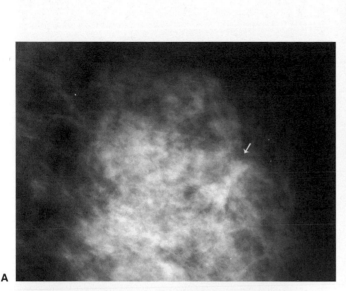

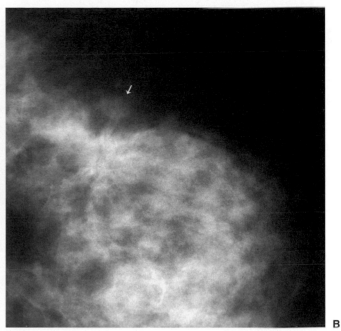

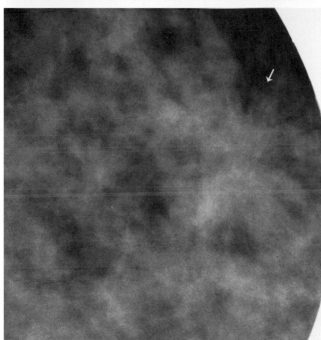

Figure 7.8 *Moderately differentiated, invasive ductal carcinoma, not otherwise specified.* Mediolateral oblique (*A*) and craniocaudal (*B*) views. Screening study in a 52-year-old patient. Possible distortion is noted (*arrows*). As discussed for calcifications, detection of these areas in a background of dense tissue requires a specific search for distortion. Category 0: additional imaging evaluation is indicated. *C.* Spot compression and rolled views (only one shown) confirm the presence of distortion (*arrow*). Note straight lines at arrow tip. Category 4. Imaging-guided biopsy is undertaken under ultrasound (not shown) guidance.

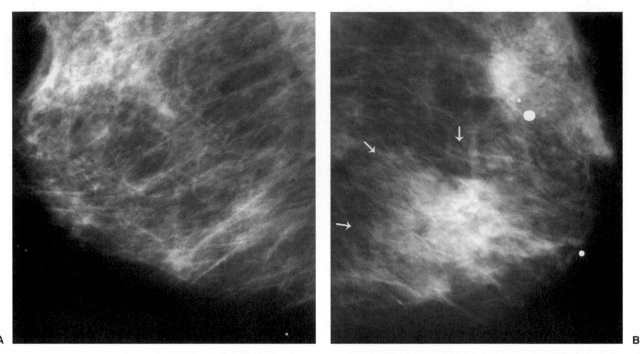

Figure 7.9 *Well-differentiated, invasive ductal carcinoma with associated intermediate-grade ductal carcinoma* in situ. Right (A) and left (B) mediolateral oblique views in a 67-year-old patient presenting with a palpable, global area of parenchymal asymmetry in the left breast. This breast is less compressible than the right and is perceived as smaller. Diffuse changes, with a global area of parenchymal asymmetry (*arrows*), are imaged at the palpable site (metallic BB).

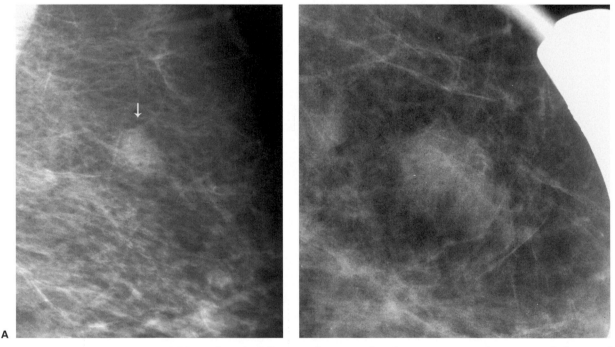

Figure 7.10 *Moderately differentiated, invasive ductal carcinoma, not otherwise specified.* A. Mediolateral oblique view in a 71-year-old patient. Low-density, round mass (*arrow*) is identified as new compared with the prior study. Category 0: incomplete; additional imaging evaluation is indicated. B. Spot compression views confirm the presence of a low-density mass (orthogonal view not shown) with indistinct margins. Category 4: biopsy is indicated. Although more commonly high in density, breast cancer can be low in density.

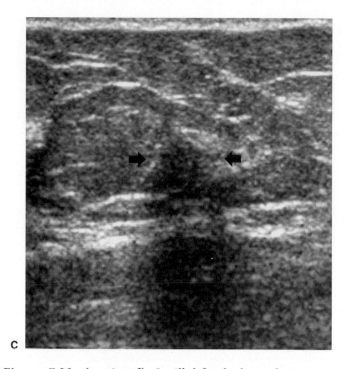

C

Figure 7.10 (continued) *C.* Ill-defined, hypoechoic mass (*arrows*) with associated shadowing corresponding to the mammographic finding. Incorporating information from prior studies, spot compression views, physical examination, and ultrasound is helpful in determining appropriate recommendations. Imaging-guided biopsy is undertaken.

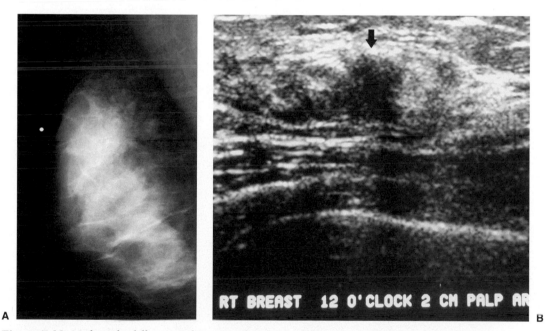

A   B

Figure 7.11 *Moderately differentiated invasive ductal carcinoma, not otherwise specified (NOS). A.* Mediolateral oblique (MLO) view in a 37-year-old patient presenting with a palpable mass; metallic BB marks the area. MLO and spot views (not shown) demonstrate dense glandular tissue. On physical examination, a hard mass is readily palpated at the site of concern to the patient. *B.* Irregular, hypoechoic mass (*arrow*) with angular margins is imaged corresponding to the area of clinical concern. Imaging-guided biopsy is done. In patients with a discrete palpable abnormality and dense tissue mammographically, ultrasound is indicated for further evaluation.

(continued on next page)

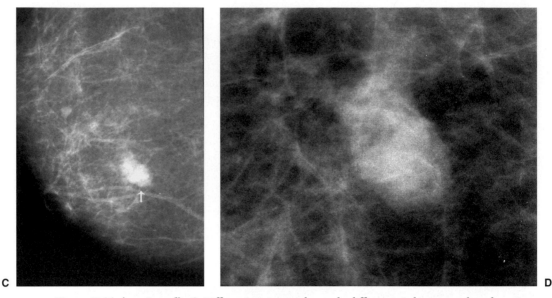

C   **D**

Figure 7.11 (continued) *C.* Different patient with poorly differentiated invasive ductal carcinoma, NOS. Craniocaudal view demonstrates oval mass (*arrow*) in medial aspect of the breast. *D.* Spot compression view confirms oval mass with indistinct margins. Seemingly normal tissue is seen on ultrasound. Because no cyst is imaged, it is presumed that the mass seen mammographically is solid and isoechoic with surrounding tissue. Stereotactically guided biopsy is done to establish the diagnosis.

dular tissue, the ultrasound study may be normal because the lesion is isoechoic to the surrounding tissue (Figure 7.11C, D). Many of our patients with invasive ductal carcinoma NOS presenting with a round mass (expansile margins), posterior acoustic enhancement and marked hypoechogenicity, have poorly differentiated, rapidly growing tumors (Figure 7.6B).

It is important to recognize that patients with breast cancer are at significantly higher risk for other lesions. *Multifocal* lesions are defined as multiple cancers occurring in the same quadrant (Figure 7.12), whereas *multicentric* cancers are those occurring in different quadrants of the involved breast. Bilateral cancers are *synchronous* (Figure 7.13) when diagnosed at the same time, or within 6 months of each other, and

> Dynamic contrast-enhanced MRI is emerging as a powerful tool that, when used in conjunction with mammography and ultrasound, can help establish the presence of clinically occult multifocal and multicentric disease.

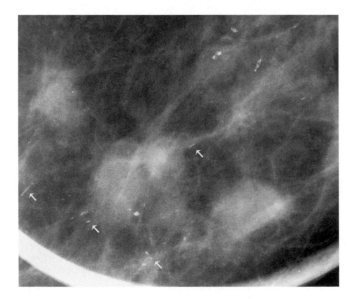

Figure 7.12 *Multifocal, poorly differentiated invasive ductal carcinoma with associated high-nuclear-grade ductal carcinoma in situ.* In a 67-year-old patient, a spot compression view demonstrates three masses with ill-defined margins and associated linear (casting) calcifications (*arrows*) consistent with the diagnosis of multifocal (same quadrant) invasive ductal carcinoma with associated intraductal carcinoma. Multicentricity is suggested when lesions highly suggestive of cancer are seen in separate quadrants.

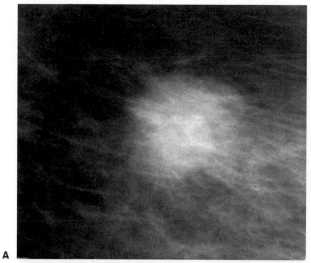

A

Figure 7.13 *Synchronous lesions, invasive ductal carcinomas, not otherwise specified; moderately and well-differentiated left and right breast, respectively.* A. Left breast. Mediolateral oblique spot compression view demonstrates mass with ill-defined margins. Having detected one lesion, *keep looking!* Remember that these patients are at increased risk for multifocal, multicentric, and bilateral disease. Mediolateral oblique (B) and craniocaudal (C) views of the right breast (only anterior portion of breast is shown). Anterior tissue is not well compressed, and there is the suggestion of "straight lines" (*arrows*). With what degree of certainty would you say there is a lesion at this site? Mediolateral oblique (D) and craniocaudal (E) spot compression views greatly simplify the situation. These demonstrate a spiculated mass (*arrows*). Bilateral ultrasound-guided (not shown) core biopsies are done.

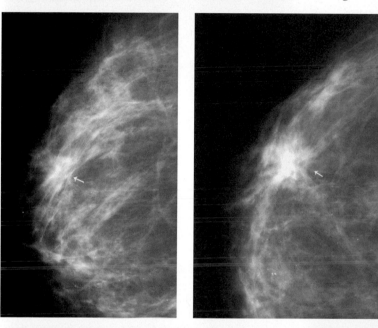

B

C

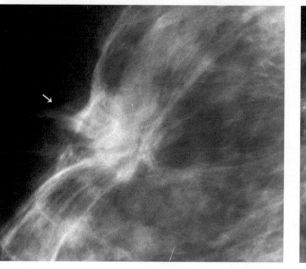

D

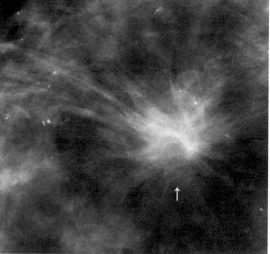

E

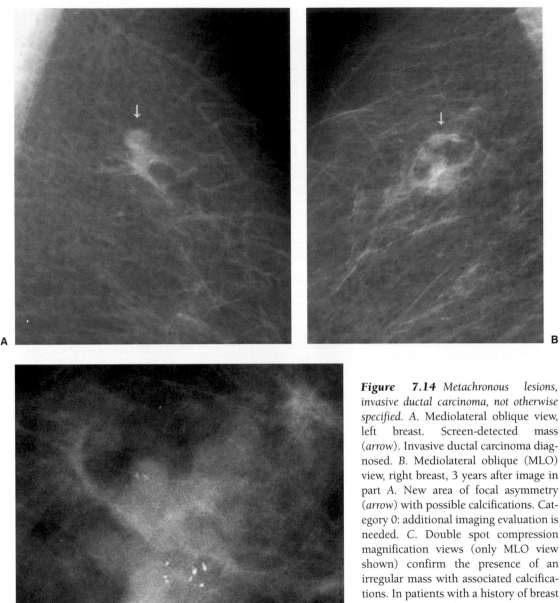

Figure 7.14 *Metachronous lesions, invasive ductal carcinoma, not otherwise specified. A.* Mediolateral oblique view, left breast. Screen-detected mass (*arrow*). Invasive ductal carcinoma diagnosed. *B.* Mediolateral oblique (MLO) view, right breast, 3 years after image in part A. New area of focal asymmetry (*arrow*) with possible calcifications. Category 0: additional imaging evaluation is needed. *C.* Double spot compression magnification views (only MLO view shown) confirm the presence of an irregular mass with associated calcifications. In patients with a history of breast cancer, aggressively pursue any perceived changes in the contralateral breast. In this patient, the second lesion is arising within tissue and has associated ductal carcinoma *in situ* consistent with second primary and not metastasis from the prior cancer.

metachronous (Figure 7.14) when they occur bilaterally at different times (diagnosed more than 6 months apart). The reported frequency of multifocality varies, depending on study design and meticulousness of histologic evaluation, and may be as high as 33% to 50% (5,6).

The described frequency of synchronous lesions is 0.1% to 2%, compared with 1% to 12% for metachronous lesions. The risk for subsequent breast cancer development among patients with a history of breast cancer is significant, and some of the factors to consider

---

Box 7.1: *Factors to Consider in Assessing Risk for Subsequent Breast Cancer Development in Patients with Personal History of Breast Cancer*

....

Tumor size
Degree of anaplasia
Location
Clinical stage
Family history
Multicentricity
Ductal carcinoma *in situ*
Premenopausal (younger patients)
Genetics: *BRCA1* and *BRCA2*
Peutz-Jeghers syndrome
Histology of lesion (greater incidence with tubular or invasive lobular carcinomas)

---

in assessing this risk are listed in Box 7.1. In the general population, 0.1% of women per year are expected to develop breast cancer. In comparison, the frequency of developing a second breast cancer among patients with a history of breast cancer is 0.53% to 0.8% per year (6). Nielsen and colleagues reported on 86 women with a diagnosis of invasive ductal carcinoma, in whom, at autopsy, invasive and *in situ* lesions were identified in the contralateral breast in 33% and 35% of patients, respectively (7). In a separate study done by the same investigators in an age-matched population, autopsy results identified 14 patients with *in situ* lesions and only 1 patient with invasive cancer among 77 women with no history of breast cancer (8).

When a patient with breast cancer develops a lesion in the contralateral breast, the second lesion may represent a second primary or a metastasis from the prior lesion (6). In considering prognosis and treatment options for the patient, it is important to distinguish between these two considerations (Figure 7.14). The features suggestive of a second primary are contrasted with the features suggestive of metastatic disease in Table 7.1.

In women with known invasive breast primary tumors, we routinely scan the ipsilateral axilla. Ultrasound evaluation in patients with suspected axillary adenopathy can be useful because it provides access to an area that may be difficult to evaluate mammographically. Ultrasonographic features of axillary lymph nodes that raise our concern include marked hypoechogenicity (in some patients, nearly anechoic) with through transmission, bulging cortex, mass effect, attenuation or obliteration of the

Table 7.1: *Features of Second Primary Tumor Compared with Metastasis from Contralateral Breast*

New Primary Tumor	Metastasis
Develops in tissue	Develop in fatty tissue (axillary tail)
Single lesion	Often multiple lesions
Spiculated mass (scirrhous, infiltrative margins)	Round mass (expansile margins)
Associated ductal carcinoma *in situ*	No associated ductal carcinoma *in situ*
Nuclear differentiation higher than previous primary tumor	

hyperechoic fatty hilum (Figure 7.6C, D), and increased blood flow. If a suspicious node is identified, a core biopsy or fine-needle aspiration is done at the time of the primary breast lesion biopsy. Patients identified with metastatic disease bypass sentinel lymph node biopsy and go on to have full axillary dissections at the time of the lumpectomy. When an abnormal intramammary lymph node is identified and found to be positive for metastatic disease, consider preoperative wire localization of the intramammary lymph node. These nodes are not routinely excised during axillary dissections.

Histologically, invasive ductal carcinomas, NOS, demonstrate variable growth patterns (infiltrative, expansile), cellular morphology, and no special features. Several grading systems are available based on tubule formation, nuclear morphology, and mitotic activity. Estrogen receptors are reportedly positive in 55% to 72% of lesions; however, poorly differentiated lesions are less likely to have estrogen receptors. Progesterone receptors occur in 33% to 70% of lesions, and about 15% of lesions are estrogen receptor positive and progesterone receptor negative (1,2,6).

EXTENSIVE INTRADUCTAL COMPONENT

Patients with invasive ductal carcinomas and extensive areas of associated intraductal carcinoma were initially thought to have a worse prognosis and were described as having a higher incidence of local recurrence after conservative treatment. This is probably related to incomplete resection of the lesion and residual disease in the breast (9). When lesions with an extensive intraductal component (EIC) are adequately resected, prognosis is not significantly different from that of women with lesions lacking EIC (10,11). When malignant-type calcifications are seen extending for a distance away from a clinically or mammographically detected mass (Figure 7.15), it is important to alert the sur-

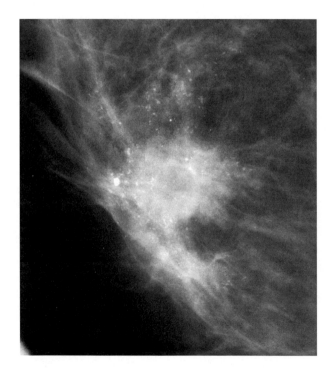

Figure 7.15 *Invasive ductal carcinoma, not otherwise specified, with associated high-nuclear-grade ductal carcinoma* in situ *(e.g., extensive intraductal component). A 55-year-old patient. When a mass is seen with associated pleomorphic and linear calcifications, an invasive ductal carcinoma (the mass) with an associated intraductal component (the calcifications) is the likely diagnosis. If extending away from the mass, it is important that the extent of the calcifications be determined with appropriate magnification views and that this be communicated to the surgeon and pathologist. Localization of the calcifications may be indicated for adequate excision.*

geon and localize the area (bracketing may be needed) so that the intraductal disease is resected with the invasive component. Definitions of EIC have varied. Currently, EIC is diagnosed when ductal carcinoma *in situ* (DCIS) constitutes 25% or more of the invasive tumor or when DCIS is present within and extends beyond the invasive component (1,2,6,12).

Ductal Carcinoma In Situ

As discussed in Chapter 5, DCIS is now most commonly diagnosed in asymptomatic women after the detection of calcifications on screening mammograms. Before the widespread use of screening mammography, however, DCIS was uncommon and constituted less than 5% of all breast cancers; patients presented with a palpable mass, spontaneous nipple discharge, or Paget's disease (13). Although uncommon (so much so that DCIS is rarely included in the differential of an uncalcified, mammographically detected mass), DCIS can be detected mammographically as an uncalcified, macrolobulated mass with partially distinct margins (Figure 7.16), a spiculated mass (Figure 7.17), distortion (Figure 7.18), or parenchymal asymmetry (Figure 7.19). These findings are attributable to the presence of markedly distended, cancer-containing ducts, in aggregate, and an associated periductal inflammatory process. Histologically, central necrosis may be present.

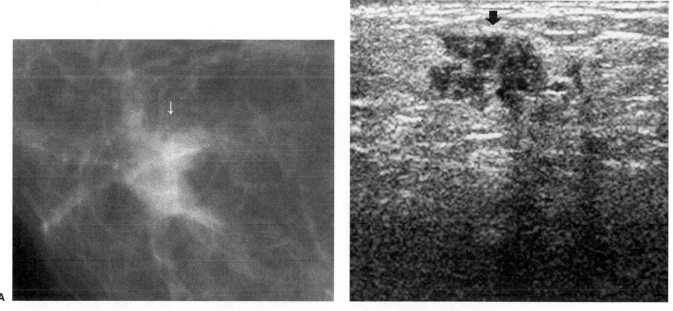

A   **B**

Figure 7.16 *Multifocal, high-nuclear-grade ductal carcinoma* in situ *(DCIS).* A. A 73-year-old patient with a screen-detected abnormality. Spot compression view demonstrates irregular, ill-defined mass (*arrow*) with lobulation in the medial aspect of the right breast. B. An irregular mass (*arrow*) with a heterogeneous echotexture is imaged in the upper inner quadrant of the right breast corresponding to the area of mammographic concern. Core biopsy under ultrasound guidance is done. Diagnosis of DCIS with no associated invasive disease is confirmed on excisional biopsy. Rarely, DCIS presents with a mass and no calcifications.

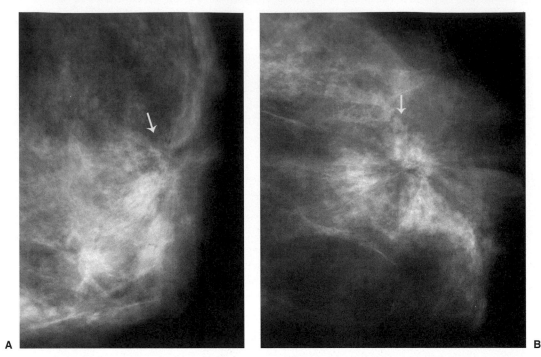
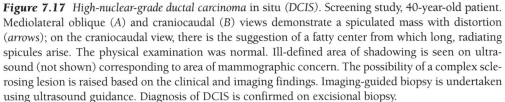

Figure 7.17 *High-nuclear-grade ductal carcinoma* in situ *(DCIS)*. Screening study, 40-year-old patient. Mediolateral oblique (*A*) and craniocaudal (*B*) views demonstrate a spiculated mass with distortion (*arrows*); on the craniocaudal view, there is the suggestion of a fatty center from which long, radiating spicules arise. The physical examination was normal. Ill-defined area of shadowing is seen on ultrasound (not shown) corresponding to area of mammographic concern. The possibility of a complex sclerosing lesion is raised based on the clinical and imaging findings. Imaging-guided biopsy is undertaken using ultrasound guidance. Diagnosis of DCIS is confirmed on excisional biopsy.

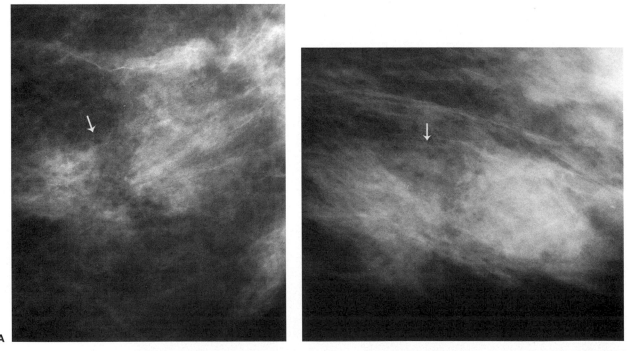

Figure 7.18 *High-nuclear-grade ductal carcinoma* in situ *(4.7 cm)*. Craniocaudal (*A*) and mediolateral oblique (*B*) views from a screening study in a 67-year-old patient. Distortion (*arrows*) is detected and confirmed on spot compression views with no history of surgery or trauma to this area. On the craniocaudal view, a fatty center with long, radiating spicules is noted. Physical examination and ultrasound targeted to the area of mammographic concern are normal. Given the mammographic appearance of the lesion in conjunction with a normal physical examination and ultrasound, a complex sclerosing lesion is the primary diagnostic consideration; however, a large area of ductal carcinoma *in situ* is diagnosed on excisional biopsy.

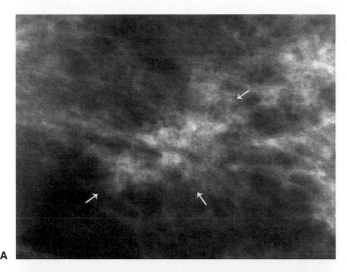

A

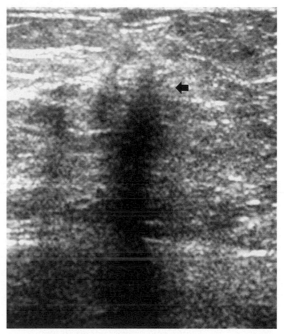

Figure 7.19 *High-nuclear-grade ductal carcinoma in situ.* Mediolateral oblique (*A*) and spot compression (*B*) views in craniocaudal projection demonstrate island of parenchymal asymmetry (*arrows*) with some distortion in a 58-year-old patient. *C.* Ill-defined mass (*arrow*) with shadowing corresponding to the area of mammographic concern. Imaging-guided biopsy is done using ultrasound guidance. Extensive DCIS with a 2-mm focus of microinvasion is reported on the excisional biopsy.

B

C

TUBULAR CARCINOMA

Tubular carcinomas are uncommon lesions representing less than 2% of all breast cancers. These are well-differentiated lesions considered as a subtype of invasive ductal carcinoma. The lesions are commonly diagnosed as small spiculated masses (Figure 7.20) or distortion (Figure 7.21) in asymptomatic women (14–18). Rarely, these lesions are palpable. Associated amorphous, pleomorphic, round, and oval calcifications (Figure 7.22) may be present because low-nuclear-grade DCIS lacking central necrosis is reported in as many as 65% of patients with tubular carcinomas. The pure form of tubular carcinoma is associated with an excellent prognosis: only about 10% of patients are found to have axillary metastasis at the time of diagnosis.

Histologically, there is proliferation of angulated, oval, and elongated tubules lined with a single cell layer. No myoepithelial cells are present. Mitoses are uncommon. Histologically, these lesions need to be distinguished from sclerosing adenosis and complex sclerosing lesions.

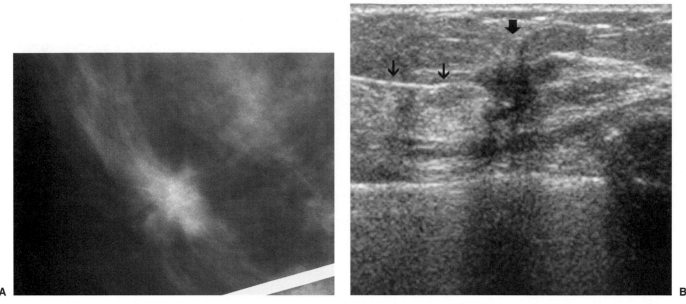

Figure 7.20 *Tubular carcinoma. A.* Double spot compression magnification view in the medial aspect of the right breast demonstrates a spiculated mass with no associated calcifications. *B.* Irregular, hypoechoic mass (*thick arrow*) with spiculation, angular margins, variable amounts of shadowing, and vertical orientation with disruption of ligament (*thin arrows*). Imaging-guided core biopsy diagnosis is confirmed on excisional biopsy.

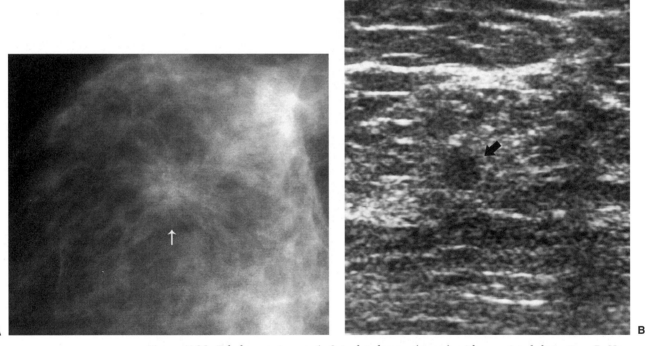

Figure 7.21 *Tubular carcinoma. A.* Spiculated mass (*arrow*) with associated distortion. *B.* Hypoechoic, vertically oriented mass corresponding to area of mammographic concern (*arrow*).

Figure 7.22 *Tubular carcinoma with associated low-nuclear-grade ductal carcinoma* in situ (*cribriform*). Craniocaudal (*A*) and mediolateral oblique (*B*) views from a screening study in a 55-year-old woman. Possible mass with associated calcifications (*arrows*). Category 0: additional imaging evaluation is indicated. *C.* Spot compression magnification view confirms the presence of a spiculated mass with associated distortion and punctate calcifications (*arrow*). *D.* Specimen radiograph demonstrating spiculation, distortion, and morphology of calcifications (*arrows*). Localization wire is partially seen. *E.* Different patient. Mediolateral oblique view from screening study in a 51-year-old patient demonstrates rounding of upper tissue cone (*arrow*); calcifications may also be present. Category 0: additional evaluation is indicated. *F.* Spot compression magnification view confirming the presence of a spiculated mass (*white arrow*) with low-density amorphous calcifications (*black arrows*).

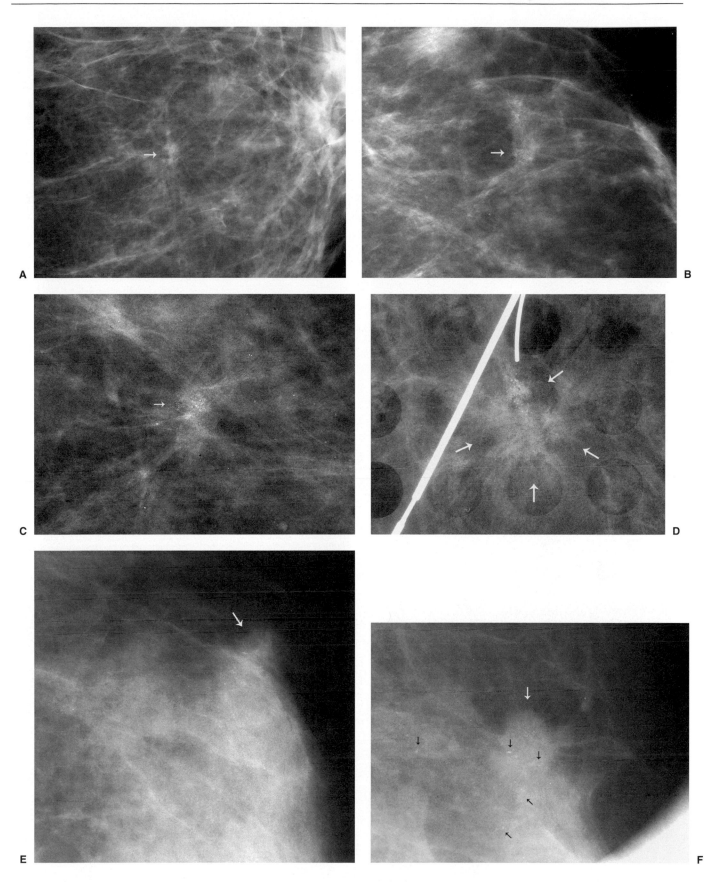

MUCINOUS CARCINOMA

Mucinous carcinomas are a subtype of invasive ductal carcinoma. Although these tumors can present at any age, they are more commonly seen in older postmenopausal women. Patients can present with a palpable mass (Figure 7.23); alternatively, if asymptomatic, a round mass with well-circumscribed to ill-defined margins (Figure 7.24) is identified mammographically (19–21). Rarely, spiculation (Figure 7.25) or focal parenchymal asymmetry (Figure 7.26) may be seen. Many of these lesions are slow growing and as such may be seen on prior studies. A minimal increase in volume and loss of margin definition in a small, round mass in an older patient should suggest the diagnosis of mucinous carcinoma. Ultrasonographically, these lesions are well-defined, hypoechoic, or nearly isoe-

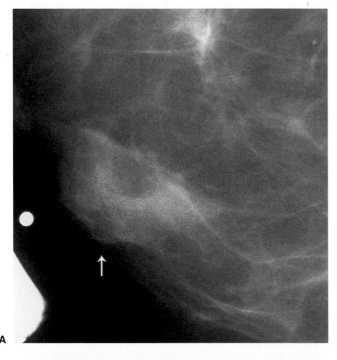

Figure 7.23 *Mucinous carcinoma. A.* Right breast. Spot tangential view of a palpable mass (metallic BB marks site) in an 84-year-old patient shows an oval mass (*arrow*) with indistinct margins. *B.* Ultrasound demonstrates a nearly isoechoic, superficial mass (*short arrow*) corresponding to palpable area. Pseudolesion is seen (*long arrow*) deep to actual mass; fatty lobulation changes and elongates as transducer is rotated over the site. *C.* Orthogonal ultrasound image demonstrating mass (*short arrow*) with a small anechoic area and elongation of pseudolesion consistent with fatty lobulation (*long arrow*). Imaging-guided biopsy is done.

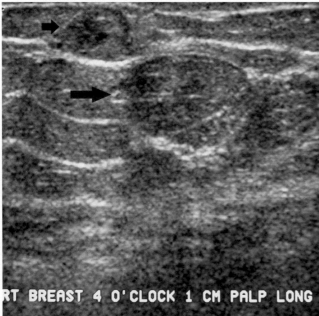

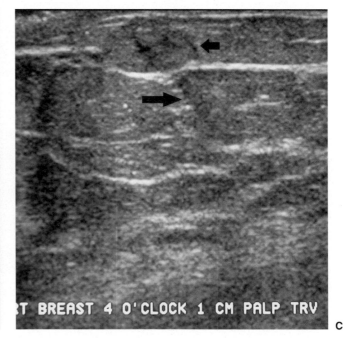

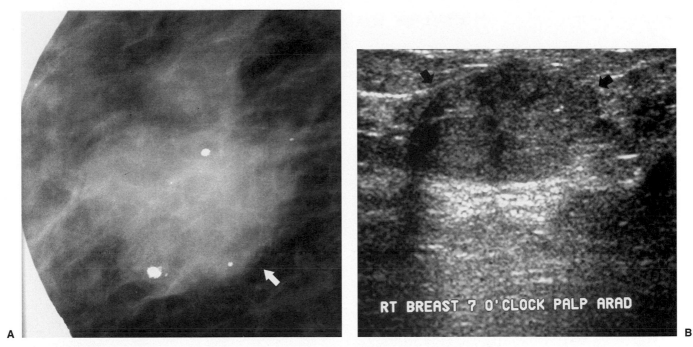

A
B

Figure 7.24 *Mucinous carcinoma.* A. Right breast. Spot compression view demonstrates an irregular mass (*white arrow*) with ill-defined margins in a 77-year-old patient. B. Oval mass (*black arrows*) with ill-defined margins, heterogeneous echotexture, and posterior acoustic enhancement. Imaging-guided core biopsy is done.

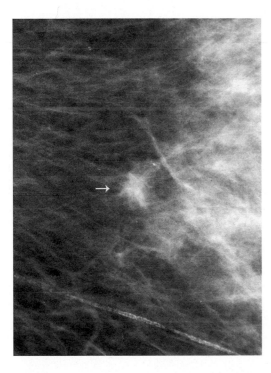

Figure 7.25 *Mucinous carcinoma.* Spiculated mass (*arrow*) with distortion in 79-year-old patient.

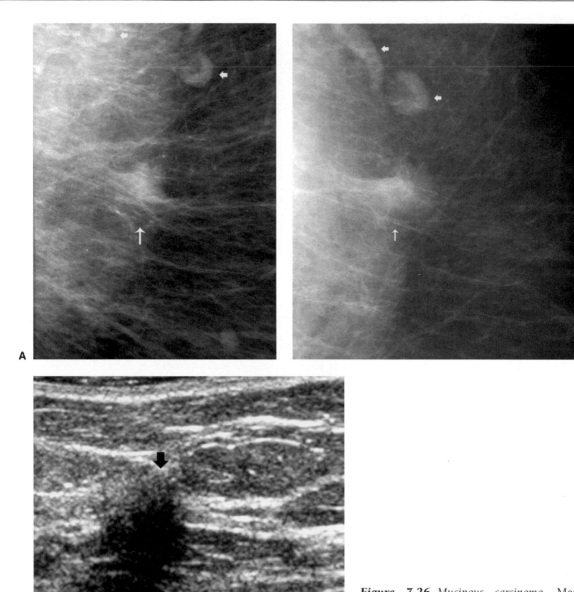

Figure 7.26 *Mucinous carcinoma.* Mediolateral oblique (*A*) and exaggerated craniocaudal (*B*) views demonstrate ill-defined, spiculated mass (*long, thin arrow*) in a 77-year-old patient. Benign-appearing lymph nodes with fatty hila noted (*short, thick arrows*). *C.* Ill-defined mass with vertical orientation and shadowing corresponding to mammographically detected abnormality (*black arrow*). Imaging-guided biopsy is done.

choic masses with variable amounts of posterior acoustic enhancement or shadowing. Although often homogeneous in echotexture, heterogeneity is sometimes noted. Rarely, a complex cystic mass is seen (Figure 7.27).

Grossly, core samples and the cut surface of these lesions are gelatinous and glistening in appearance. Histologically, aggregates of cancer cells floating in extracellular pools of mucin characterize mucinous carcinomas. The aggregates vary from dense to sparse cellularity, and fibrous septa separate the pools of mucin. Some mucinous carcinomas have associated low- to intermediate-grade DCIS lacking central necrosis; however, associated DCIS is not usually a prominent feature. In women with mucinous carcinomas, estrogen and progesterone receptors have been reported to be positive in 43% to 75% and 14% of patients, respectively. Necrosis is uncommon (1,2).

The cores obtained from mucinous carcinomas commonly have a distinctive appearance compared with those from other invasive lesions. These cores are gelatinous and crystal-like, and air droplets form on their outer margin after the cores are placed in 10% formalin (Chapter 11).

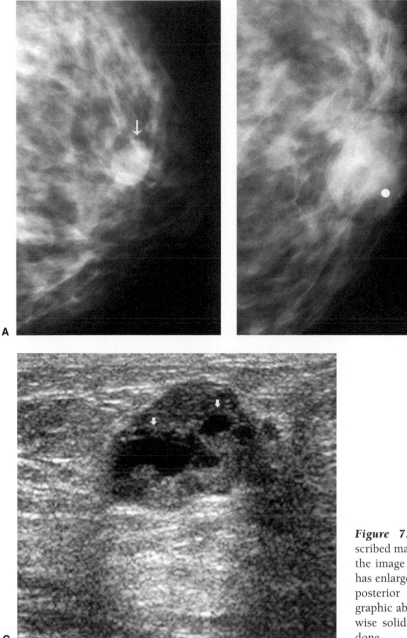

Figure 7.27 *Mucinous carcinoma. A.* Round, well-circumscribed mass (*arrow*) in a 78-year-old woman. *B.* Two years after the image in part *A*, the mass remains well circumscribed but has enlarged and is now palpable. *C.* Complex cystic mass with posterior acoustic enhancement corresponding to mammographic abnormality. Cystic spaces (*arrows*) are noted in otherwise solid mass. Imaging-guided core biopsy is subsequently done.

MEDULLARY CARCINOMA

Medullary carcinomas are a special form of invasive ductal carcinoma. The reported incidence is variable because of an overdiagnosis of this tumor type (22). When strict histologic criteria are followed, these tumors represent less than 2% of breast cancers. These tumors present as round or oval masses with well-circumscribed to ill-defined margins (Figure 7.28). On ultrasound, they are moderately to markedly hypoechoic with irregular margins; in some patients, posterior acoustic enhancement is noted (22,23). They may be palpable and can be characterized by rapid growth rates, at times presenting in young women as interval cancers.

Histologically, nests of large, high-grade epithelial cells with scant surrounding stroma form a syncytial pattern. Nuclei are pleomorphic, and there is a high mitotic rate. A significant lymphocytic and plasma cell infiltrate is present. Associated intraductal carcinoma is not common. Areas of necrosis may be present as the rapid growth of the tumor outstrips the vascular supply. Most of these tumors are estrogen and progesterone receptor negative (1,2).

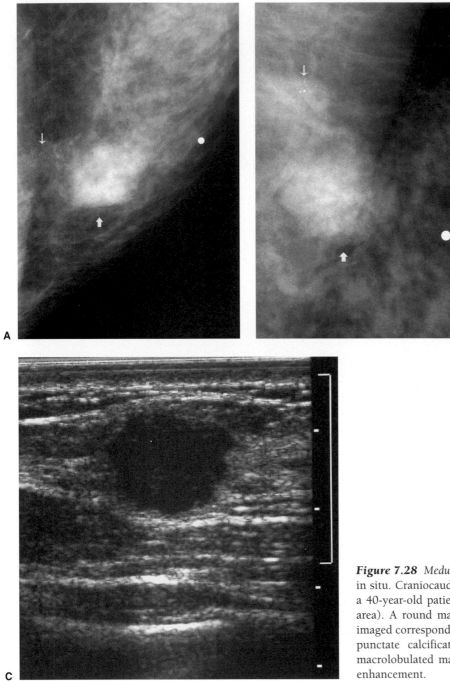

Figure 7.28 *Medullary carcinoma with adjacent ductal carcinoma* in situ. Craniocaudal (*A*) and mediolateral oblique (*B*) views in a 40-year-old patient with a palpable mass (metallic BB marks area). A round mass (*thick arrows*) with indistinct margins is imaged corresponding to the area of clinical concern. Associated punctate calcifications are noted (*thin arrows*). *C.* Round, macrolobulated mass with marked hypoechogenicity; minimal enhancement.

PAPILLARY CARCINOMA

Papillary carcinoma is common in older patients who present describing a palpable mass. In women with solitary papillary carcinomas, the mass is often subareolar in location and may cause nipple displacement and skin stretching. Mammographically, one of two patterns may be seen. Solitary papillary carcinomas are common in the subareolar area, presenting as a well-circumscribed, oval, round, or macrolobulated mass (Figure 7.29). A complex cystic mass is the most common ultrasonographic feature in these patients (24,25). Alternatively, multiple peripheral papillary carcinomas present as multiple, well-

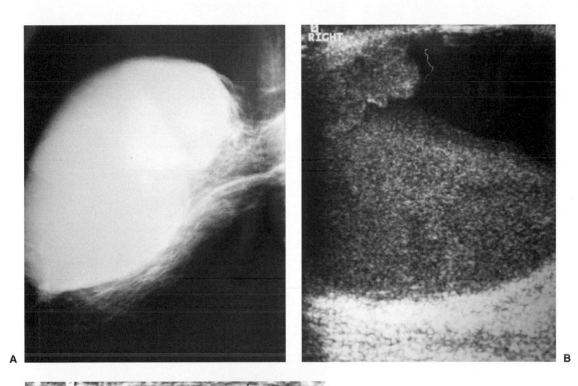

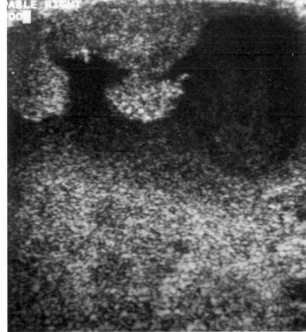

Figure 7.29 *Papillary carcinoma.* A. Medio-lateral oblique view in a patient presenting with a palpable mass that is smoothly protuberant; overlying skin thinning and stretching are noted on physical examination. Oval, well-circumscribed mass is imaged in the right breast. *B.* Complex cystic mass with posterior acoustic enhancement corresponding to palpable mass. *C.* Complex cystic mass, image through a different area of tumor.

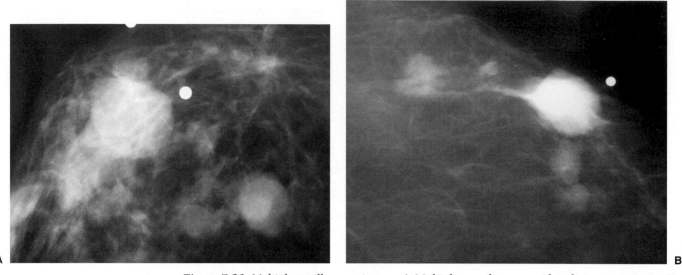

Figure 7.30 *Multiple papillary carcinomas. A.* Multiple round masses with indistinct margins in 69-year-old patient presenting with a palpable mass (metallic BB). Solid masses seen on ultrasound (not shown). *B.* A 74-year-old patient presenting with a palpable mass (metallic BB marks area). Multiple round masses with indistinct margins are present in association with the palpable area. Solid masses seen on ultrasound (not shown).

circumscribed to ill-defined, oval, round, or macrolobulated masses of varying sizes and densities (Figure 7.30). On ultrasound, these lesions are often solid and indistinguishable from any other solid mass; however, complex cystic masses may also be seen.

INVASIVE LOBULAR CARCINOMA

The incidence rates for invasive lobular carcinoma may be increasing.

Invasive lobular carcinoma represents about 10% of all breast cancers; it constitutes less than 2% of all breast cancers in women younger than 35 years of age and 11% in women older than 75 years of age. The sensitivity of detecting invasive lobular carcinomas using mammography and ultrasonography is lower than that for invasive ductal carcinoma; reported false-negative rates of interpretation range from 19% to 43% (26–28). In our experience, 66% of patients with lobular carcinoma are symptomatic at the time of presentation, and 41% have positive axillary lymph nodes at the time of diagnosis. Bilaterality is seen in as many as 28% of patients. Many of the tumors (up to 92%) are estrogen receptor positive (1,2).

Although there are variants, most lobular carcinomas are characterized by the migration of individual small cells through the stroma with little associated reaction or scirrhous change histologically. Clinically, mammographically, and histologically, the findings are subtle. The tissue feels thickened, and its consistency is different from that of surrounding tissue or the corresponding region in the contralateral breast; however, a discrete mass is not usually palpated. Histologically, the invasive cells can simulate lymphocytes, making the pathologic diagnosis difficult in some patients.

Among our patients, 41% have associated lobular neoplasia (i.e., lobular carcinoma *in situ*, or LCIS). This observation is interesting and hard to reconcile with what is reported on lobular neoplasia. LCIS is considered a premenopausal condition but not thought to be a premalignant lesion; rather, it is considered a marker lesion imparting one of the most significant lifetime risks for the subsequent development of an equal proportion of invasive ductal or lobular carcinomas in either breast. LCIS is thought to regress after menopause. Why, then, do as many as 41% of elderly patients with invasive lobular carcinoma have extensive LCIS in association with the invasive lobular carcinoma? Does LCIS not regress in all patients, or does it recur when invasive lobular carcinomas develop? Could it be a premalignant lesion in some patients?

In our experience, the mammographic presentation of invasive lobular carcinoma is variable and parallels what has been described in the literature (27–32). A spiculated mass (Figure 7.31) is seen in 40% of our patients, asymmetric densities (Figure 7.32) in 16%, architectural distortion (Figure 7.33) in 15%, and diffuse trabecular abnormalities leading to either a shrinking (Figure 7.34) or enlarging breast in 11% of patients. Less than 5% of invasive lobular carcinomas present as a round or oval mass. Although some authors have reported that some invasive lobular carcinomas present with calcifications, in our experience, calcifications do not occur in invasive lobular carcinomas. The malignant cells do not usually form any nests or spaces within which calcifications can develop. The cells invade individually. When biopsies are done for calcifications, the invasive lobular carcinoma is an incidental, unsuspected finding, and the calcifications are found in benign processes, including sclerosing adenosis, fibrocystic changes, and fibroadenomas. In about 3% of patients with invasive lobular carcinoma, the imaging studies are normal.

On ultrasound, significant shadowing can be associated with invasive lobular carcinomas. Alternatively, a hypoechoic mass with angular, ill-defined margins, spiculation, and shadowing (Figure 7.35) or a hypoechoic, lobulated mass may be seen (33). Commonly, the lesion seen ultrasonographically appears smaller than what is palpated. Some initial studies on the role of MRI show promise in helping determine the extent of disease in women with invasive lobular carcinomas. Additional studies are needed to elucidate further the role of MRI in patients with lobular carcinoma (34–36).

The metastatic pattern of invasive lobular carcinomas may be distinctive in some patients. Unlike invasive ductal carcinomas that tend to metastasize to solid organs, including liver, lungs, bones and brain, invasive lobular carcinomas may simulate ovarian carcinomas in their behavior. Studding of peritoneal and pleural surfaces is seen, with the development of ascites and pleural effusions; involvement of the leptomeninges, uterus, ovaries and stomach can also occur (37).

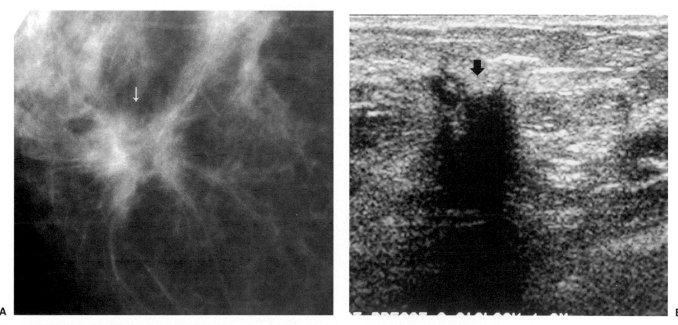

Figure 7.31 *Invasive lobular carcinoma. A.* Spot compression view demonstrating a spiculated mass (*arrow*) corresponding to a lump in a 42-year-old woman. *B.* Ill-defined mass (*arrow*) with vertical orientation, angular margins, and significant shadowing.

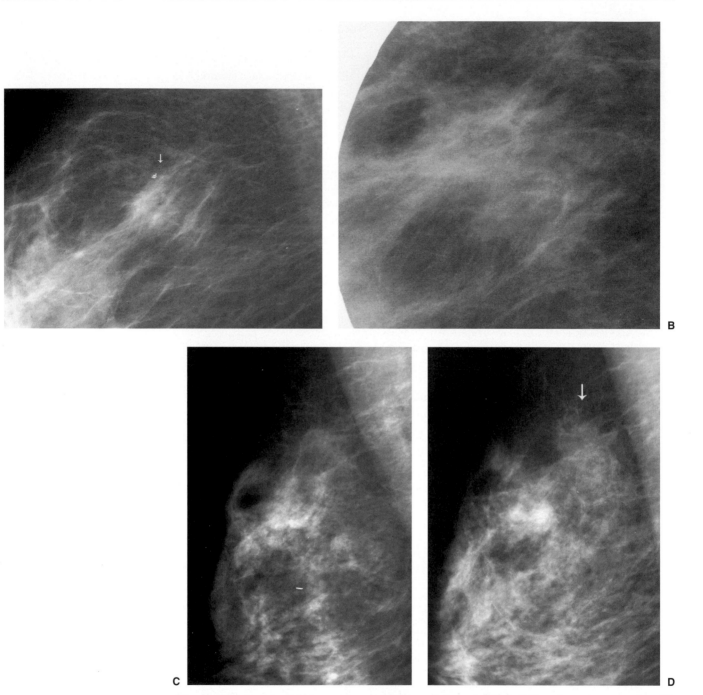

Figure 7.32 *Invasive lobular carcinoma.* Right mediolateral oblique (*A*) and spot compression (*B*) view demonstrating focal parenchymal asymmetry (*arrow*) in 74-year-old patient. As discussed previously, focal areas of parenchymal asymmetry require evaluation with spot compression views, physical examination, and ultrasound. Consider invasive lobular carcinoma when there are subtle mammographic and physical findings in older patients with focal parenchymal asymmetry. *C.* Different patient. Right mediolateral oblique view in a 54-year-old patient. Normal. *D.* Right mediolateral oblique view 1 year after image in part *C*. Island of developing asymmetry (*arrow*).

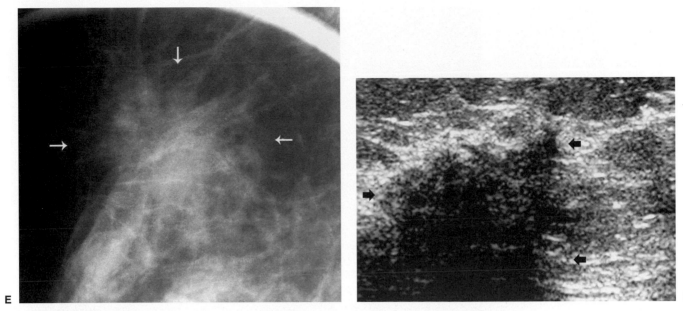

E   F

Figure 7.32 (continued) E. Spot compression view demonstrates focal parenchymal asymmetry (*arrows*) with associated distortion (*straight lines*). On physical examination, this area is thickened, and focal tenderness is elicited. F. Ultrasound in area of mammographic and clinical concern demonstrates an irregular mass with spiculation, angular margins, and significant shadowing (*arrows*). Ultrasound-guided core biopsy is done.

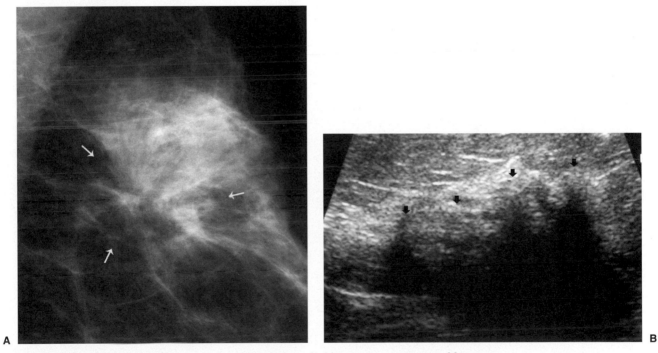

A   B

Figure 7.33 *Invasive lobular carcinoma.* A. Left mediolateral oblique view in 58-year-old patient. Architectural distortion is present (*arrows*). B. Ultrasound in area of distortion demonstrates irregular mass with significant shadowing (*arrows*). Diagnosis made on ultrasound-guided core biopsy. A 3.5-cm invasive lobular carcinoma confirmed on excisional biopsy.

(continued on next page)

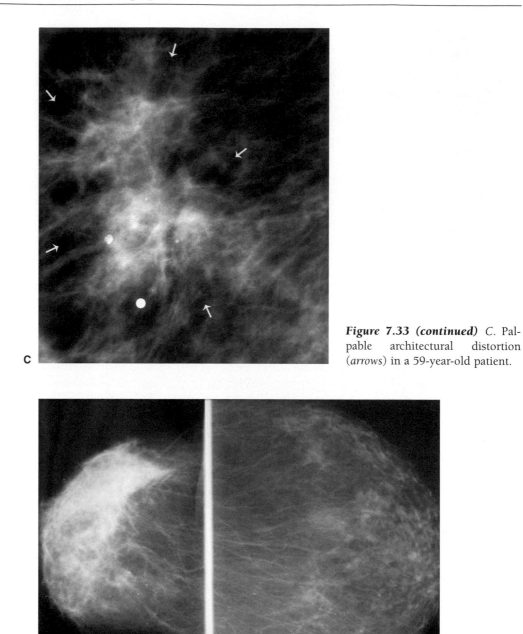

C

Figure 7.33 (continued) *C.* Palpable architectural distortion (*arrows*) in a 59-year-old patient.

A

Figure 7.34 *Invasive lobular carcinoma. A.* Right and left craniocaudal views. "Shrinking" right breast. Slowly progressive changes in density, compressibility, and perceived breast size are observed on the right.

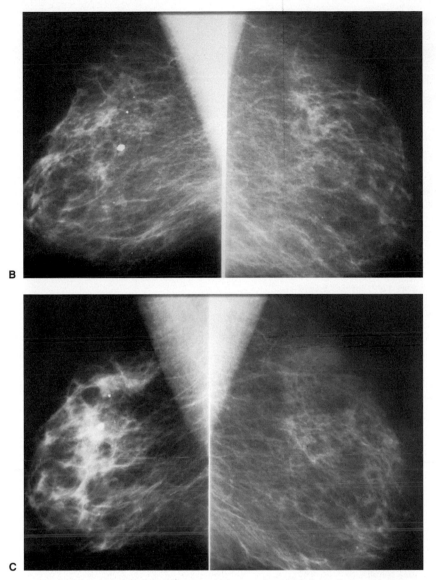

Figure 7.34 (continued) *B.* Different patient; right and left mediolateral oblique views. *C.* Right and left mediolateral oblique views 4 years after images in part B. Shrinking breast and slowly progressive changes in density, compressibility, and perceived breast size are seen. Subtle, diffuse changes are difficult to perceive from one year to the next. When comparison is made to a study from several years previously, the change is readily apparent.

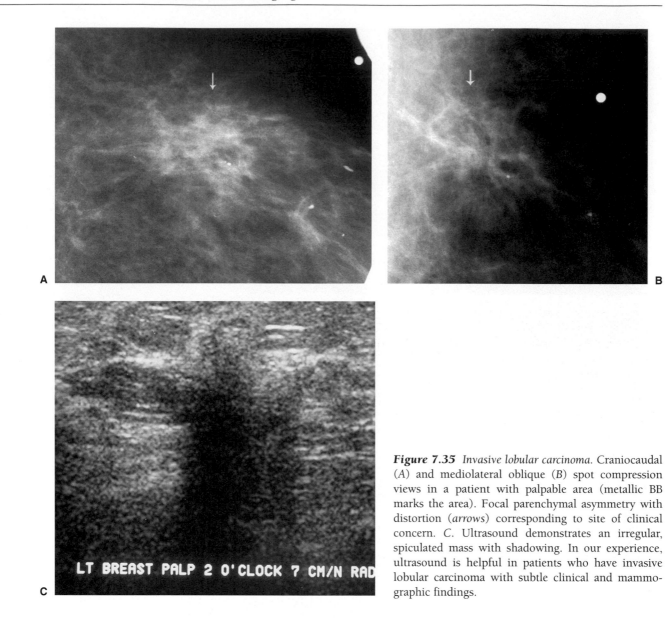

Figure 7.35 *Invasive lobular carcinoma.* Craniocaudal (*A*) and mediolateral oblique (*B*) spot compression views in a patient with palpable area (metallic BB marks the area). Focal parenchymal asymmetry with distortion (*arrows*) corresponding to site of clinical concern. *C.* Ultrasound demonstrates an irregular, spiculated mass with shadowing. In our experience, ultrasound is helpful in patients who have invasive lobular carcinoma with subtle clinical and mammographic findings.

LYMPHOMA

Lymphoma is considered primary to the breast when widespread or prior extramammary lymphoma is excluded; more commonly, lymphoma involves the breast secondarily. It represents about 0.1% of all breast malignancies. Patients present with single (Figure 7.36) or multiple masses with well-circumscribed to ill-defined margins or, rarely, diffuse changes (38). Calcifications are uncommon. At the time of presentation, axillary nodes are involved in 30% to 40% of patients (1,2). Bilateral disease is uncommon. Night sweats, fever, and weight loss have been reported in 6% to 20% of patients.

Two different patterns have been described. In the first group, a Burkitt's-type lymphoma presents during pregnancy or lactation with bilateral involvement and a rapid time course. The second pattern, usually with unilateral involvement, is a diffuse large cell lymphoma of the B-cell type involving a wider age spectrum. Primary breast lymphoma is treated like other extranodal lymphomas. After histologic diagnosis, the disease is staged, and radiation and chemotherapy are used.

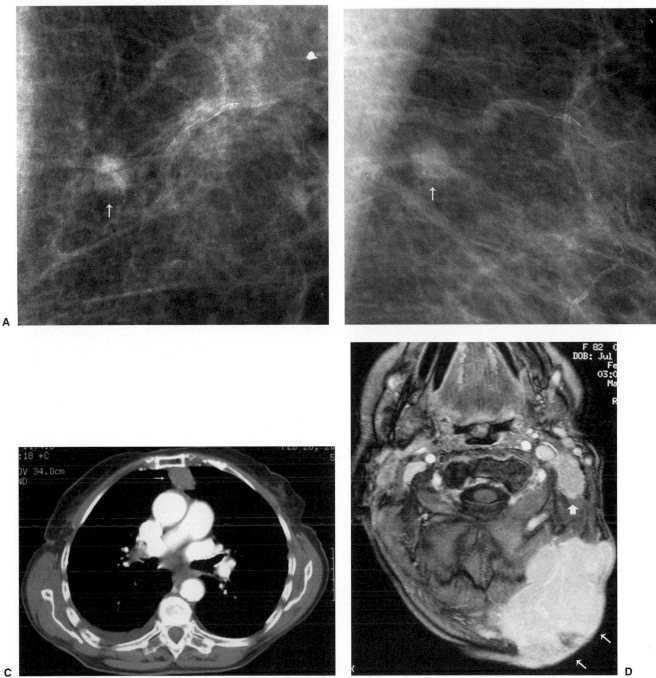

Figure 7.36 *Primary breast lymphoma.* Left craniocaudal (*A*) and mediolateral oblique (*B*) views in an 80-year-old patient. A mass (*arrows*) with indistinct margins is detected mammographically in the upper inner quadrant of the left breast. Low-grade lymphoma diagnosed on excisional biopsy of mass. Patient has no history of lymphoma, and all staging studies done at the time of diagnosis are normal. *C.* Two years after the initial diagnosis, chest computed tomography demonstrates a small pleural effusion on the right and anterior mediastinal adenopathy (*arrow*). *D.* Magnetic resonance imaging demonstrates scalp mass (*thin arrows*) and adenopathy (*thick arrow*) adjacent to left jugular vein.

(*continued on next page*)

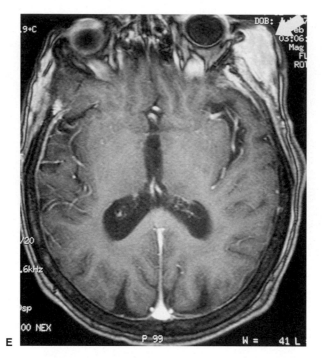

Figure 7.36 (continued) E. Additional soft tissue mass lateral to left orbit (*arrow*). Biopsy of the scalp mass is consistent with recurrent lymphoma. Lesion is now diffuse, large, B-cell type lymphoma.

SARCOMA

Malignancies involving the stromal tissues of the breast represent a heterogeneous group of lesions that are rare. Included in this group of lesions are malignant phyllodes

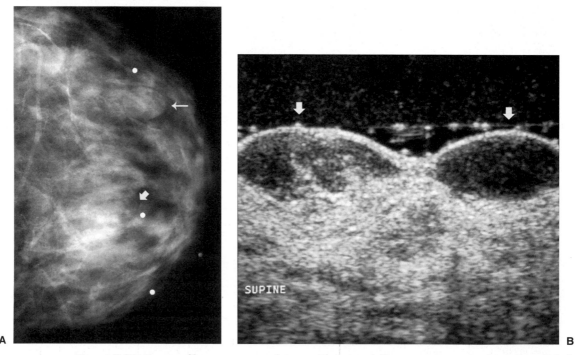

Figure 7.37 *Dermatofibrosarcoma protuberans with eventual fibrosarcomatous transformation.* A. Left craniocaudal view in a 31-year-old patient with multiple lumps. Well-circumscribed mass (*thin arrow*) corresponds to one of the palpable areas. Fibroadenoma diagnosed after excisional biopsy of this lesion. No definite mass is noted at second palpable site (*thick arrow*). B. Ultrasound using standoff pad to evaluate inner quadrant lesions. Two oval, well-circumscribed masses (*arrows*) are causing bulging of the skin. It is not possible to determine whether these lesions arise in the breast or the skin. Dermatofibrosarcoma protuberans is diagnosed on excisional biopsy. Although wider excision is strongly recommended, the patient refuses further evaluation.

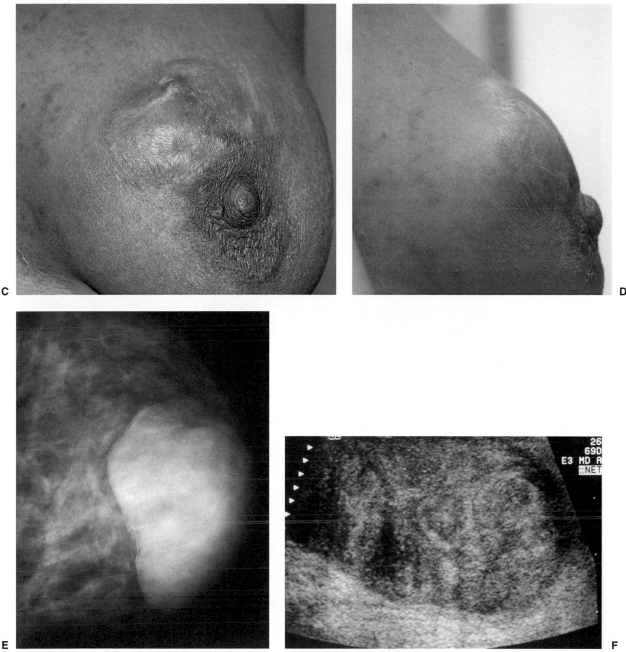

Figure 7.37 (continued) Frontal (*C*) and lateral (*D*) views of the patient 21 months after image in part *A*. A mass is visible in the upper inner quadrant of the left breast (at the site of the prior biopsy). The patient presents because of significant tenderness associated with the mass. *E*. Left craniocaudal view. Well-circumscribed mass is seen mammographically corresponding to area of clinical concern. *F*. Ultrasound demonstrates oval mass with heterogeneous echotexture and posterior acoustic enhancement. Biopsy at this time shows sarcoma (fibrosarcomatous variant) arising in dermatofibrosarcoma protuberans.

tumor, stromal sarcoma, fibrosarcoma, malignant fibrous histiocytoma, carcinosarcoma, granulocytic sarcoma (chloroma), leiomyosarcoma, liposarcoma, and angiosarcoma. Patients commonly present with a mass (39) that may be well circumscribed (Figures 7.37 and 7.38). On ultrasound, a solid mass with a heterogeneous echotexture and enhancement or shadowing may be seen. Alternatively, a complex cystic mass may be imaged. Axillary lymph nodes are usually not involved because these lesions spread hematogenously.

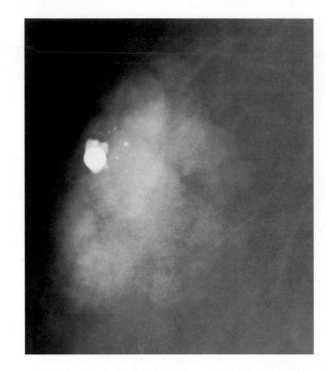

Figure 7.38 *Angiosarcoma.* Spot tangential view showing macrolobulated mass with cloudlike appearance sometimes seen with vascular lesions. Associated coarse calcifications. Some patients with angiosarcomas have bruit or bluish discoloration overlying the lesion.

METASTATIC DISEASE

The most common metastatic lesion to the breast arises from the contralateral breast through lymphatic channels on the anterior chest wall. Patients present with erythema involving the medial quadrants of the breast; some have nodules that may be ulcerative and associated with the erythema. There may be relative sparing of the skin overlying the sternum.

Extramammary metastases are usually hematogenous and represent 1% to 3% of all breast lesions. Hematopoietic and lymphoreticular lesions, such as leukemia and lymphoma; melanoma; and lung, ovarian, renal, bladder, colon (Figure 7.39), stomach, and cervical cancer have been reported. Single or multiple masses may be palpated. Rarely,

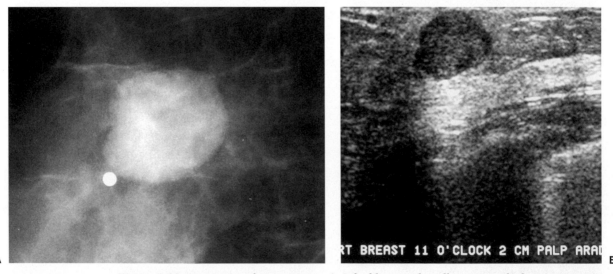

Figure 7.39 *Metastatic colon carcinoma.* A. Palpable, round, well-circumscribed mass in a patient with known colon cancer. B. Ultrasound demonstrates well-circumscribed, hypoechoic mass with posterior acoustic enhancement. Ultrasound-guided core biopsy is done.

lung carcinoma can extend through the chest wall to involve the breast secondarily (Figure 7.40).

Mammographically, single or multiple unilateral or bilateral masses are identified. The masses are usually round or oval with well-circumscribed to ill-defined margins. Solid hypoechoic masses with variable echotextures are seen on ultrasound (38). Because some of these lesions grow fairly rapidly, posterior acoustic enhancement may be seen, as may cystic spaces reflecting areas of necrosis.

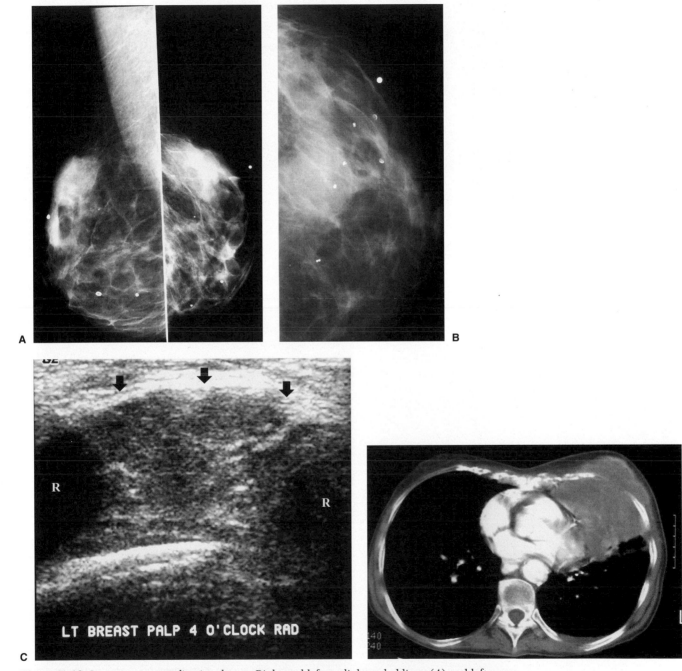

Figure 7.40 *Lung cancer extending into breast.* Right and left mediolateral oblique (A) and left craniocaudal (B) views in a 73-year-old patient presenting with a mass (metallic BB marks area) in the lower outer quadrant of the left breast. Positioning of left breast is limited secondary to presence of a mass. C. Ultrasound demonstrates soft tissue abnormality (*arrows*) between ribs (R). Site of origin is difficult to establish on ultrasound. Core biopsy suggests small cell histology. D. Chest computed tomography scan demonstrates lung cancer extending into left breast.

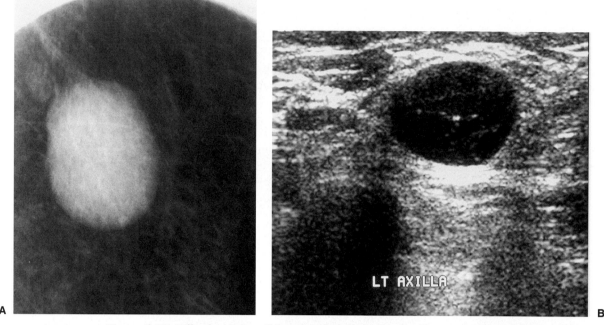

Figure 7.41 *Follicular center cell lymphoma, grade III (large cell).* A. A 74-year-old patient with new enlarged lymph nodes in the left axilla. Spot compression view demonstrates a well-circumscribed, oval mass. No fatty hilum is seen. *B.* A palpable round, markedly hypoechoic mass with posterior acoustic enhancement is imaged in the left axilla. No hyperechoic notch is seen. Additional enlarged lymph nodes are palpated in the left neck, and two masses are present in the scalp. Biopsy is indicated. Category 4.

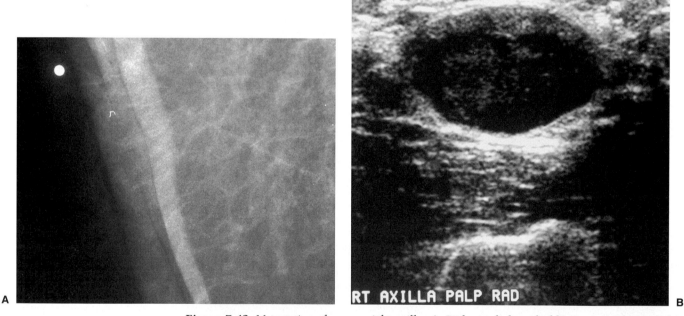

Figure 7.42 *Metastatic melanoma, right axilla. A.* Right mediolateral oblique view. Photographic cone of right axilla in a 35-year-old patient presenting with mass in right axilla (BB marks area). No focal abnormality is seen mammographically. Past medical history is notable for malignant melanoma removed from abdominal wall 3 years previously. *B.* Ultrasound evaluation of palpable area demonstrates oval, well-circumscribed, solid mass with nearly anechoic areas and posterior acoustic enhancement. Ultrasound is particularly useful in evaluating sites of clinical concern in areas difficult to image with mammography (e.g., axilla, upper inner quadrants, lesions close to the chest wall).

METASTATIC DISEASE TO AXILLARY LYMPH NODES

Lymphoproliferative disorders, including lymphoma and leukemia, can involve the intramammary or axillary lymph nodes. Although the lymph nodes are enlarged and dense, they may remain well circumscribed (Figure 7.41). Metastatic breast cancer usually results in ipsilateral enlargement of the axillary lymph nodes with ill-defined margins, spiculation, and matting. Metastases from nonbreast primary tumors, including melanoma, lung cancer, and ovarian cancer, can also involve the axillary lymph nodes (40–44). Rarely, unsuspected malignancies are detected because of enlarged lymph nodes (Figure 7.42). Although pleomorphic calcifications related to metastatic breast cancer have been reported, this is unusual and may reflect the presence of tumor necrosis from a breast primary tumor (Figure 7.43) or calcifications related to psammoma body formation from ovarian (45) or thyroid primary tumors (Figure 7.44).

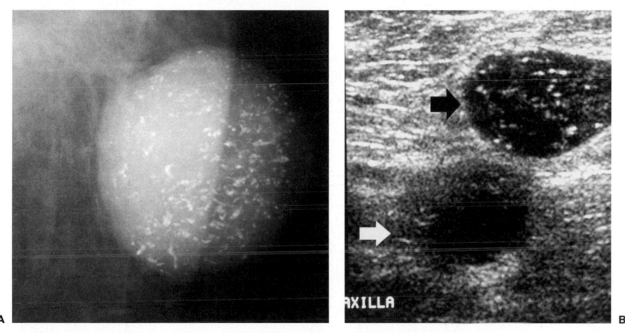

A   B

Figure 7.43 *Metastatic breast cancer from contralateral breast with calcifications in tumor necrosis.* A. A 50-year-old patient who underwent contralateral mastectomy (right breast) for inflammatory carcinoma 2 years previously. New, well-circumscribed, round mass with pleomorphic calcifications. Differential considerations include metastasis from the contralateral cancer or a new primary in the left breast with associated ductal carcinoma *in situ* (DCIS). B. Two masses are imaged on ultrasound. One of these has hyperechogenic foci consistent with the calcifications seen mammographically (*black arrow*). A deeper, irregular hypoechoic mass is seen with a nearly anechoic center (*white arrow*). An ultrasound-guided needle biopsy of the calcified mass is done. Metastatic breast cancer (similar features to contralateral inflammatory carcinoma) with calcifications in areas of necrosis is diagnosed histologically. No DCIS is seen. Also, note that the mass is arising high in the axillary tail of the breast with no surrounding tissue; this is consistent with metastatic disease (as opposed to a second primary tumor).

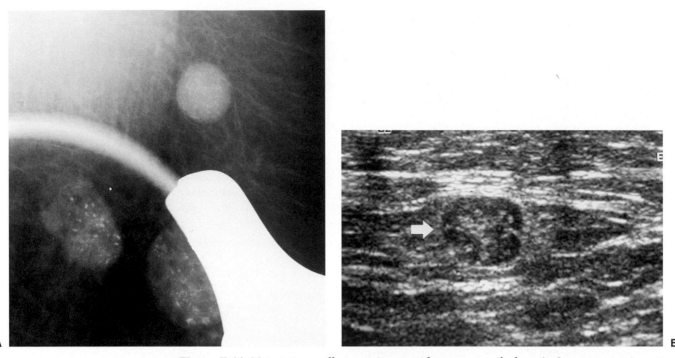

Figure 7.44 *Metastatic papillary carcinoma with psammoma bodies. A.* Spot compression view. Enlarged axillary lymph nodes with calcifications noted on screening mammogram in a 71-year-old patient. Spot compression views of the left axilla demonstrate three well-circumscribed masses with round, punctate, and amorphous calcifications. *B.* A hypoechoic mass with areas of hyperechogenicity consistent with calcifications is noted on ultrasound (*arrow*). Metastatic papillary carcinoma with psammoma bodies is identified; features suggest gynecologic serous papillary carcinoma or primary serous carcinoma of the peritoneum, which is diagnosed after ultrasound-guided core biopsy.

REFERENCES

1. Rosen PP. *Rosen's breast pathology,* 2nd ed. Philadelphia: Lippincott Williams & Wilkins, 2001.
2. Tavassoli FA. *Pathology of the breast,* 2nd ed. Stamford: Appleton & Lange, 1999.
3. Orel SG, Weinstein SP, Schnall MD, et al. Breast MR imaging in patients with axillary node metastases and unknown primary malignancy. *Radiology* 1999;212:543–549.
4. Stavros AT, Thickman D, Rapp CL, et al. Solid breast nodules: use of sonography to distinguish benign and malignant lesions. *Radiology* 1995;196:123–134.
5. Tinnemans JGM, Wobbes T, van der Sluis RF. Multicentricity in nonpalpable breast carcinoma and its implications for treatment. *Am J Surg* 1986;151:334–338.
6. Donegan WL, Spratt JS. *Cancer of the breast,* 5th ed. Philadelphia: WB Saunders, 2002.
7. Nielsen M, Christensen L, Andersen J. Contralateral cancerous breast lesions in women with clinical invasive breast carcinoma. *Cancer* 1986;57:897–903.
8. Nielsen M, Christensen L, Andersen J. Precancerous and cancerous breast lesions during lifetime and at autopsy. *Cancer* 1984;54:612–615.
9. Holland R, Connolly JL, Gelman R, et al. The presence of an extensive intraductal component following a limited excision correlates with prominent residual disease in the remainder of the breast. *J Clin Oncol* 1990;8:113–118.
10. Schnitt SJ, Connolly JL, Khettry U, et al. Pathologic findings on reexcision of the primary site in breast cancer patients considered for treatment by primary radiation therapy. *Cancer* 1987;59: 675.
11. Gage I, Schnitt SJ, Nixon AJ. Pathologic margin involvement and the risk of recurrence in patients treated with breast conserving therapy. *Cancer* 1996;78:1921.
12. Harris JR, Lippman ME, Morrow M, et al., eds. *Disease of the breast,* 2nd ed. Philadelphia: Lippincott Williams & Wilkins, 2000.

13. Haagensen CD. *Diseases of the breast,* 3rd ed. Philadelphia: WB Saunders, 1986.
14. Leibman AJ, Lewis M, Kruse B. Tubular carcinoma of the breast: mammographic appearance. *AJR Am J Roentgenol* 1993;160:263–265.
15. Helvie MA, Paramagul C, Oberman HA, et al. Invasive tubular carcinoma: imaging features and clinical detection. *Invest Radiol* 1993;28:202–207.
16. Elson BC, Helvie MA, Frank TS, et al. Tubular carcinoma of the breast: mode of presentation, mammographic appearance and frequency of nodal metastases. *AJR Am J Roentgenol* 1993;161: 1173–1176.
17. Sheppard DG, Whitman GJ, Huynh PT, et al. Tubular carcinoma of the breast: mammographic and sonographic features. *AJR Am J Roentgenol* 2000;174:253–257.
18. Mitnick JS, Gianutsos R, Pollack AH, et al. Tubular carcinoma of the breast: sensitivity of diagnostic techniques and correlation with histopathology. *AJR Am J Roentgenol* 1999;172:319–323.
19. Conant EF, Dillon RL, Palazzo J, et al. Imaging findings in mucin-containing carcinomas of the breast: correlation with pathologic features. *AJR Am J Roentgenol* 1994;163:821–824.
20. Wilson TE, Helvie MA, Oberman HA, et al. Pure and mixed mucinous carcinoma of the breast: pathologic basis for differences in mammographic appearance. *AJR Am J Roentgenol* 1995;165: 285–289.
21. Cardenosa G, Doudna C, Eklund GW. Mucinous (colloid) breast cancer: clinical and mammographic findings in 10 patients. *AJR Am J Roentgenol* 1994;162:1077–1079.
22. Liberman L, LaTrenta LR, Samli B, et al. Overdiagnosis of medullary carcinoma: a mammographic-pathologic correlative study. *Radiology* 1996;201:443–446.
23. Meyer JE, Amin E, Lindfors KK, et al. Medullary carcinoma of the breast: mammographic and US appearance. *Radiology* 1989;170:79–82.
24. Schneider JA. Invasive papillary breast carcinoma: mammographic and sonographic appearance. *Radiology* 1989;171:377–379.
25. Soo MS, Williford ME, Walsh R, et al. Papillary carcinoma of the breast: imaging findings. *AJR Am J Roentgenol* 1995;164:321–326.
26. Gisvold JJ. Imaging of the breast: techniques and results. *Mayo Clin Proc* 1990;65:56–66.
27. Krecke KN, Gisvold JJ. Invasive lobular carcinoma of the breast: mammographic findings and extent of disease at diagnosis in 184 patients. *AJR Am J Roentgenol* 1993;161:957–960.
28. Hilleren DJ, Anderson IT, Lindholm K, et al. Invasive lobular carcinoma: mammographic findings in a 10 year experience. *Radiology* 1991;178:149–154.
29. Le Gal M, Ollivier L, Assclain B, et al. Mammographic features of 455 invasive lobular carcinomas. *Radiology* 1992;185:705–708.
30. Newstead GM, Baute PB, Toth HK. Invasive lobular and ductal carcinoma: mammographic findings and stage at diagnosis. *Radiology* 1992;184:623–627.
31. Harvey JA, Fechner RE, Moore MM. Apparent ipsilateral decrease in breast size at mammography: a sign of infiltrating lobular carcinoma. *Radiology* 2000;214:883–889.
32. Evans WP, Burhenne LJW, Louba L, et al. Invasive lobular carcinoma of the breast: mammographic characteristics and computer-aided detection. *Radiology* 2002;225:182–189.
33. Butler RS, Venta LA, Wiley EL, et al. Sonographic evaluation of infiltrating lobular carcinoma. *AJR Am J Roentgenol* 1999;172:325–330.
34. Qayyum A, Birdwell RL, Daniel BL, et al. MR imaging features of infiltrating lobular carcinoma of the breast: histopathologic correlation. *AJR Am J Roentgenol* 2002;178:1227–1232.
35. Weinstein SP, Orel SG, Heller R, et al. MR imaging of the breast in patients with invasive lobular carcinoma. *AJR Am J Roentgenol* 2001;176:399–406.
36. Rodenko GN, Harms SE, Pruneda JM, et al. MR imaging in the management before surgery of lobular carcinoma of the breast: correlation with pathology.
37. Winston CB, Hadar O, Teitcher JB, et al. Metastatic lobular carcinoma of the breast: patterns of spread in the chest abdomen and pelvis on CT. *AJR Am J Roentgenol* 2000;175:795–800.
38. Bassett LW, Jackson VP, Jahan R, et al. *Diagnosis of disease of the breast.* Philadelphia: WB Saunders, 1997.
39. Liberman LL, Dershaw DD, Kaufman RJ, et al. Angiosarcoma of the breast. *Radiology* 1992;183: 649–654.
40. Neuman ML, Homer MJ. Association of medullary carcinoma with reactive axillary adenopathy. *AJR Am J Roentgenol* 1996;167:185–186.
41. Yang WT, Metreweli, Lam PKW, et al. Benign and malignant breast masses and axillary nodes: evaluation with echo-enhanced color power Doppler US. *Radiology* 2001;220:795–802.
42. Leibman AJ, Wong R. Findings on mammography in the axilla. *AJR Am J Roentgenol* 1997;169: 1385–1390.

43. Murphy TJ, Mowad CM, Feig SA, et al. Breast imaging case of the day (dermatopathic lymphadenopathy). *Radiographics* 1998;18:536–539.

44. Zack JR, Trevisan SG, Gupta M. Primary breast lymphoma originating in a benign intramammary lymph node. *AJR Am J Roentgenol* 2001;177:177–178.

45. Singer C, Blankstein E, Koenigsberg T, et al. Mammographic appearance of axillary lymph node calcification in patients with metastatic ovarian carcinoma. *AJR Am J Roentgenol* 2001;176: 1437–1440.

MISCELLANEOUS

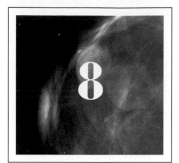

8

- Diffuse Breast Changes
- Dilated Vasculature
- Solitary Dilated Duct
- Mondor's Disease
- Parenchymal Asymmetry
- Paget's Disease
- Lobular Neoplasia

DIFFUSE BREAST CHANGES

Changes that affect the breast diffusely can be difficult to perceive mammographically, particularly if the process is bilateral and evolving slowly. Comparison with prior films can be helpful if studies are viewed in sequence. These changes are characterized by increases in the overall density of the breast parenchyma, thickening of the trabecular pattern (Kerley B lines) and thickening of the skin. In some women, increases or decreases (shrinking) in the perceived size of the breast accompany these changes. The overall compressibility of the breast may be decreased, and the techniques needed to penetrate the tissue and thickened skin increase. As the kilovoltage is increased to penetrate the tissue adequately, contrast decreases.

Ultrasonographically, skin thickening is appreciated readily, although it may require use of the standoff pad: the hypoechoic central band of the skin increases in width. The hyperechoic stripes superficial and deep to the hypoechoic band do not change in thickness. Skin thickening may be associated with dilated, anastomosing lymphatic channels seen as hypoechoic to anechoic, thin tubular structures just deep to the deep hyperechoic stripe of the skin. No flow is seen in these structures with Doppler. These changes may be associated with disruption of the normal breast architecture, increases in tissue echogenicity, and in some patients, focal findings. During real-time scanning, changes of pitting edema can be seen from the pressure applied on the breast with the transducer. Some benign causes of diffuse breast changes are listed in Box 8.1.

On physical examination, *peau d'orange* changes reflecting edema may be apparent diffusely involving the breast or, less commonly, localized to the dependent portion of the breast. Depending on the underlying cause of the diffuse change, additional findings may be apparent on physical examination.

Radiation therapy is probably one of the most common benign causes of diffuse breast changes. It is typically unilateral, limited to the treated breast. On physical examination, the breast is "tanned"; there may be associated tenderness, and surgical changes are present at the lumpectomy site and, commonly, the axilla. Distortion, spiculation, and metallic clips at the lumpectomy site (Figure 8.1) accompany the skin and trabecular thickening. Diffuse changes are typically seen in the acute setting and slowly resolve over the first 2 years following completion of therapy. Residual skin thickening is seen in 20% to 40% of patients 2 years after the lumpectomy (1,2). Increases in density, combined with trabecular and skin thickening, that develop after the first 2 years following radiation therapy need to be evaluated carefully and may warrant a biopsy to exclude recurrent disease.

Diffuse breast changes include increases and decreases in the perceived size of the breast and are often reflected by differences in the technique needed for adequate exposure.

Box 8.1: Benign Causes of Diffuse Breast Changes

Radiation therapy
Congestive heart failure
Superior vena cava (SVC) obstruction (SVC syndrome)
Axillary adenopathy with lymphatic obstruction
Trauma
Mastitis
Granulomatous mastitis (rare)
Giant cell arteritis (rare)
Scleroderma (rare)

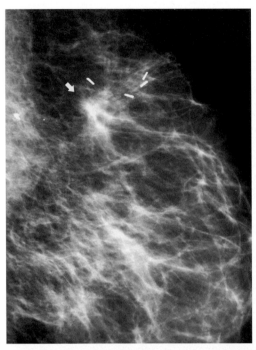

A

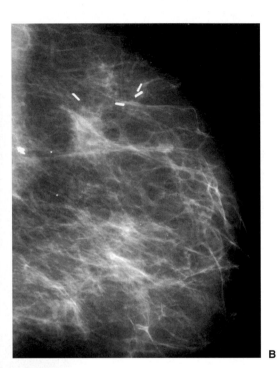

B

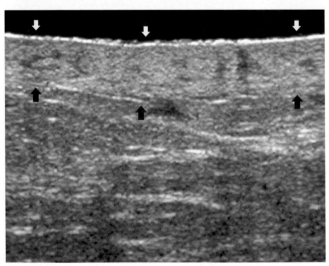

C

Figure 8.1 *Radiation therapy. A.* Increased density, diffuse trabecular thickening, distortion (*arrow*), and surgical clips at the lumpectomy site. *B.* One year later, the overall density of the parenchyma is decreased, and the trabecular pattern is less striking. The distortion at the lumpectomy site has decreased in size and density; surgical clips are again noted. *C.* Different patient. A standoff pad is used to evaluate skin. Skin thickening is seen on ultrasound (*all arrows*), and the hypoechoic band is thickened. The superficial and deep hyperechoic stripes are unchanged. Except in the acute setting, dilated lymphatics may not be seen in patients with a history of radiation therapy.

Patients with congestive heart failure can present with unilateral (Figure 8.2) or, more commonly, bilateral (Figure 8.3) diffuse breast changes, findings of peripheral edema, and shortness of breath. Obtaining technically acceptable images with no blurring is made even more difficult in these patients because of the shortness of breath. The breast is not usually very tender on exam. With successful treatment of the congestive heart failure and peripheral edema, the changes noted in the breast can resolve rapidly. If the patient is lying preferentially on one side for long periods of time, the edema may be more pronounced or limited to the dependent breast. With significant congestive heart failure, the periareolar region can become quite dense on the mammogram (Figure 8.3D); this is a finding we have not seen with many other conditions.

In more than 80% of patients, complete or partial obstruction of the superior vena cava is caused by superior mediastinal tumors, including adenocarcinoma of the lung, lymphoma, thyroid carcinoma, thymomas, and teratomas. Less common causes include chronic fibrotic mediastinitis that is idiopathic or secondary to tuberculosis, histoplasmosis, or drugs (e.g., methysergide); thrombophlebitis related to indwelling central venous catheters or pacemaker wires; aortic arch aneurysms; and constrictive pericarditis. Symptoms include swelling of the neck and face, headaches, visual disturbances, and obstructive venous drainage of the head, neck, and upper extremities. Facial flushing and dilation of anterior chest wall veins secondary to collateral flow may develop. Diffuse breast changes and dilated venous structures may be seen mammographically in these patients, more commonly involving the right breast; however, it can be a bilateral process. With a

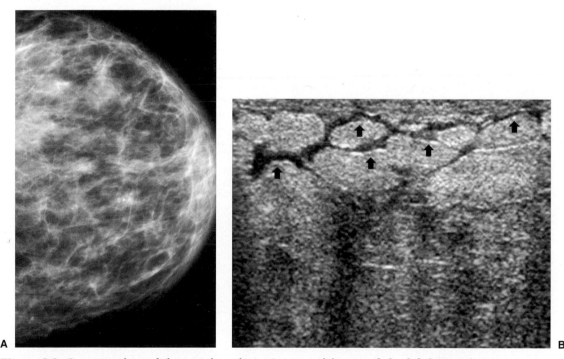

A   B

Figure 8.2 Congestive heart failure, unilateral. A. Craniocaudal view of the left breast shows increased density, diffuse trabecular thickening, and skin thickening (seen with a bright light) diffusely involving the left breast. The patient presents with shortness of breath, pitting edema, and enlargement of her left breast. She has a history of congestive heart failure. After questioning the patient, she describes favoring her left side because of a recent right hip fracture. B. Ultrasound shows anastomosing lymphatic channels (*arrows*) just deep to the dermis, which is a common finding in patients with edema related to congestive heart failure. The surrounding tissue appears hyperechoic.

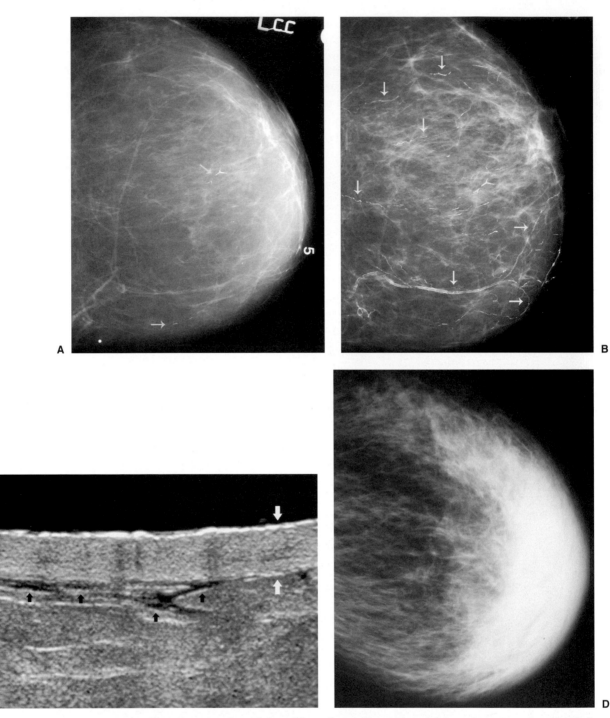

Figure 8.3 *Congestive heart failure, bilateral. A.* Left craniocaudal view shows a predominantly fatty pattern with some scattered, benign, large, rodlike calcifications (*arrows*) and no vascular calcification. The cassette number (5) can be seen on this view. *B.* Left craniocaudal view 4 years after image in part A. The patient presents with shortness of breath. Trabecular pattern is prominent compared with prior study, and extensive vascular calcification (*arrows* mark some of the calcified vessels) is now seen. No additional rodlike calcifications have developed. Although the right films are not shown, this is a bilateral process. *C.* A standoff pad is used to evaluate skin and subcutaneous tissue. Ultrasound demonstrates skin thickening (*white arrows*). Hypoechoic band is thickened. Superficial and deep hyperechoic stripes seen at the tip of the *white arrows* are unchanged. Anastomosing lymphatic channels (*black arrows*) are seen just deep to skin. *D.* Different patient. This 89-year-old patient presented with left breast swelling. Increased density, diffuse trabecular thickening, and marked thickness and density are noted in the periareolar region and anterior portion of the breast. Findings are bilateral, although less pronounced on the right (not shown).

similar mechanism, axillary adenopathy with lymphatic obstruction can lead to diffuse breast changes limited to the ipsilateral breast.

Patients with acute bacterial mastitis present with diffuse breast tenderness that may preclude an adequate mammogram because the patient is unable to tolerate significant compression. Diffuse changes may be present (Figure 8.4). On physical examination, the breast is erythematous and warmer than the contralateral breast. On ultrasound, skin thickening may not be a prominent feature; however, dilated lymphatics and disruption of

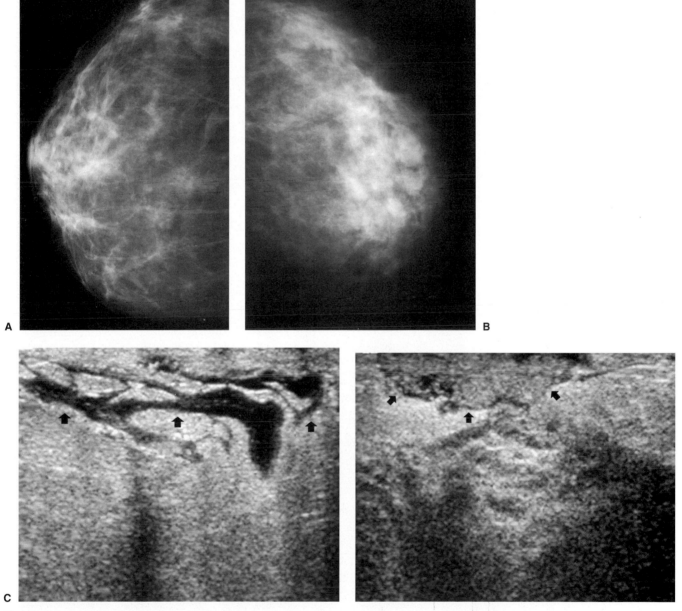

Figure 8.4 *Acute bacterial mastitis.* Right [kV(p), 26; mAs, 68; compression, 4 cm] (*A*) and left [kV(p), 34; mAs, 143; compression, 7 cm] (*B*) craniocaudal views in a diabetic patient presenting with the rapid onset of left breast pain, swelling, and redness. Increased density with decreased compressibility of breast. As the kilovoltage is increased to obtain an adequate exposure on the left, contrast decreases. *C.* Dilated lymphatic channels (*arrows*) are seen throughout all four quadrants. Surrounding tissue is hyperechoic, possibly reflecting edematous changes. *D.* In other areas of the breast, tubular-like areas of hypoechogenicity and hyperechogenicity (*arrows*) are seen. Surrounding tissue architecture is disrupted; tissue is hyperechoic. Significant amounts of pus are obtained during surgical excision and drainage.

the normal breast architecture with areas of hyperechogenicity and hypoechogenicity may be seen. Although mastitis is more commonly seen in patients who are lactating, it can be seen in women of all ages. An antibiotic that covers aerobic and anaerobic organisms is used in patients who are not lactating. We follow these patients closely to ensure that an abscess requiring drainage does not develop and that there is complete resolution of the symptoms and findings after antibiotic therapy. Some patients require two courses of antibiotics for complete resolution.

Granulomatous mastitis is an uncommon cause of diffuse breast changes (Figure 8.5) and is usually unilateral. Clinically, patients present with a mass that may be tender or, less commonly, with diffuse breast tenderness in the absence of focal findings. Patients are relatively young, and in many, the disease presents within 6 years of pregnancy. The etiology

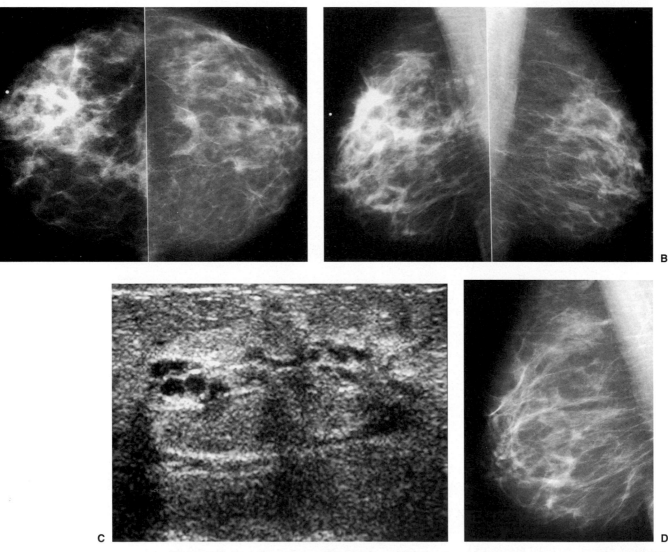

Figure 8.5 *Granulomatous mastitis.* Right and left craniocaudal views [technique used for right CC: kV(p), 28; mAs, 205; compression, 6.6 cm; for left CC: kV(p), 26; mAs, 95; compression, 4.8 cm] (*A*) and mediolateral oblique (*B*) views. This 52-year-old patient presented with swelling and hardness of her right breast for 1 month. Some resolution of tenderness and erythema was achieved after a trial of antibiotics. Screening mammogram 8 months previously was normal. *C.* Ultrasound evaluation is diffusely abnormal with disruption of normal tissue planes, areas of hyperechogenicity, and tubular, serpiginous hypoechoic structures. *D.* Right mediolateral oblique view obtained 5 months after image in part *B.* After surgical resection, symptoms resolved.

is unknown; however, some have suggested an autoimmune reaction, undetected organisms, or the use of oral contraceptives. Histologically, granulomatous mastitis is characterized by noncaseating granulomas limited to the perilobular regions; no microorganisms are identified in the tissue. In addition to diffuse breast changes, other reported mammographic findings include one or multiple masses and large, focal areas of asymmetry. On ultrasound, findings in granulomatous mastitis include multiple, relatively circumscribed lesions with a tubular configuration or irregular hypoechoic lesions with shadowing (3).

Giant cell or temporal arteritis is another rare cause of diffuse breast changes (Figure 8.6). It may be a unilateral or bilateral process, and biopsy usually demonstrates granulomatous inflammatory changes surrounding the arteries (4). This is a systemic panarteritis involving medium and large vessels in patients older than 50 years of age. The temporal arteries and other extracranial branches of the carotid artery are usually involved. Patients present with headaches, scalp tenderness, visual symptoms, jaw claudication, throat pain,

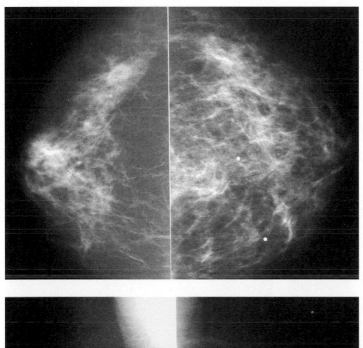

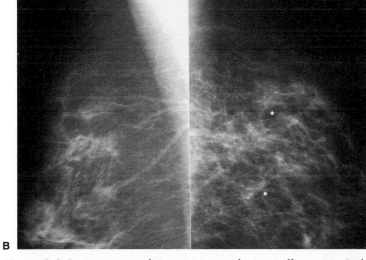

Figure 8.6 *Prominent vasculitis consistent with giant cell arteritis.* Right and left craniocaudal (A) and mediolateral oblique (B) views. This 70-year-old patient presented with diffuse left breast tenderness and swelling. The left breast appears larger than the right. Diagnosis is made on excisional biopsy.

Box 8.2: Malignant Causes of Diffuse Breast Changes

Inflammatory carcinoma (infiltrating ductal carcinoma)
Infiltrating ductal carcinoma, not otherwise specified
Infiltrating lobular carcinoma (shrinking or enlarging breast)
Lymphoma

Clinically, inflammatory carcinoma is characterized by *peau d'orange* skin changes reflecting edema, erythema, and warmth of the involved breast. Aggressive treatment with neoadjuvant therapy is used in these patients, followed by surgery for local and regional control.

and asymmetry of arm pulses. If blindness occurs, it is often irreversible. Patients have an elevated sedimentation rate with a normal white blood cell count, and about half have associated polymyalgia rheumatica. Elevated doses of prednisone are used in the treatment of symptoms and are helpful in minimizing visual disturbances.

Malignant causes of diffuse breast changes are listed in Box 8.2.

Inflammatory carcinoma is an uncommon form of breast cancer constituting about 1% of all breast cancers; it is a stage IIIB cancer at the time of presentation. The diagnosis of inflammatory carcinoma is made based on clinical findings. Patients describe the rapid onset of breast warmth, erythema, and edema. As implied by its name, inflammatory carcinoma simulates mastitis in presentation; however, the involved breast is not usually as tender as that seen in women with diffuse acute bacterial mastitis. Although patients with inflammatory carcinoma may improve initially with antibiotics, the symptoms persist and eventually worsen. Histologically, inflammatory carcinomas are usually poorly differentiated invasive ductal carcinomas characterized by tumor emboli in dilated dermal lymphatics and a lymphocytic reaction surrounding dilated vasculature in the dermis. These

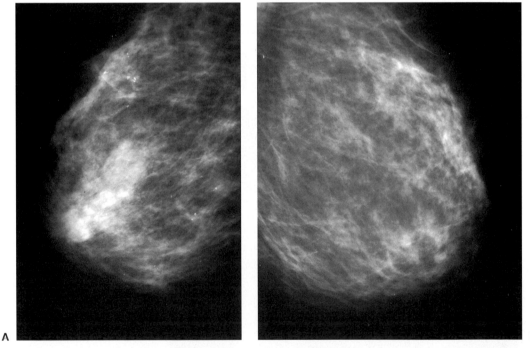

A   B

Figure 8.7 *Inflammatory carcinoma.* Right (*A*) and left (*B*) mediolateral oblique (MLO) views in a 49-year-old patient presenting with the rapid onset of erythema and edema involving the right breast; minimal tenderness [technique used for right MLO: kV(p), 30; mAs, 295; compression, 8.1 cm; for left MLO: kV(p), 29; mAs, 122; compression, 6.4 cm]. Increased density, thickening of the trabecular pattern and skin (seen with bright light), and decreased compressibility of breast are observed. The right breast appears smaller than the left. Enlarged and dense axillary lymph nodes (not shown) are noted in the axilla on the right MLO view.

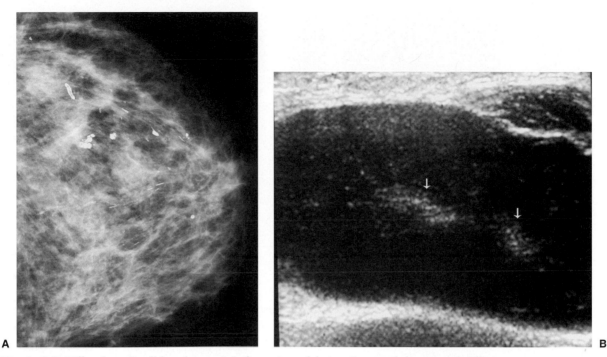

Figure 8.8 *Diffuse large B-cell lymphoma. A.* Left craniocaudal view. Increased density and diffuse prominence of the trabecular markings are seen. Dystrophic and some scattered rodlike calcifications are present. *B.* Enlarged lymph nodes in the ipsilateral axilla. The cortex is thickened, bulging, and markedly hypoechoic, and there is posterior acoustic enhancement. There is mass effect with attenuation (*arrows*) of the central hyperechoic hilum.

histologic findings occur in about 80% of patients with the clinical diagnosis of inflammatory carcinoma, and the histologic findings associated with inflammatory carcinoma occur in about 4% of patients who do not have the described clinical findings (4,5).

Mammographically, skin thickening and diffusely increased parenchymal density are the most common findings (Figure 8.7). Axillary adenopathy has been reported in as many as 58% of patients at the time of presentation. Ultrasonographically, there is skin thickening, dilated lymphatics, and disruption of the normal breast architecture (6,7). In some patients, a focal finding, including a mass, distortion, or calcifications, may be seen; these patients may have locally advanced breast cancer with secondary skin involvement rather than inflammatory carcinoma (6). Patients with inflammatory carcinoma are treated aggressively with neoadjuvant chemotherapy for systemic disease followed by surgery for local control. The prognosis for these patients is poor.

Lymphoma is primary to the breast when widespread or prior extramammary lymphoma is excluded. More commonly, lymphoma involves the breast secondarily. It may present with localized findings as discussed in Chapter 7 or with a more diffuse pattern of involvement (Figure 8.8). Axillary and intramammary adenopathy are found in 30% to 40% of patients at the time of presentation (4,5).

DILATED VASCULATURE

Dilated venous structures (Figure 8.9) can sometimes be seen in patients with fluid overload (Figure 8.10) or in situations in which collateral flow develops, such as discussed earlier in patients with superior vena cava syndrome. In many patients, no underlying cause is identified. Dilated venous structures can be seen on the anterior chest wall extending into the breasts bilaterally.

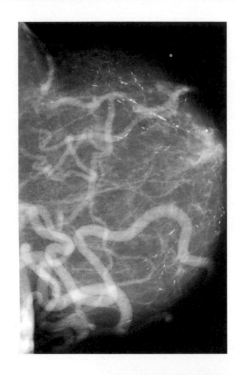

Figure 8.9 *Dilated anterior chest wall veins.* Bilateral process (only left craniocaudal view shown) of unknown etiology. Large, rodlike calcifications are present.

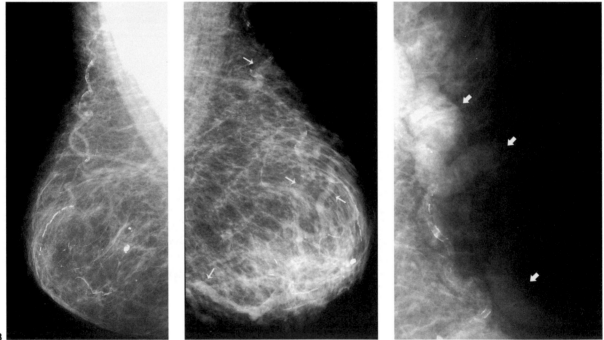

A,B   C

Figure 8.10 *Unilateral diffuse changes and dilated anterior chest wall veins.* A. Right mediolateral oblique view [kV(p), 27; mAs, 95.3; compression, 4.4 cm] for comparison. Arterial and dystrophic calcifications are present. Venous structures are normal in appearance. B. Left mediolateral oblique view [kV(p), 27; mAs, 348.3; compression, 6.3 cm] demonstrates diffuse trabecular thickening and dilated venous structures (*arrows*). The left breast appears larger than the right. This 63-year-old patient with chronic renal failure is on dialysis; the dialysis shunt is on the upper portion of the left arm. Increased flow is thought to be related to the shunt. C. Dilated venous structures (*arrows*) extending into the left axilla. Vascular calcifications are also present.

SOLITARY DILATED DUCT

Although initially thought to be a secondary sign of breast cancer, some women have a solitary dilated duct with no underlying breast cancer or other significant pathology. Some patients with papillomas may present with a solitary dilated duct (Figure 8.11). On physical examination, nipple discharge may be elicited. Dystrophic calcifications related to the papilloma can sometimes be seen in the dilated duct (Figure 8.12). In some patients, no etiology for the dilated duct is identified (Figure 8.13). Ultrasonographically, the dilated duct can be followed for a variable distance away from the nipple and, in some patients, can be used to identify an intraductal lesion.

It has been suggested that a solitary dilated duct in an asymptomatic woman should be considered a probably benign finding and follow-up studies done at 6, 12, and 24 months (8). Our approach to these patients includes performing a physical examination to determine whether there is any nipple discharge, followed by an ultrasound looking for an intraductal lesion. In the absence of discharge or an intraductal lesion, we recommend annual screening studies. If discharge is found to be copious and arising from a single duct opening, we do a ductogram.

MONDOR'S DISEASE

Mondor's disease is an uncommon, self-limited thrombophlebitis involving a superficial vein of the breast. The thoracoepigastric vein, coursing obliquely over the lateral quadrants of the breasts from the epigastrium to the anterior axillary line, is the most commonly affected; the lateral thoracic vein coursing along the lateral margin of the pectoralis major muscle is involved less frequently. Patients describe a cord of tenderness corresponding to the course of the vein. Linear dimpling can be seen in some patients when they raise their arm (Figure 8.14A). In some women, superficial, linear, serpiginous nodularity (e.g., simulating the appearance of varicose veins in the leg) can be seen corre-

> Mondor's disease is a self-limited thrombophlebitis involving the thoracoepigastric and, less commonly, the lateral thoracic vein.

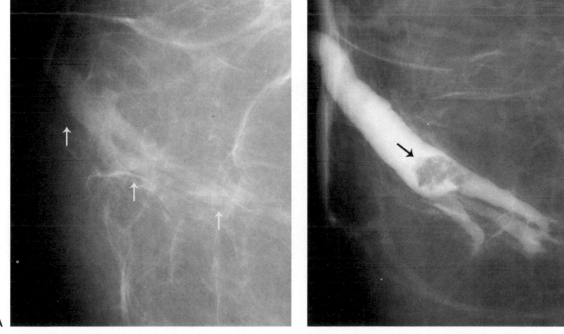

A   B

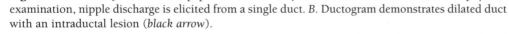

Figure 8.11 *Solitary dilated duct; papilloma. A. Solitary dilated duct (white arrows). On physical examination, nipple discharge is elicited from a single duct. B. Ductogram demonstrates dilated duct with an intraductal lesion (black arrow).*

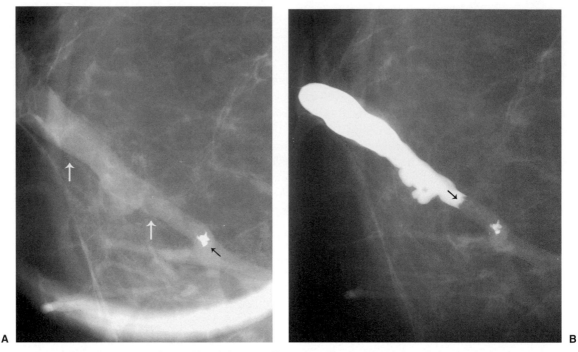

Figure 8.12 *Solitary dilated duct; papilloma. A.* Solitary dilated duct (*white arrows*) with associated coarse calcification (*black arrow*). On physical examination, nipple discharge is easily elicited from a single duct opening. *B.* Ductogram demonstrates duct obstruction by an intraductal lesion at the site of the calcification (*black arrow*).

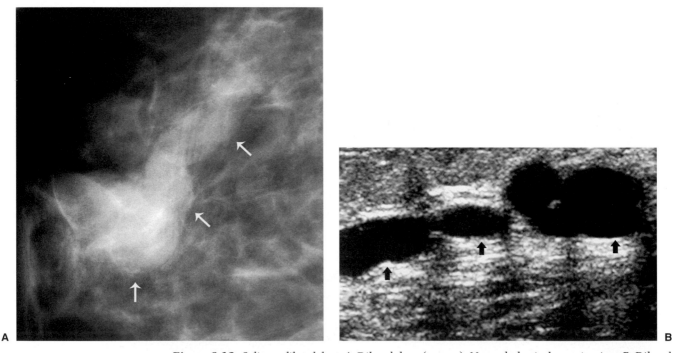

Figure 8.13 *Solitary dilated duct. A.* Dilated duct (*arrows*). Normal physical examination. *B.* Dilated duct (*arrows*) with no intraductal lesion identified during real-time scanning. Stable finding for 4 years.

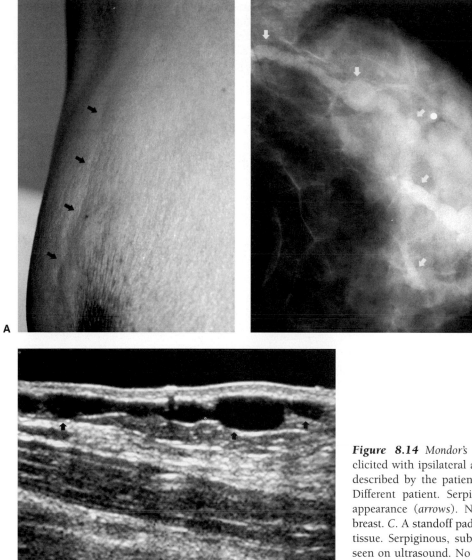

Figure 8.14 Mondor's disease. *A.* Linear dimpling (*arrows*) elicited with ipsilateral arm raising correlates to the tender cord described by the patient developing after vigorous exercise. *B.* Different patient. Serpiginous, tubular structure with beaded appearance (*arrows*). Nodularity could be seen on surface of breast. *C.* A standoff pad used to evaluate skin and subcutaneous tissue. Serpiginous, subcutaneous tubular structure (*arrows*) is seen on ultrasound. No flow is seen with Doppler. Normal skin thickness is observed on ultrasound. Complete resolution of symptoms and findings occurs 8 weeks after presentation.

sponding to the thrombosed vein. This condition usually resolves spontaneously and requires no aggressive intervention. Patients need to be reassured of the likely benign etiology of this condition and supported with nonsteroidal antiinflammatory agents as needed for symptomatic relief. The cause of this condition is not identified in most patients; however, a list of some reported causes is provided in Box 8.3.

Box 8.3: Causes of Mondor's Disease

Idiopathic
Breast trauma
Breast surgery
Breast cancer
Extensive physical activity
Dehydration
Core needle biopsy (9)

Mammographically, a vein or ropelike density is imaged corresponding to the area of dimpling; this may be associated with subcutaneous thickening (10). In women with nodularity, the vein may have a beadlike appearance (Figure 8.14B). Ultrasonographically, a superficial, serpiginous, tubular structure (10) can be imaged corresponding to the area of dimpling in some patients (Figure 8.14C). No flow is usually seen acutely with Doppler. In some patients, the sonogram is normal. On follow-up studies 6 to 8 weeks after presentation, the imaged venous structure may not be apparent mammographically or ultrasonographically. Rarely, the thrombosed vein may calcify (11).

PARENCHYMAL ASYMMETRY

In most women, breast tissue is symmetric. Asymmetry may be localized (Figures 8.15 and 8.16) and focal or involve larger islands of tissue (Figure 8.17). In many women, these patterns represent normal variation. It is important to examine the patient and evaluate the area of asymmetry ultrasonographically. Intervention is usually not warranted if the asymmetry is not palpable and ultrasound is normal. If the area of asymmetry is hard or indurated, or if an abnormality is seen ultrasonographically, biopsy may be indicated unless the history provides a good explanation for the findings.

Some causes of parenchymal asymmetry are listed in Box 8.4.

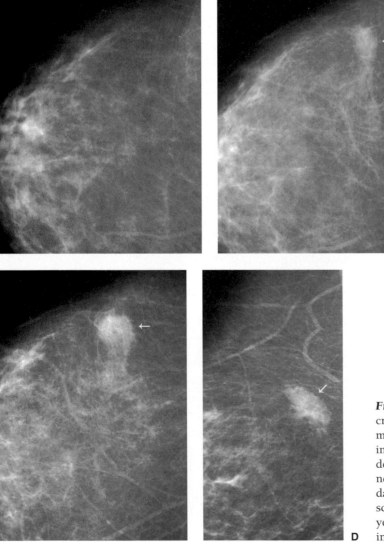

Figure 8.15 *Focal parenchymal asymmetry. A.* Right craniocaudal view. No focal finding. *B.* Screening mammogram 1 year later. Focal asymmetry is developing (*arrow*). Although not shown, a corresponding density is seen on the mediolateral oblique view, and no corresponding area is seen on the left. Craniocaudal (*C*) and mediolateral oblique (*D*) views from screening study. Four years after image in part *A*, 3 years after image in part *B*. Focal asymmetry is increasing in size and density (*arrows*).

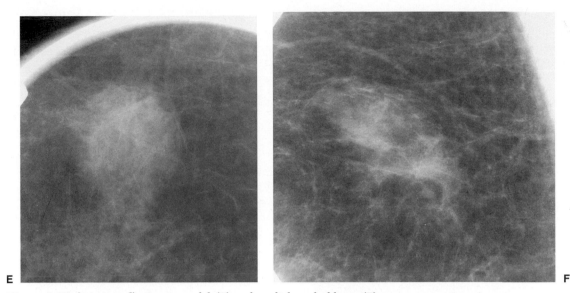

Figure 8.15 (continued) Craniocaudal (E) and mediolateral oblique (F) spot compression views. Although round on the craniocaudal view, this area spreads out on the mediolateral oblique view. No associated distortion or calcification is identified. Given its progressive development, however, physical examination and ultrasound are undertaken without a corresponding abnormality on either test. Focal fibrosis is a common finding when developing islands of asymmetry are stereotactically sampled.

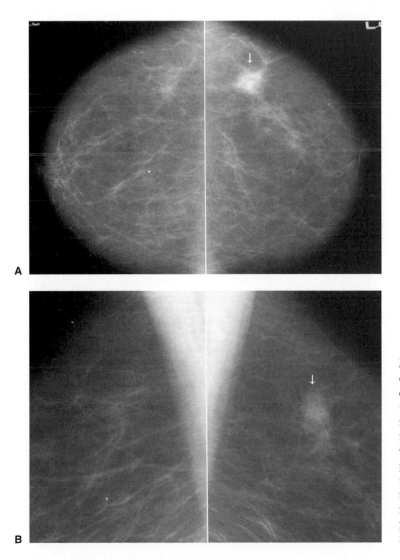

Figure 8.16 *Focal parenchymal asymmetry*. Right and left craniocaudal (A) and mediolateral oblique (B) views demonstrating a round island of parenchymal tissue (*arrows*). No corresponding density is evident on the right. It is important to evaluate focal areas of parenchymal asymmetry. Evaluation includes spot compression views to ensure that no underlying distortion or unsuspected mass is present, ultrasound and physical examination to ensure that no corresponding palpable abnormality is present. Invasive lesions, particularly lobular carcinomas, can sometimes present with innocuous areas of parenchymal asymmetry. This finding has been stable for 5 years.

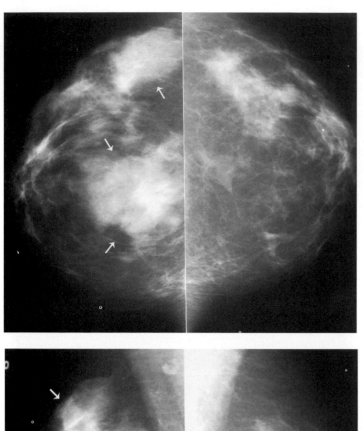

A

B

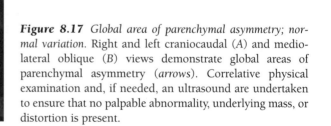

Figure 8.17 *Global area of parenchymal asymmetry; normal variation.* Right and left craniocaudal (*A*) and mediolateral oblique (*B*) views demonstrate global areas of parenchymal asymmetry (*arrows*). Correlative physical examination and, if needed, an ultrasound are undertaken to ensure that no palpable abnormality, underlying mass, or distortion is present.

Box 8.4: Causes of Parenchymal Asymmetry

Normal variation
Prior surgery with removal of tissue in contralateral breast
Estrogen effect
Focal fibrosis
Trauma
Mastitis (granulomatous mastitis)
Invasive lobular carcinoma
Invasive ductal carcinoma
Lymphoma

PAGET'S DISEASE

Paget's disease of the nipple represents 1% to 5% of all breast cancers. Initial findings are limited to the nipple and include reddening with associated pruritus. As the disease progresses, the nipple surface may be moist (oozing, gummy), and there may be scaling and eczematoid changes leading to ulceration, erosions (Figure 8.18A), and crusting (Figure 8.18B) of the nipple surface. It is usually a unilateral process related to an underlying intraductal or invasive ductal carcinoma. Patients may have an underlying palpable abnormality; however, the nipple findings may be all that is apparent in the patients with intraductal disease. In some patients, the mammogram is normal. Alternatively, nipple retraction, nipple and areolar thickening, calcifications in the nipple and subareolar area, or a mass may be present (Figure 8.18C, D). Histologically, large cells with abundant cytoplasm and large nuclei with prominent nucleoli (Paget's cells) infiltrate the epidermis of the nipple (12,13).

Paget's disease always involves the nipple.

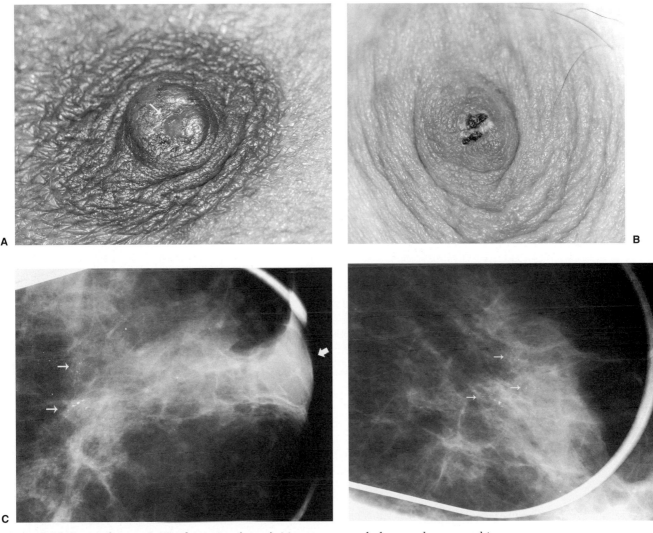

Figure 8.18 *Paget's disease. A.* Nipple erosion (*arrow*). Mammogram and ultrasound are normal in this patient. *B.* Different patient. Crusting on nipple surface. *C.* Double spot compression magnification view of the left subareolar area demonstrates thickening and retraction of the nipple (*thick arrow*) with associated linear calcifications (*thin arrows*). *D.* Double spot compression magnification view in the upper outer quadrant of the left breast demonstrates calcifications (*arrows*) consistent with intraductal disease and associated invasive disease with distortion.

Dermatitis may be difficult to distinguish from Paget's disease. This condition is commonly associated with a rapid time course and sparing of the nipple (always involved in Paget's disease). Rarely, intraductal papillomas can intermittently protrude onto the nipple surface, simulating Paget's disease. Papillomas, however, can be reduced back into the duct so that the nipple surface can be evaluated and is normal in appearance.

LOBULAR NEOPLASIA

Lobular carcinoma *in situ* is a marker lesion imparting one of the greatest risks for the subsequent development of breast cancer. The risk involves both breasts, and the cancers that develop are equally divided between invasive ductal and lobular types.

Lobular neoplasia is also known as lobular carcinoma *in situ* (LCIS). Although this entity imparts one of the greatest risks for subsequent breast cancer development, the lesion itself is not considered premalignant. Given this, Haagensen and others have suggested the term *lobular neoplasia* to get away from the use of the word *carcinoma* with its associated implications (14). The term lobular neoplasia has associated detractors because some authors use it to refer to lobular hyperplasia and atypical lobular hyperplasia.

Lobular neoplasia is an incidental finding on biopsy done for clinical findings, most commonly, a palpable mass, or after biopsy done for mammographic findings, usually calcifications. Although there have been some reports of calcifications associated directly with lobular carcinoma *in situ* (15), this is unusual. Unless the pathologist specifically states that calcifications are in areas of LCIS, we do not consider LCIS a congruent histologic finding of biopsy done for calcifications (see Chapter 11).

Lobular neoplasia is often a bilateral, multifocal process affecting premenopausal women. Biologically, this process is considered different from some forms of ductal carcinoma *in situ*. This is a marker lesion. The risk for subsequent breast cancer involves the breasts bilaterally, and the cancers that develop are equally divided between invasive ductal and lobular carcinomas. The management of these patients can be controversial. Periodic clinical and mammographic follow-up is advocated by some, yet others recommend bilateral mastectomy. Unilateral mastectomy is not appropriate because the increased breast cancer risk applies equally to both breasts.

REFERENCES

1. Mendelson EB. Imaging the postoperative breast. *Radiol Clin North Am* 1992;30:107–138.
2. Dershaw DD. Evaluation of the breast undergoing lumpectomy and radiation therapy. *Radiol Clin North Am* 1995;33:1147–1160.
3. Han BK, Choe YH, Park JM, et al. Granulomatous mastitis: mammographic and sonographic appearances. *AJR Am J Roentgenol* 1999;173:317–320.
4. Rosen PP. *Rosen's breast pathology,* 2nd ed. Philadelphia: Lippincott Williams & Wilkins, 2001.
5. Tavassoli FA. *Pathology of the breast,* 2nd ed. Stamford: Appleton & Lange, 1999.
6. Kushwaha AC, Whitman GJ, Stelling CB, et al. Primary inflammatory carcinoma of the breast: retrospective review of the mammographic findings. *AJR Am J Roentgenol* 2000;174:535–538.
7. Günhan-Bilgen I, Üstün EE, Memis A. Inflammatory breast carcinoma: mammographic, ultrasonographic, clinical and pathological findings in 142 cases. *Radiology* 2002;223:829–838.
8. Sickles EA. Management of probably benign breast lesions. *Radiol Clin North Am* 1995;33: 1123–1130.
9. Jaberi M, Willey SC, Brem RF. Stereotactic vacuum-assisted breast biopsy: an unusual cause of Mondor's disease. *AJR Am J Roentgenol* 2002;179:185–186.
10. Conant EF, Wilkes AN, Mendelson EB, et al. Superficial thrombophlebitis of the breast (Mondor's disease): mammographic findings. *AJR Am J Roentgenol* 1993;160:1201–1203.
11. Bassett LW, Jackson VP, Jahan R, et al. *Diagnosis of disease of the breast.* Philadelphia: WB Saunders, 1997.
12. Burke ET, Braeuning MP, McLelland R, et al. Paget disease of the breast: a pictorial essay. *Radiographics* 1998;18:1459–1464.
13. Ikeda DM, Helvie MA, Frank TS, et al. Paget disease of the nipple: radiologic-pathologic correlation. *Radiology* 1993;189:89–94.
14. Haagensen CD. *Diseases of the breast,* 3rd ed. Philadelphia: WB Saunders, 1986.
15. Georgian-Smith D, Lawton TJ. Calcifications of lobular carcinoma in situ of the breast: radiologic-pathologic correlation. *AJR Am J Roentgenol* 2001;176:1255–1259.

THE MALE BREAST

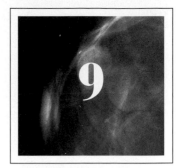

■ Gynecomastia
■ Benign Lesions
■ Breast Cancer
■ Metastatic Disease

Our approach to male patients presenting with breast-related symptoms includes marking the area of concern with a metallic BB and obtaining craniocaudal and mediolateral oblique views of the symptomatic side. After reviewing of these images, we may obtain views of the contralateral breast for comparison. If benign changes are diagnosed, no further evaluation is undertaken. Spot compression and magnification views are obtained as needed for evaluation of findings suggestive of an underlying cancer.

Mammographically, the normal male breast is predominantly fatty with prominent pectoral muscles and a small nipple. Male breast tissue is primarily composed of subareolar ducts with no significant branching and sparse surrounding stroma. Lobular units are rare in men. Consequently, lesions arising in the lobules such as cysts, fibroadenomas, and sclerosing adenosis are unusual in men not taking exogenous estrogen (e.g., for prostate cancer treatment). All of the lesions discussed for female patients can occur in male patients, however, with a significantly lower incidence (particularly the lobular-derived lesions).

The principles for positioning the breast described for female patients apply to male patients. The compression paddle used routinely for screening studies can make it difficult for the technologist to hold the male breast in place as compression is applied. The technologist may find it difficult to slide her hand out from under the paddle as compression is applied without scraping her knuckles or letting go of the breast prematurely. Some equipment manufacturers provide a paddle that is half the width of the standard compression paddle for imaging male patients (these paddles are also useful in women with implants for the implant-displaced views).

Breast imaging studies in men are scheduled as diagnostics because the patients present with breast-related symptoms. Cooper and associates (1) suggest that mammography is not necessary in male patients younger than 50 years of age who present with diffuse breast enlargement or a palpable nonindurated central subareolar mass, unless there are other strong clinical indications such as skin changes or bloody nipple discharge. In their series, none of 43 male patients younger than 50 years of age were found to have breast cancer (1). Although there are no significant data supporting screening mammography in men, it may be something to consider in men who have a personal history of breast cancer or in families with male breast cancer and the *BRCA2* gene.

GYNECOMASTIA

Gynecomastia is common, reportedly occurring in 57% of men older than 44 years of age (2). Gynecomastia is the enlargement of the male breast with secondary branching of the

Enlargement of the male breast with secondary branching of subareolar ducts and proliferation of the surrounding stroma is termed *gynecomastia*. This process can be unilateral or bilateral, symmetric or asymmetric.

subareolar ducts and proliferation of the surrounding stroma. Patients present with a subareolar mass that may be tender. The process may be unilateral or bilateral, symmetric or asymmetric. Cooper and colleagues (1) described unilateral involvement in 33% of their patients with gynecomastia, and in another 33% involvement was asymmetric. Appelbaum and co-workers (2) reported 61 patients with gynecomastia, 55 of whom had bilateral mammograms. In 84% of the patients, the gynecomastia was asymmetric; in 2%, it was symmetric; and in 14%, it was unilateral. Increases in serum estradiol levels, combined with decreases in testosterone levels, are thought to be the etiologic factors governing the development of gynecomastia. At this time, there is no known association between gynecomastia and male breast cancers. Some of the causes of gynecomastia are listed in Box 9.1.

Three patterns have been described for gynecomastia mammographically (1–5). The *nodular* pattern is characterized by increased tissue focally in the subareolar area (Figure 9.1) that fans out symmetrically from the nipple. It has been suggested that this represents the early phase of gynecomastia and corresponds to florid gynecomastia histologically. The epithelial lining of the ducts is hyperplastic, and the surrounding stroma is edematous, loose, and cellular. The *fibrous* or *dendritic* pattern appears as retroglandular tissue with prominent fibrous extensions that radiate out into the fatty tissue (Figure 9.2). Histologically, this is fibrous gynecomastia and reflects long-standing changes; there is ductal proliferation with dense fibrotic stroma. *Diffuse* glandular gynecomastia is the third pattern; it simulates the heterogeneously dense female breast pattern (Figure 9.3). Appelbaum and

---

Box 9.1: Causes of Gynecomastia

Idiopathic
Physiologic
- Neonatal (placental estrogens)
- Puberty (imbalance in androgen-to-estrogen ratio)
- Elderly (decreases in plasma testosterone levels)

Diseases with estrogen excess
- Testicular tumors (Leydig cell, Sertoli cell, testicular germ cell)
- Nontesticular tumors (lung, liver, renal, adrenocortical, hepatocellular)
- Cirrhosis
- Endocrine abnormalities (hypothyroidism or hyperthyroidism)
- Nutritional deprivation

Androgen deficiency
- Aging
- Primary hypogonadism; Klinefelter's syndrome (XXY)
- Secondary hypogonadism (trauma, orchitis, cryptorchidism, irradiation, hydrocele)
- Renal failure (and hemodialysis)

Drugs
- Estrogenic activity (anabolic steroids, exogenous estrogen—diethylstilbestrol for prostate cancer, digitalis, heroin, marijuana, alcohol)
- Inhibition of testosterone action or synthesis (cimetidine, diazepam, phenytoin, spironolactone, vincristine, methotrexate)
- Idiopathic mechanism (furosemide, isoniazid, methyldopa, nifedipine, reserpine, theophylline, verapamil)

Systemic disorders (unknown mechanism)
- Nonneoplastic diseases of the lung
- Chest wall trauma
- Human immunodeficiency virus

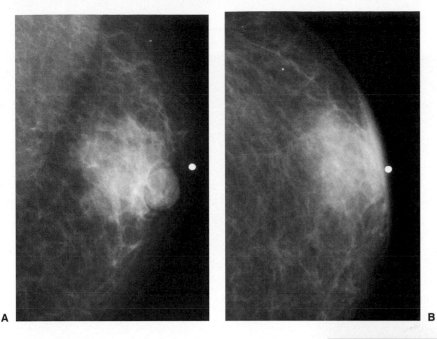

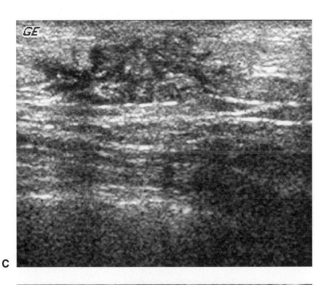

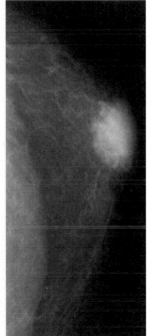

Figure 9.1 *Gynecomastia, nodular pattern.* Mediolateral oblique (*A*) and craniocaudal (*B*) views in a 94-year-old male patient presenting with a palpable mass. Metallic BB marks the area. Round glandular tissue is imaged corresponding to the mass. Scalloping of the density is noted, consistent with tissue. *C*. Ultrasound demonstrates hypoechoic, serpiginous, tubular-like tissue radiating out symmetrically from under the nipple. No cystic or solid masses are imaged when correlating clinical and imaging findings. *D*. In this 72-year-old male patient, the craniocaudal view demonstrates round glandular tissue, symmetrically centered on the nipple. *E*. Ultrasound demonstrates hypoechoic, serpiginous, tubular-like tissue radiating out symmetrically from under the nipple and corresponding to the area of concern in the patient.

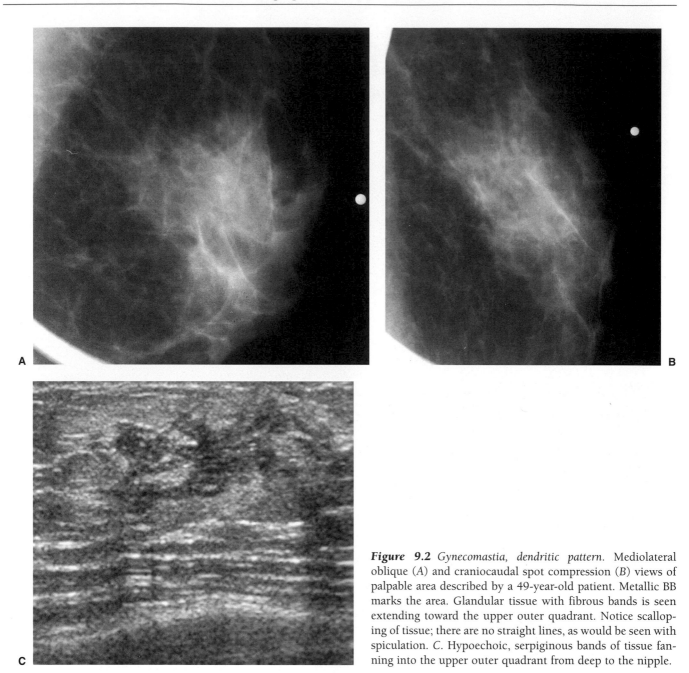

Figure 9.2 *Gynecomastia, dendritic pattern.* Mediolateral oblique (*A*) and craniocaudal spot compression (*B*) views of palpable area described by a 49-year-old patient. Metallic BB marks the area. Glandular tissue with fibrous bands is seen extending toward the upper outer quadrant. Notice scalloping of tissue; there are no straight lines, as would be seen with spiculation. *C.* Hypoechoic, serpiginous bands of tissue fanning into the upper outer quadrant from deep to the nipple.

co-workers (2) described 61 patients with histologically proven gynecomastia: 77% had nodular, 20% dendritic, and 3% diffuse patterns mammographically. In some men presenting with breast enlargement and tenderness, fatty tissue alone is imaged mammographically (Figure 9.4).

On ultrasound, the findings in gynecomastia are nonspecific. Normal-appearing tissue is imaged corresponding to the palpable abnormality fanning out from under the nipple. Ultrasound is useful in distinguishing gynecomastia from other underlying focal lesions.

The management of gynecomastia is variable. In patients with drug-related gynecomastia, attempts can be made to eliminate the causative agent, or if this is not possible, another drug can be tried. Those patients with significant symptoms may undergo surgi-

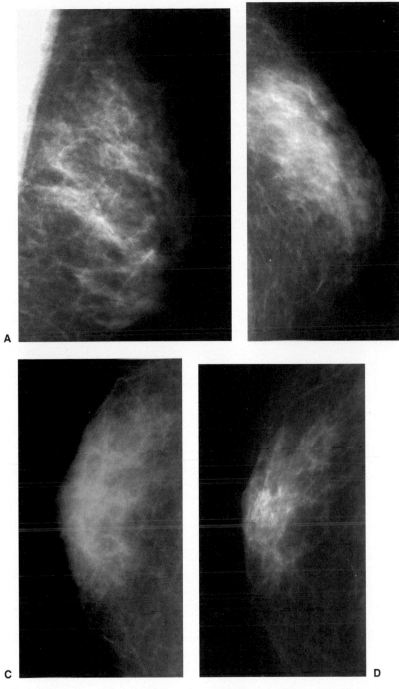

Figure 9.3 *Gynecomastia, diffuse pattern.* Mediolateral oblique (*A*) and craniocaudal (*B*) views demonstrating glandular tissue in a pattern similar to that seen in the female breast. *C.* Different patient; 84-year-old male, craniocaudal view. *D.* Craniocaudal view taken 1 year after image in part *C*. Diffuse glandular tissue with some resolution on the follow-up mammogram. Once developed, gynecomastia may decrease in prominence (and fluctuate); however, it does not usually resolve completely.

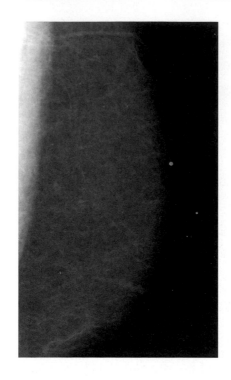

Figure 9.4 *Fatty tissue.* Fatty breast, sometimes called *pseudogynecomastia.*

cal excision of the tissue. If symptoms are not severe and the patient is not bothered by the change in his breast, no intervention is absolutely indicated. Unless there is a significant change in the physical findings, no imaging follow-up is recommended. Once it has developed, gynecomastia does not usually resolve, particularly if the underlying cause is not identified (e.g., idiopathic).

BENIGN LESIONS

Lobular units are rare in men; hence, lesions derived from lobular elements (e.g., fibroadenomas, cysts, sclerosing adenosis) are unusual in male patients.

Fat-containing masses in the male breast are benign and have appearances similar to those described for women. These include lipomas, lymph nodes (Figure 9.5), hematomas, and fat necrosis (Figures 9.6 and 9.7). Water-density masses seen in men include epidermal inclusion cysts, abscesses, papillomas, pseudoangiomatous stromal hyperplasia, and focal fibrosis (diabetic mastopathy).

BREAST CANCER

Invasive ductal carcinoma, not otherwise specified is the most common type of breast cancer diagnosed in male patients.

Male breast cancer represents less than 0.5% of all breast cancers and 0.17% of all cancers diagnosed in men. About 300 breast cancer–related deaths occur in men annually; it is thought to be unrelated to gynecomastia. Risk factors for breast cancer in men are listed in Box 9.2.

Clinically, male patients present at an older age than female patents with a painless, hard mass most commonly in the subareolar area or, second in frequency, in the upper outer quadrant of the breast; they can, however, occur anywhere in the breast. Skin or nipple retraction may be present, and some patients present with spontaneous nipple discharge. Axillary adenopathy is identified in about half of patients at the time of presentation. As with female breast cancer, prognosis depends on the status of the axillary lymph nodes and the size of the tumor at the time of diagnosis. Unfortunately, many men delay seeking medical attention for breast cancer–related signs and symptoms.

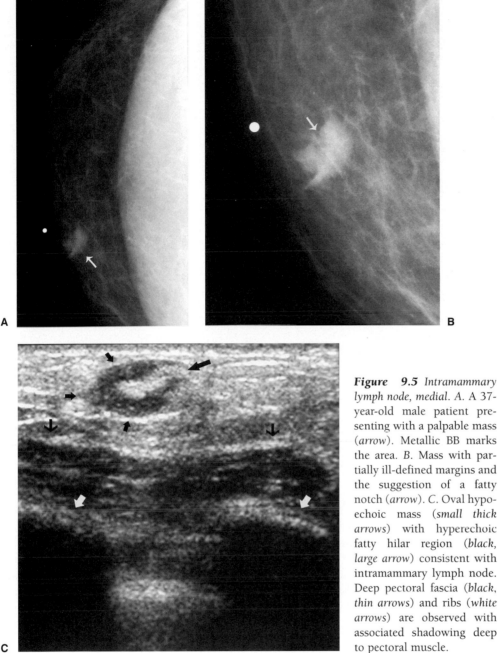

Figure 9.5 *Intramammary lymph node, medial. A. A 37-year-old male patient presenting with a palpable mass (arrow). Metallic BB marks the area. B. Mass with partially ill-defined margins and the suggestion of a fatty notch (arrow). C. Oval hypoechoic mass (small thick arrows) with hyperechoic fatty hilar region (black, large arrow) consistent with intramammary lymph node. Deep pectoral fascia (black, thin arrows) and ribs (white arrows) are observed with associated shadowing deep to pectoral muscle.*

Invasive ductal carcinomas represent 85% of all the cancers diagnosed in male patients. Associated ductal carcinoma *in situ* (DCIS) is found in 35% to 50% of patients (6–8). DCIS, in the absence of an infiltrative component, is much less common, representing about 5% of all breast cancers in male patients. Papillary-type DCIS is the most common subtype diagnosed in male patients (6).

A retroareolar, noncalcified, round or oval mass with well-circumscribed to indistinct margins that is slightly eccentric in position is the most common mammographic finding in male patients with breast cancer (Figure 9.8). A spiculated mass (Figure 9.9) that may be associated with skin or nipple retraction may also be seen. Calcifications reflecting DCIS (Figure 9.10) may be associated with the mass, possibly extending beyond the mass.

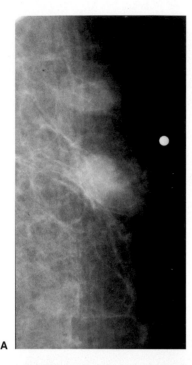

A

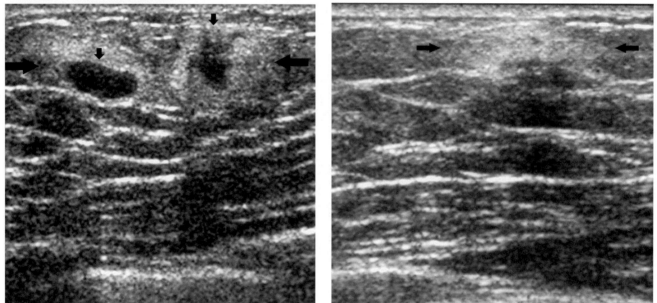

B
C

Figure 9.6 *Fat necrosis.* A. A 74-year-old male patient presenting with a palpable area in the left breast. Metallic BB marks the area. Two adjacent masses with ill-defined margins are imaged mammographically. *B.* Hyperechoic, lobulated mass (*large arrows*) with central hypoechoic areas (*small arrows*). Ultrasound findings are consistent with fat necrosis. *C.* Follow-up ultrasound 6 weeks later demonstrates nearly complete resolution with some residual hyperechogenicity (*arrows*).

When present, calcifications have been described as coarser, fewer in number, less commonly linear and more scattered than those seen with female breast cancers.

Ultrasonographically, a complex cystic mass and a hypoechoic mass with a heterogeneous echotexture are the two most common appearances (6). The margins can be irregular, indistinct, microlobulated, or well circumscribed. The complex cystic pattern is commonly seen with papillary-type lesions (6).

Male breast cancer is usually treated with mastectomy and either sentinel lymph node biopsy or axillary dissection. Radiation therapy may be given to the chest wall for larger lesions, and chemotherapy may be added as indicated by the status of the axillary lymph nodes. Although there are no data in the literature to support the use of screening mammography on the contralateral breast, we recommend this for our male patients with breast cancer.

Chapter 9: The Male Breast

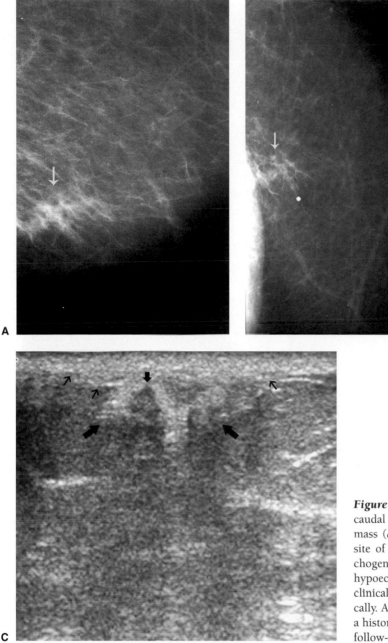

Figure 9.7 *Fat necrosis.* Mediolateral oblique (*A*) and cranio-caudal (*B*) views in a male patient presenting with a palpable mass (*arrow*). Metallic BB marks the area. Irregular density at site of clinical concern (*arrow*). *C.* Ill-defined area of hypere-chogenicity (*thick, long arrows*) with heterogeneity and area of hypoechogenicity (*thick, short arrow*) corresponding to area of clinical concern consistent with fat necrosis ultrasonographi-cally. Associated skin thickening is noted (*thin arrows*). There is a history of trauma to this site. Resolution of findings is seen on follow-up.

Box 9.2: Risk Factors for Male Breast Cancer

Advanced age
History of chest radiation (ionizing)
Occupational exposure (electromagnetic field radiation)
Cryptorchism
Testicular injury
Mumps (after 20 years of age)
Klinefelter's syndrome
Liver dysfunction (cirrhosis, schistosomiasis, malnutrition)
Family history of breast cancer (*BRCA2*)
Men of Jewish descent
Exogenous estrogen use

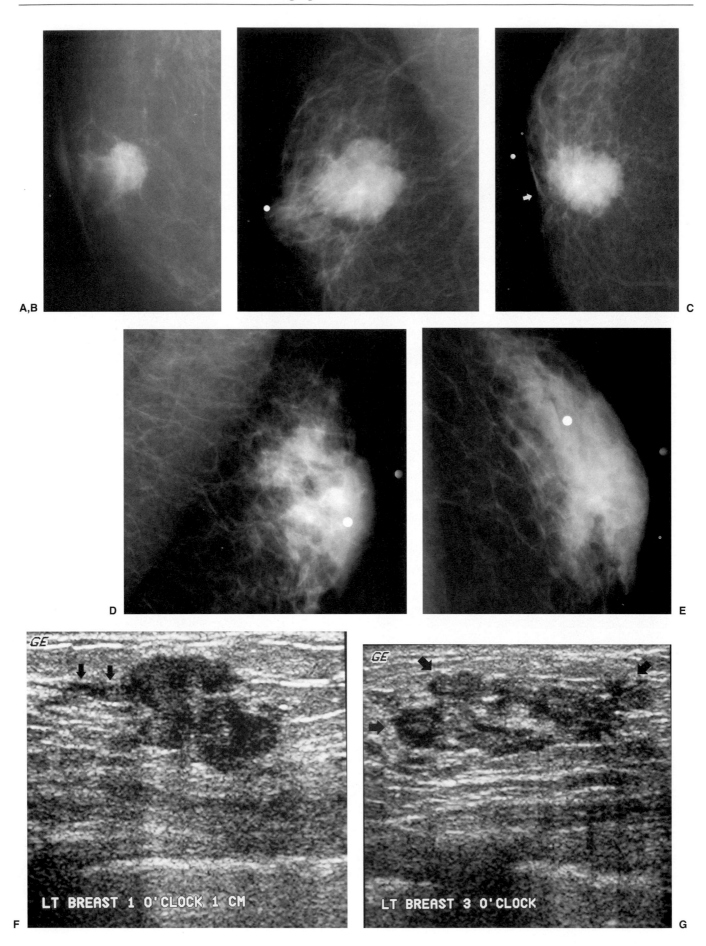

LT BREAST 1 O'CLOCK 1 CM

LT BREAST 3 O'CLOCK

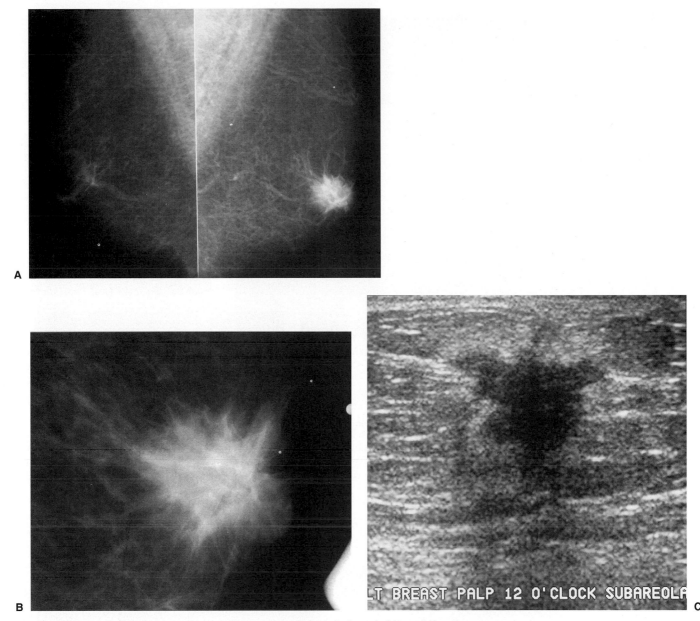

Figure 9.9 *Invasive ductal carcinoma, not otherwise specified.* Mediolateral oblique (*A*) and spot compression (*B*) views of a 75-year-old male patient presenting with a palpable mass. Metallic BB marks the area. A spiculated mass is seen in the subareolar area. *C.* Hypoechoic mass with irregular and angular margins that is taller than wide (crossing a ligament) and some shadowing consistent with breast cancer is observed.

Figure 9.8 *Invasive ductal carcinomas, not otherwise specified.* A. Oval mass with ill-defined margins; eccentrically positioned in subareolar area. *B.* Mediolateral oblique (MLO) view in a different patient. This 57-year-old male presented with a palpable mass and history of chronic renal failure on dialysis. Metallic BB marks the area. A dense, round mass with ill-defined margins is seen. *C.* On the craniocaudal (CC) view, a dense, round mass with spiculated margins is seen, along with associated skin thickening and subtle skin retraction (*arrow*). *D.* MLO and CC views (*E*) on the same patient 2 years later, now with two palpable masses in the remaining left breast. *E.* Craniocaudal view. Metallic BBs mark the areas. Dense glandular tissue, but no definite abnormality, is seen mammographically. *F.* Heterogeneously, a hypoechoic mass with ill-defined, angular margins and duct extension (*arrows*) is identified on ultrasound at the 1-o'clock position. *G.* Ill-defined mass with heterogeneous echotexture and microlobulation at the 3-o'clock position (*arrows*). These are synchronous lesions in a male patient with a history of contralateral breast cancer.

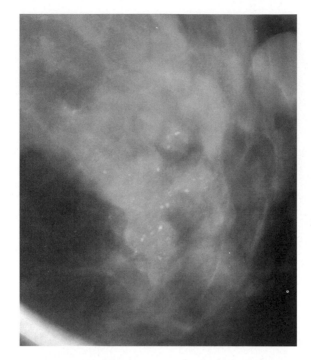

Figure 9.10 Invasive ductal carcinoma, not otherwise specified with associated ductal carcinoma in situ. Spot compression magnification view demonstrating an ill-defined, macrolobulated mass with associated pleomorphic calcifications.

METASTATIC DISEASE

Metastatic carcinoma to the male breast is rare. Prostate cancer is most commonly reported (7,8); hematopoietic (Figure 9.11), lymphoreticular, melanoma, and lung (Figure 9.12) cancers occur less frequently. Mammographically, a round mass with well-circumscribed

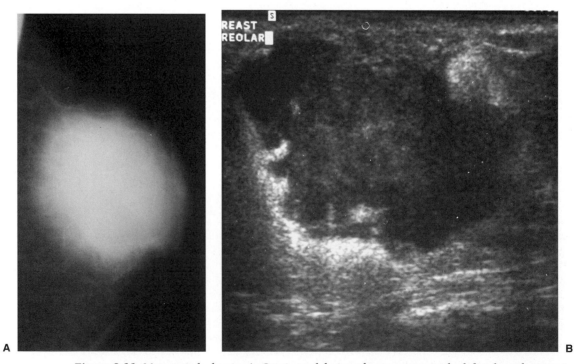

Figure 9.11 Metastatic leukemia. *A.* Craniocaudal view shows a mass in the left subareolar area in a 21-year-old male patient with a history of leukemia. *B.* Irregular mass with heterogeneous echotexture corresponds to palpable subareolar mass.

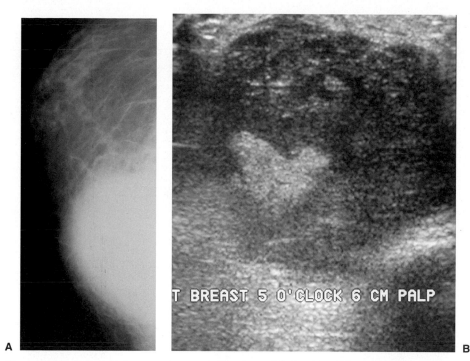

Figure 9.12 *Metastatic lung carcinoma.* A. Craniocaudal view. Partially visualized, round mass with indistinct margins is seen in the medial aspect of the right breast of a 77-year-old male patient with history of lung cancer. B. Irregular mass with heterogeneous echotexture and posterior acoustic enhancement.

to indistinct margins is the most common finding. Ultrasonographically, a well-circumscribed to ill-defined mass with a homogeneous (Figure 9.13) or heterogeneously hypoechoic echotexture may be seen. A complex cystic mass is seen when there is associated tumor necrosis. Posterior acoustic enhancement may be seen with some of the more rapidly growing lesions.

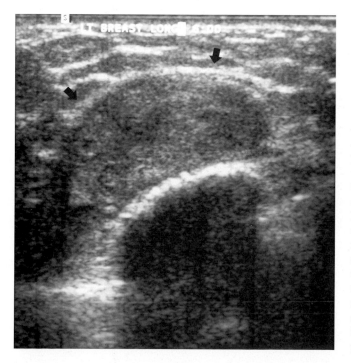

Figure 9.13 *Pleomorphic liposarcoma.* An 86-year-old male presenting with a palpable mass that could not be imaged mammographically. An oval, well-circumscribed mass that is homogeneously hypoechoic is corresponding to the palpable mass (*arrows*). Rib with associated shadowing is imaged deep to the mass. As illustrated in this patient and previously discussed, ultrasound is helpful in evaluating areas that may be difficult to image with mammography.

REFERENCES

1. Cooper RA, Gunter BA, Ramamurthy L. Mammography in men. *Radiology* 1994;191:651–656.
2. Appelbaum AH, Evans GFF, Levy KR, et al. Mammographic appearances of male breast disease. *Radiographics* 1999;19:559–568.
3. Dershaw D. Male mammography. *AJR Am J Roentgenol* 1986;146:127–131.
4. Chantra PK, So GJ, Wollman JS, et al. Mammography of the male breast. *AJR Am J Roentgenol* 1995;164:853–858.
5. Hendrix TM, Tobin CE, Resnikoff LB, et al. Breast imaging case of the day. *Radiographics* 1996;16:452–455.
6. Yang WT, Whitman GJ, Yuen EHY, et al. Sonographic features of primary breast cancer in men. *AJR Am J Roentgenol* 2001;176:413–416.
7. Tavassoli FA. *Pathology of the breast,* 2nd ed. Stamford: Appleton & Lange. 1999:829–855.
8. Rosen PP. *Rosen's breast pathology,* 2nd ed. Philadelphia: Lippincott Williams & Wilkins. 2001:703–728.

THE ALTERED BREAST

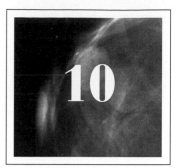

EXCISIONAL BIOPSY CHANGES

Accurate preoperative wire localization methods now facilitate minimal volume biopsies, and an increasing number of minimally invasive imaging-guided needle biopsies have reduced the need for excisional biopsies. Consequently, the likelihood of an excisional biopsy creating a permanent change that affects subsequent mammographic interpretations has decreased significantly. When postoperative changes occur, they often resolve in the first several months after the procedure. Unless a mammogram is done in the first 6 months after the biopsy, annual mammograms are normal in more than half of these women (1–3).

The technologists take a careful history, inspect the breast, and document on the patient's history sheet the site of any scars . This allows the interpreting radiologist to correlate any findings on the mammogram with prior biopsy sites. Although we do not routinely mark biopsy scars at the time screening studies are done, thin wires or metallic BBs can be used (2). Given the expense associated with these markers, in conjunction with the high number of women who have had at least one breast biopsy, we reserve the use of markers for the few patients a year in whom there is a question about an area of mammographic concern correlating with a biopsy site. Also, having one or multiple linear markers on a study is a source of distraction that is not necessary for most patients (Figure 10.1).

Changes that may be seen on a mammogram correlating with excisional biopsy sites include skin thickening, parenchymal distortion (Figure 10.2A–D), asymmetry, and a spiculated (Figure 10.2 E, F), round or oval mass. Except for parenchymal asymmetry, resulting from the removal of tissue from one breast, these changes usually resolve completely, remain stable after the first year, or slowly evolve with time (Figure 10.3). Increasing amounts of fat, dispersion of the density, oil cyst formation, and the development of dystrophic calcifications are changes that can be seen on follow-up (1–3). Occasionally, retained fragments from the localization wire or foreign bodies (Figure 10.4) may be seen at prior biopsy sites.

If a postoperative finding does not resolve completely, stability or progressive resolution needs to be established on annual studies. This is particularly important in patients with a personal or significant family history of breast cancer or if, histologically, the biopsy yielded a high-risk lesion (atypical ductal hyperplasia, lobular neoplasia, and multiple peripheral papillomas). In patients with a high-risk lesion diagnosed on excisional breast biopsy, we recommend a mammogram 6 months after the biopsy to establish the presence of any biopsy change (e.g., a new baseline for the patient). Changes seen 6 months after biopsy are unlikely to represent recurrent or interval cancer. On subsequent studies, we

Postoperative changes remain stable or resolve progressively on annual studies. Repeat biopsy should be considered if there is increasing distortion or density at a prior biopsy site.

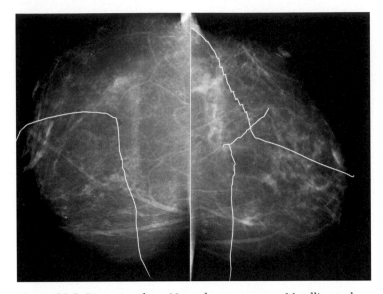

Figure 10.1 *Biopsy markers.* Normal mammogram. Metallic markers used on prior biopsy sites can be distracting and in most patients add no useful information. Given the potential source of distraction, the cost of the markers, and the lack of changes related to prior biopsies, in more than half of patients, we do not routinely mark prior biopsy sites. Even in patients with postbiopsy changes, the findings are distinctive enough that a confident diagnosis can be made without the use of markers, in most patients.

expect these changes to remain stable or, more commonly, evolve, becoming less prominent with time. Increases in distortion or density at a biopsy site after the initial 6-month postoperative study warrant a biopsy recommendation and a review of the original pathology. As yearly studies accrue, comparison is made to the earliest postoperative study available. Subtle progressive changes may not be readily apparent from year to year but can be quite obvious when comparison is made to the earliest available postoperative study (Figure 10.5).

VACUUM-ASSISTED IMAGING-GUIDED BIOPSY

Vacuum-assisted imaging-guided breast biopsies with an 11-gauge (less commonly, 14-gauge) needle can result in complete removal of small lesions. In these patients, a metallic (titanium) clip is deployed to mark the site of the lesion. If a malignancy is diagnosed,

Figure 10.2 *Biopsy change; fat necrosis.* Craniocaudal (CC) (*A*) and mediolateral oblique (MLO) (*B*) views in a patient who has had an excisional biopsy in the left subareolar area. Distortion (*short, thin arrow*) and long, curvilinear spicules (*thick arrows*) are noted at the biopsy site. Skin retraction and thickening are best seen on the left MLO view (*long, thin arrows*). CC (*C*) and MLO (*D*) views in a different patient. Distortion (*arrows*) is present at a prior site. Long spicules are present in association with the distortion. *E.* Different patient; spiculated mass at prior site. *F.* On a follow-up study, fat is now present in the center of the lesion. This may stabilize or, if the soft tissue continues to resolve, an oil cyst and dystrophic calcifications may develop. Use postbiopsy changes, such as these to test your ability to detect subtle areas of distortion and spiculation. If you can detect these findings in patients who have had a biopsy, you will probably detect small, subtle breast cancers on screening studies.

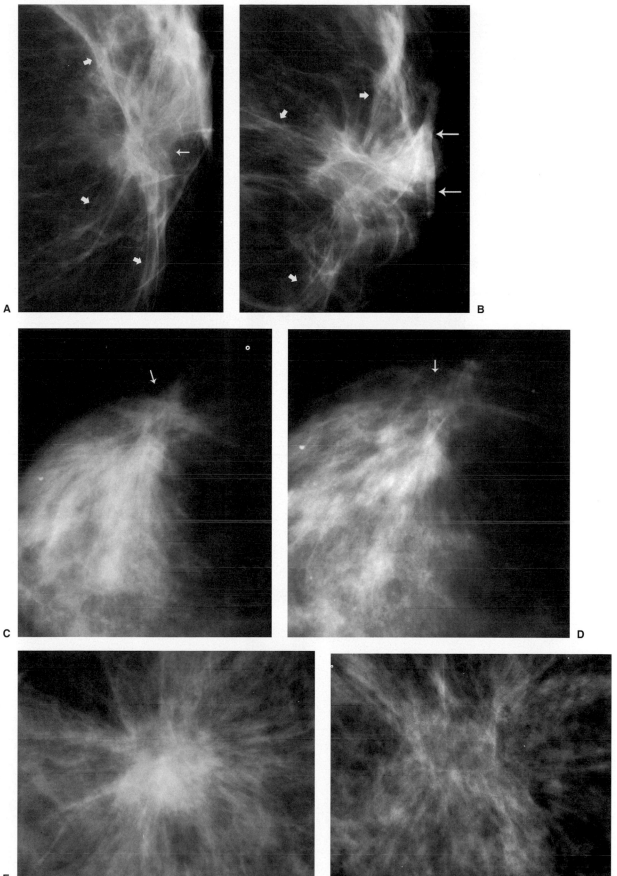

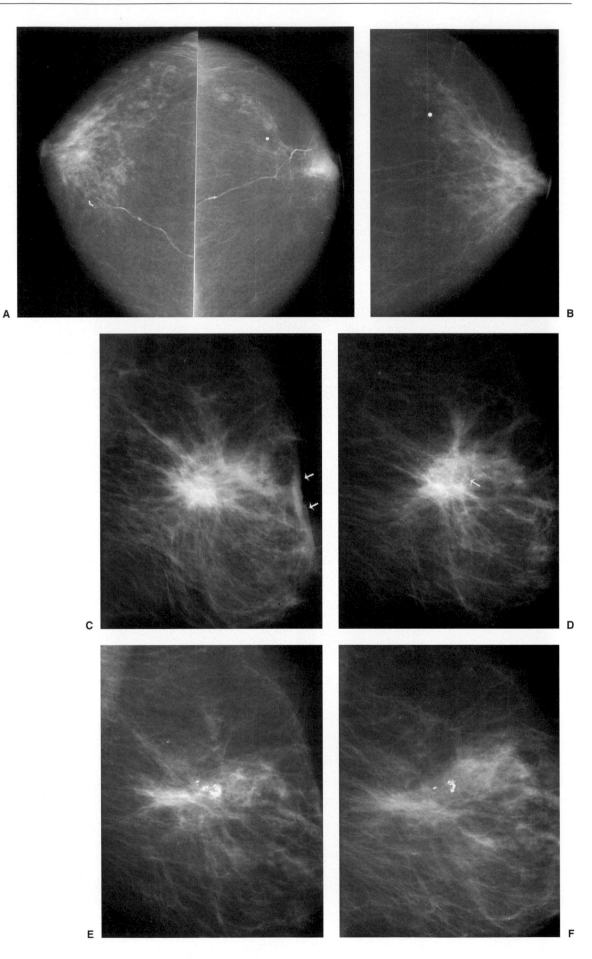

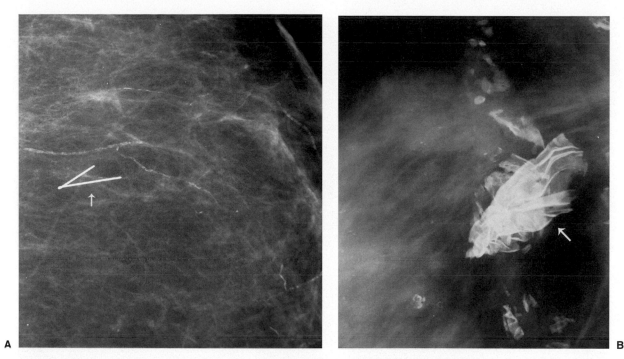

A   B

Figure 10.4 *Retained localization wire fragment and foreign body*. A. Transection of the localization wire intraoperatively can result in retained wire fragments in the breast (*arrow*). Vascular calcification is present. B. Different patient. Foreign body at prior biopsy site (*arrow*).

the metallic clip is used to guide a preoperative wire localization so that a wide excision of the tumor site can be accomplished. These imaging-guided procedures, however, do not produce long-term changes in the mammographic appearance of the breast tissue. When a metallic clip is deployed at the time of the biopsy, and the patient does not undergo surgery, the clip is seen on follow-up studies. The clip usually remains, at or close, to the biopsy site; however, migration of the clip has been reported (4,5).

At the completion of the biopsy procedure, orthogonal images are obtained to document the location of the titanium clip. On these images, one or more air locules may be seen at the biopsy site with an associated area of increased density (Figure 10.6). The air and density are usually absorbed within the first several days after the biopsy. Rarely, increased density may be seen at the biopsy site secondary to hematoma formation. In some patients, this takes a tubular appearance, suggesting it is occurring along the needle track (Figure 10.7).

Figure 10.3 *Biopsy changes*. A. Craniocaudal (CC) views show asymmetry in the appearance of the glandular tissue. More tissue is seen in the right breast than the left. This is the result of an excisional biopsy on the left. B. Left CC view before excisional biopsy. The amount and distribution of tissue is symmetric with the right breast (see image in part A). Vascular calcification is incidentally noted bilaterally. C. Different patient. Left mediolateral oblique view obtained 2 months after an excisional biopsy. Increased density, distortion, and spiculation are noted at the biopsy site. Skin thickening, distortion, and retraction are present (*arrows*). D. Six months after image in part C, 8 months after the biopsy. Increased density, distortion, and spiculation remain; however, the size and overall density are decreasing. A small lucent area is seen in the center of the density (*arrow*), and some small calcifications have developed. Skin changes are less prominent. E. One year after biopsy. Overall density is significantly decreased. Some distortion persists. Dense, coarse calcifications are now present centrally. F. Two years after biopsy. Overall density of parenchymal asymmetry continues to decrease. Dystrophic calcifications are less prominent than 1 year previously.

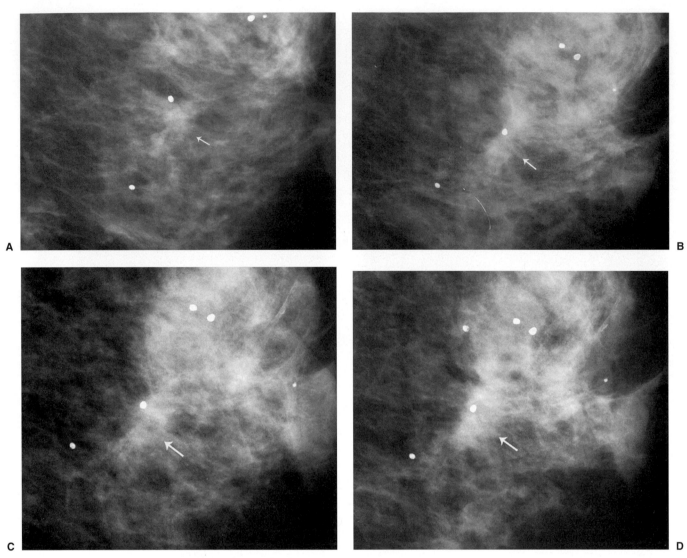

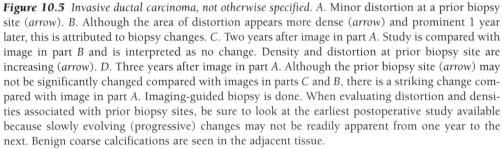

Figure 10.5 *Invasive ductal carcinoma, not otherwise specified. A.* Minor distortion at a prior biopsy site (*arrow*). *B.* Although the area of distortion appears more dense (*arrow*) and prominent 1 year later, this is attributed to biopsy changes. *C.* Two years after image in part *A.* Study is compared with image in part *B* and is interpreted as no change. Density and distortion at prior biopsy site are increasing (*arrow*). *D.* Three years after image in part *A.* Although the prior biopsy site (*arrow*) may not be significantly changed compared with images in parts *C* and *B*, there is a striking change compared with image in part *A.* Imaging-guided biopsy is done. When evaluating distortion and densities associated with prior biopsy sites, be sure to look at the earliest postoperative study available because slowly evolving (progressive) changes may not be readily apparent from one year to the next. Benign coarse calcifications are seen in the adjacent tissue.

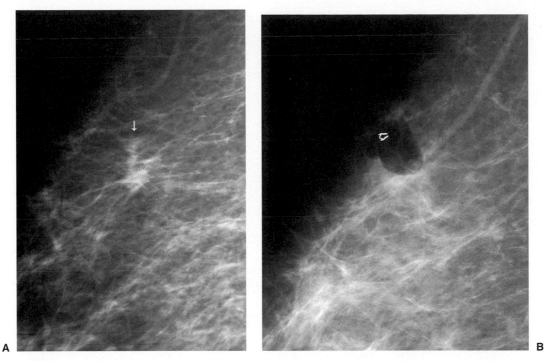

Figure 10.6 *Post–vacuum-assisted breast biopsy; invasive ductal carcinoma, not otherwise specified. A.* Small spiculated mass (*arrow*) is present. *B.* After 11-gauge vacuum-assisted core biopsies, a titanium micromark clip is deployed to mark the location of the lesion. On the day of the patient's definite surgical procedure (lumpectomy and sentinel lymph node biopsy), the clip is localized and excised with surrounding tissue. The clip and air locule are seen on orthogonal views (only one view shown) at the biopsy site.

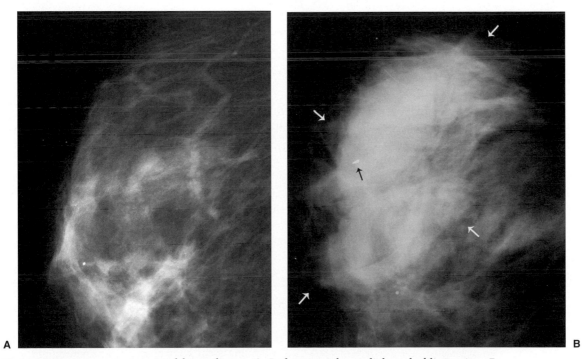

Figure 10.7 *Post–vacuum-assisted breast biopsy. A.* Prebiopsy right mediolateral oblique view. *B.* Post–vacuum-assisted breast biopsy (11-gauge) for calcifications (benign changes histologically). Micromark clip is deployed (*black arrow*). Increased density is related to a hematoma (*white arrows*). Although not common, hematomas can occur. These typically resolve spontaneously. Rarely, surgical evacuation may be needed.

(*continued on next page*)

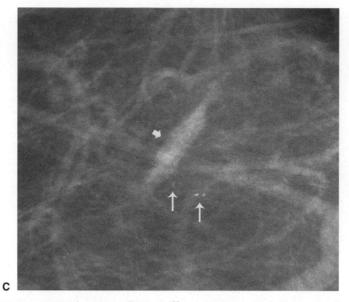

C

Figure 10.7 (continued) *C.* Different patient. Tubular area of increased density (*thick arrow*) is seen along the course of the 11-gauge needle. A clip is not deployed because residual calcifications (*thin arrows*) remain at the biopsy site after the procedure (ductal carcinoma *in situ* is diagnosed on core samples and confirmed on excision).

TRAUMA

After trauma to the breast, patients may present acutely with an ecchymosis at the site of the trauma. Irregular areas of increased density, or mixed-density masses reflecting the presence of a hematoma and fat necrosis are seen mammographically (Figure 10.8). In some patients, parenchymal asymmetry or focal prominence of the trabecular markings is seen (Figure 10.9). Hyperechoic areas with associated hypoechoic to anechoic areas are commonly seen on ultrasound (Chapters 4 and 6). On follow-up, the ecchymosis resolves. Mammographic and ultrasonographic findings usually resolve completely; some patients develop a mass that is hard and palpable on physical exam, with a mixed-density lesion seen mammographically. Alternatively, an oil cyst and dystrophic calcifications may develop at the site of trauma.

After a seat-belt injury, patients may present with a bandlike area of increased density corresponding to the course of the belt. The findings are localized to the upper inner or central quadrants of the left breast or the lower inner quadrant of the right breast when the patient is the driver. Findings in the upper inner quadrant of the right breast or lower inner quadrant of the left breast may be identified when the patient is the front-seat passenger (6).

CONSERVATIVE BREAST CANCER TREATMENT

The primary aim of breast-conserving treatment is adequate local control of breast cancer. Wide surgical margins are desired in minimizing local recurrences. The cosmetic results, however, are an important secondary consideration. If a substantial amount of tissue needs to be removed to obtain clear margins in a patient with a small breast, cosmesis may not be acceptable. Radiation therapy is used to control any residual occult breast cancer. It is begun 2 to 5 weeks after the lumpectomy. Treatment is given 5 days a week for a total of

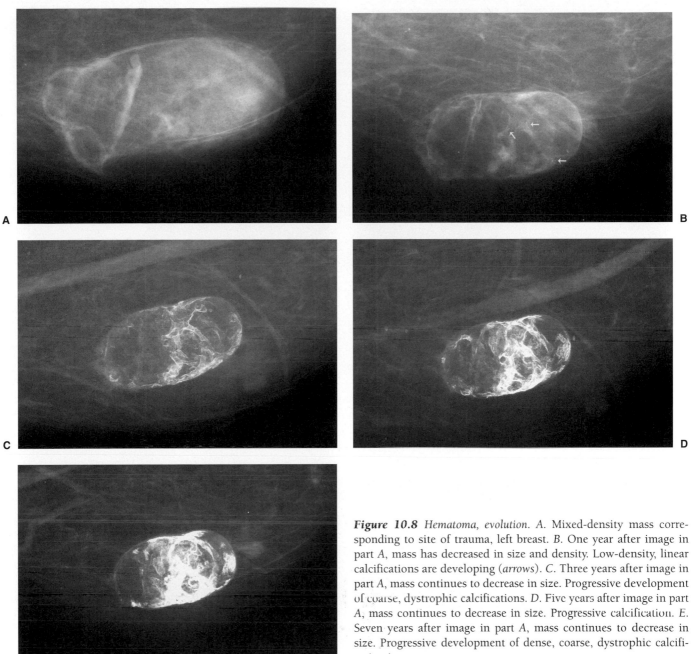

Figure 10.8 *Hematoma, evolution. A.* Mixed-density mass corresponding to site of trauma, left breast. *B.* One year after image in part *A*, mass has decreased in size and density. Low-density, linear calcifications are developing (*arrows*). *C.* Three years after image in part *A*, mass continues to decrease in size. Progressive development of coarse, dystrophic calcifications. *D.* Five years after image in part *A*, mass continues to decrease in size. Progressive calcification. *E.* Seven years after image in part *A*, mass continues to decrease in size. Progressive development of dense, coarse, dystrophic calcification is seen.

5 weeks and delivers 45 to 50 Gy of radiation to the affected breast. A boost to the lumpectomy site may be given using an electron beam or iridium implant, increasing the total dose delivered to 60 to 66 Gy (2).

Mammographic changes after lumpectomy and radiation therapy are variable and usually evolve with time. Present acutely, edema is manifested by skin and trabecular thickening leading to diffuse increases in parenchymal density and reduced breast compressibility; it usually resolves within the first 2 years after treatment (Figure 10.10). Technical factors for adequate exposure of the remaining breast tissue need to be adjusted accordingly. Ultrasonographic changes in the acute setting include skin thickening, dilated lymphatics, and increased tissue echogenicity (Chapter 4). Residual skin thickening is seen in about 20% of women 2 years after radiation therapy (2).

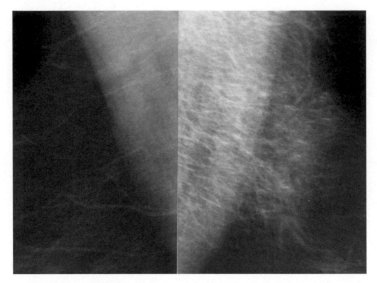

Figure 10.9 *Hematoma.* Thickening and increased density of the trabecular markings at the site of an ecchymosis in the upper portion of the left breast after trauma to the breast.

Fat necrosis at the lumpectomy site is variably characterized by a spiculated mass or distortion (Figure 10.11). These changes contract and may resolve completely with time. As the spiculated mass or area of distortion resolves, oil cysts or dystrophic calcifications (Figure 10.12) can be seen developing at the lumpectomy site in some patients (2,7–12).

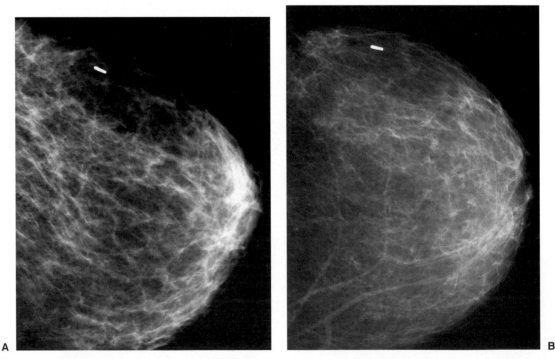

Figure 10.10 *Radiation therapy effect.* A. Increased prominence and density of the trabecular markings acutely, after completion of radiation therapy. Skin thickening is seen, if a bright light is used. B. One year later, there is significant resolution of radiation effects compared with image in part A. Edematous changes related to radiation therapy typically resolve in nearly 80% of patients, within the first 2 years after completion of radiation therapy.

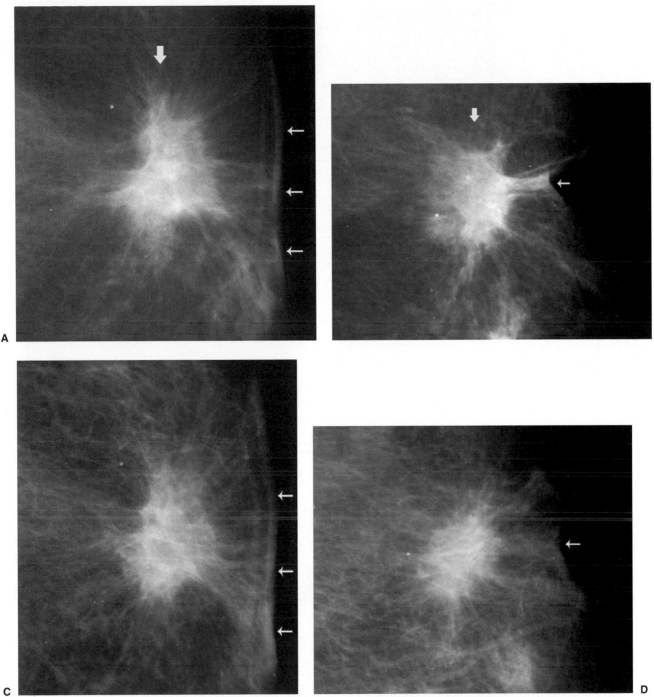

Figure 10.11 *Postlumpectomy, preirradiation and postirradiation.* Craniocaudal (CC) (*A*) and mediolateral oblique (MLO) (*B*) views in a patient after lumpectomy for an area of ductal carcinoma *in situ* who presented with calcifications. No residual linear calcifications are present at the lumpectomy site. Spiculated mass (*thick arrows*) with retraction, distortion, and thickening of the skin (*thin arrows*) are observed. CC (*C*) and MLO (*D*) views after radiation therapy. Spiculated mass and distortion at lumpectomy site are decreasing in size and density. Skin thickening (*thin arrows*) is more prominent than on the preirradiation films. The size and density of surrounding trabecular markings are increased, consistent with radiation therapy effects.

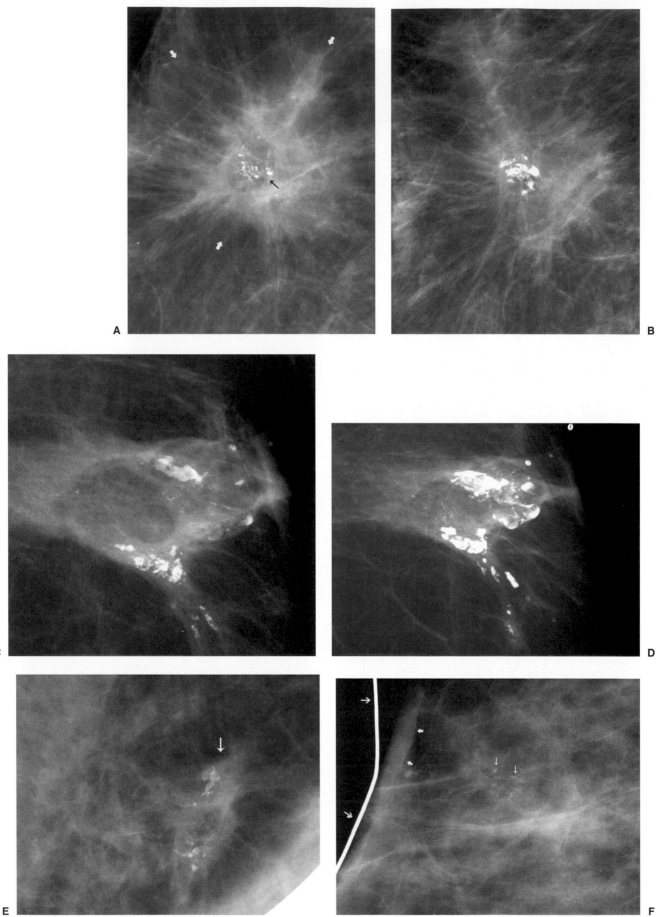

Fluid collections are seen in as many as half of patients within the first 4 weeks after the lumpectomy (2). Oval or round (Figure 10.13), well-circumscribed to ill-defined (Figure 10.14) or spiculated masses (Figure 10.15) at the lumpectomy site are variable in density and may have lucent locules or fluid–fluid levels. An internal halo partially outlining the inner margin may be present (Figure 10.16). Ultrasonographically, complex cystic masses that are predominantly cystic with septations, thickened walls, or echogenic nodules are imaged corresponding to the masses seen mammographically. Less commonly, a complex cystic mass that is predominantly solid with cystic spaces can be seen (Figure 10.17). Most fluid collections resolve within the first 2 years after the lumpectomy; however, some may persist for years. If the patient is asymptomatic, aspiration is not indicated. Reaccumulation of fluid is common after percutaneous drainage, and chronic draining sinuses can develop after aspirations (Figure 10.18). Draining sinuses can be hard to manage and often affect a patient's quality of life significantly.

Currently, there is no consensus on an appropriate follow-up protocol for patients after lumpectomy. Some facilities recommend 6-month follow-ups of the treated breast for 3, 5, or 7 years and annual imaging of the contralateral, presumably normal breast (2). We obtain a preirradiation mammogram in patients who presented with an extensive area of calcifications. Rarely, we identify patients with residual calcifications at the lumpectomy site (9). These patients may benefit from reexcision before radiation therapy is started. After completion of radiation therapy, we recommend annual bilateral diagnostic studies (9). We do not routinely obtain 6-month follow-ups of the treated breast.

After conservative breast cancer surgery, patients are scheduled annually for diagnostic studies. In addition to routine views, we obtain a double spot compression magnification view of the lumpectomy site in tangent to the x-ray beam. When evaluating these patients, it is helpful to have information on those features of the initial tumor that may influence the likelihood of recurrence, including tumor size and grade, proximity of tumor to margins, presence of an extensive intraductal component, lymphovascular space involvement, and lymph node status. Additionally, it is helpful to know whether the patient had radiation treatment or chemotherapy and if she is being treated with tamoxifen. Ideally, the patient's imaging evaluation at the time of diagnosis is available for review because recurrences often resemble the appearance of the primary tumor. The likelihood of recurrence is low in the first 2 years after treatment; it may be that some of the lesions identified within this time period reflect residual (inadequately treated) disease and not necessarily a recurrence. In the first 7 years after treatment, recurrences are likely to arise at or close to the lumpectomy site; after this, recurrences or second primary lesions develop with an equal frequency anywhere in the breast (not limited to the lumpectomy site) (13–15). The development of clustered, pleomorphic, linear or

Recurrence rates for adequately treated breast cancers are 5% to 10% within the first 5 years and 10% to 15% at 10 years.

Figure 10.12 *Lumpectomy and radiation therapy changes, fat necrosis. A.* Spiculated mass (*white arrows*) with central lucency consistent with fat necrosis and oil cyst. Developing coarse calcifications are noted in the oil cyst (*black arrow*). *B.* One year later, the overall density and associated spiculation of the mass are decreased. Dystrophic calcifications are increased in size and density. *C.* Different patient. Subareolar, mixed-density, oval mass with dystrophic calcifications corresponding to lumpectomy site; consistent with evolving fat necrosis. *D.* One year later, mass has decreased in size. Calcifications are increasing in size and density. *E.* Different patient. Dystrophic calcifications developing at lumpectomy site (*arrow*). In some patients, these calcifications have a bubbly appearance. *F.* Different patient. Early in the development of calcifications in areas of fat necrosis, the calcification can be pleomorphic, linear, and curvilinear (*short, thin arrows*), as seen in this patient after lumpectomy and radiation therapy. Skin thickening and retraction are present (*thick arrow*). Metallic marker is used at some facilities to mark biopsy and lumpectomy sites (*thin arrows*).

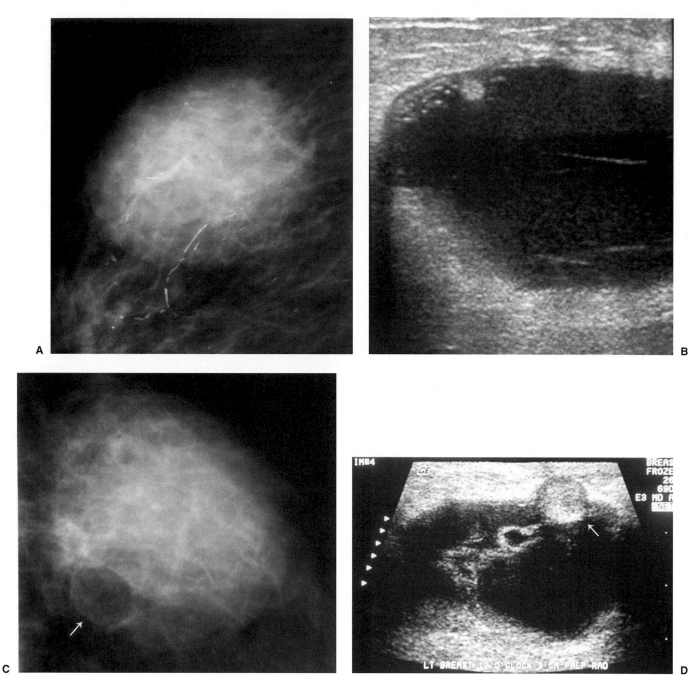

Figure 10.13 *Postlumpectomy fluid collections.* A. Round mass with indistinct margins corresponding to the lumpectomy site. Large, rodlike calcifications (secretory) are incidentally noted. B. Complex cystic mass with echogenic nodules, septations, a fluid–fluid level, and posterior acoustic enhancement. Findings consistent with a postoperative fluid collection. No aspiration is indicated unless an infection is suspected clinically. C. Different patient. Round, mixed-density lesion with indistinct margins at the lumpectomy site. Associated oil cyst is present (*arrow*). D. Complex cystic mass. Echogenic mass (*arrow*) corresponds to the attached oil cyst seen mammographically. Septations and posterior acoustic enhancement are noted. No intervention is warranted unless infection is suspected.

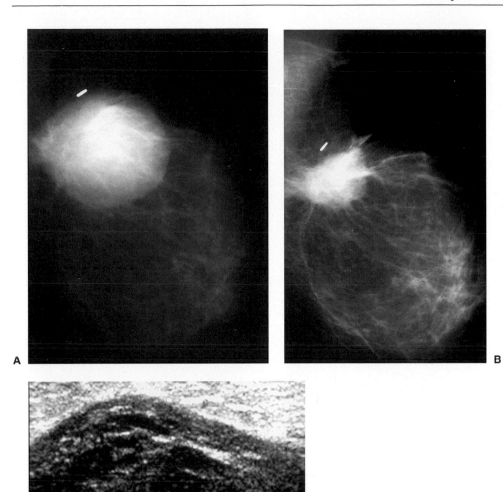

Figure 10.14 *Postlumpectomy fluid collection.* *A.* Well-circumscribed, round mass at lumpectomy site. *B.* On follow-up, the mass is smaller, and the margins are now irregular, and there is spiculation and distortion. *C.* A complex cystic mass is seen ultrasonographically. No intervention is warranted unless superimposed infection is suspected. When aspirated, these recur, and a draining sinus that can be hard to manage may develop.

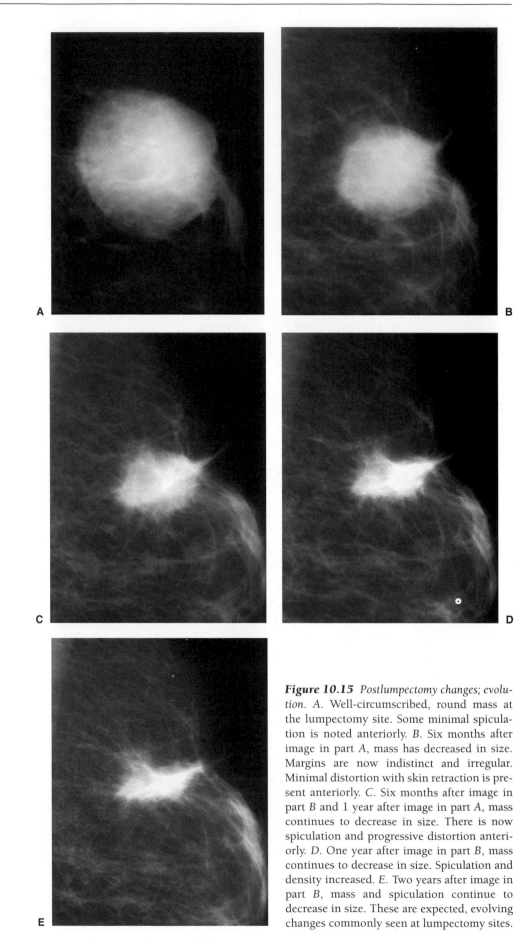

Figure 10.15 *Postlumpectomy changes; evolution.* A. Well-circumscribed, round mass at the lumpectomy site. Some minimal spiculation is noted anteriorly. B. Six months after image in part A, mass has decreased in size. Margins are now indistinct and irregular. Minimal distortion with skin retraction is present anteriorly. C. Six months after image in part B and 1 year after image in part A, mass continues to decrease in size. There is now spiculation and progressive distortion anteriorly. D. One year after image in part B, mass continues to decrease in size. Spiculation and density increased. E. Two years after image in part B, mass and spiculation continue to decrease in size. These are expected, evolving changes commonly seen at lumpectomy sites.

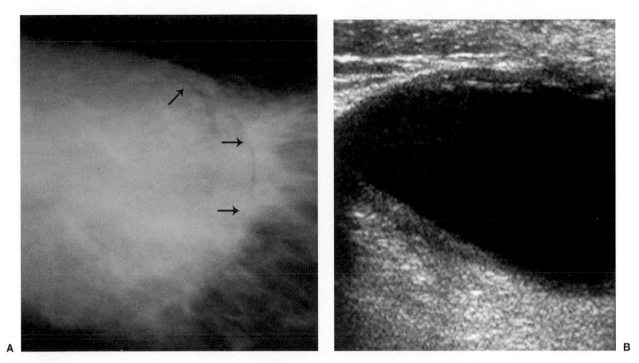

A **B**

Figure 10.16 *Postlumpectomy fluid collection, internal halo.* A. Oval mass at a lumpectomy site. Most of the mass has well-circumscribed margins (not shown). Anteriorly, there is spiculation, and an internal halo is present (*arrows*). B. Predominantly cystic mass on ultrasound. Minimal wall irregularity is noted. Mass completely resolved 1 year after the lumpectomy, 6 months after this study.

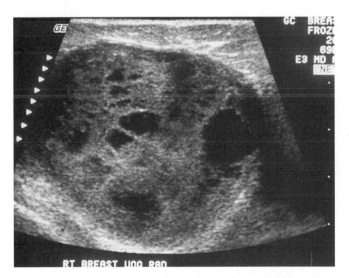

Figure 10.17 *Postlumpectomy fluid collection.* Complex cystic mass that appears predominantly solid with cystic spaces at the lumpectomy site. Unless superimposed infection is suspected, no intervention is warranted in these patients. As illustrated, most postlumpectomy fluid collections resolve with time.

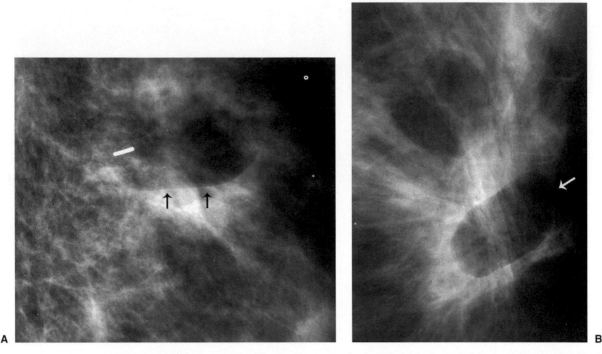

Figure 10.18 *Postlumpectomy fluid collections, after aspirations now with draining sinus. A.* Air–fluid level (*arrows*) at the lumpectomy site from the development of a draining sinus after aspirations of a fluid collection at the lumpectomy site. *B.* Different patient. Air locule is present, associated with an area of spiculation at the lumpectomy site. Draining sinus after aspiration of a postoperative fluid collection.

linearly oriented, round, punctate or amorphous (Figure 5.47 in Chapter 5) calcifications at prior lumpectomy sites should warrant biopsy (Figure 10.19). Developing masses (Figure 10.20) and increases in size and the overall density of areas of architectural distortion may also indicate recurrence. Rarely, recurrences present with diffuse changes (Figure 10.21).

Figure 10.19 *Ductal carcinoma* in situ *(DCIS); recurrences. A.* Magnification view for evaluation of screening-detected calcifications in a 39-year-old patient. A cluster of calcifications with linear forms is confirmed (*arrows*). DCIS with central necrosis is diagnosed and treated with lumpectomy and radiation therapy. *B.* Double spot compression magnification of lumpectomy site, 1 year after treatment, demonstrates low-density calcifications (*arrows*) with linear forms extending 3 cm beyond one of the clips at the lumpectomy site. These could not be seen even in retrospect on the nonmagnification views taken. Recurrent disease is diagnosed on stereotactically guided biopsy. It is unclear whether this represents recurrent or incompletely excised (and not effectively treated) DCIS. As in this patient, in women whose initial presentation is malignant-type calcifications, we obtain a double spot compression magnification view of the lumpectomy site. *C.* Different patient. Double spot compression magnification view 1 year after lumpectomy in a 57-year-old patient. The patient refused radiation therapy. Pleomorphic calcifications, including linear forms, are now present at the lumpectomy site (not seen, even in retrospect, on the postlumpectomy study). This probably represents recurrent disease; however, residual disease is an alternative explanation, particularly because the patient did not receive radiation therapy. Mediolateral oblique (*D*) and craniocaudal (*E*) views in a 69-year-old patient, 6 years after lumpectomy and radiation therapy. New cluster of calcifications is detected (*arrows*). *F.* Double spot compression magnification view demonstrate linear calcifications with linear orientation consistent with DCIS associated with central necrosis. Confirmed on stereotactically guided biopsy.

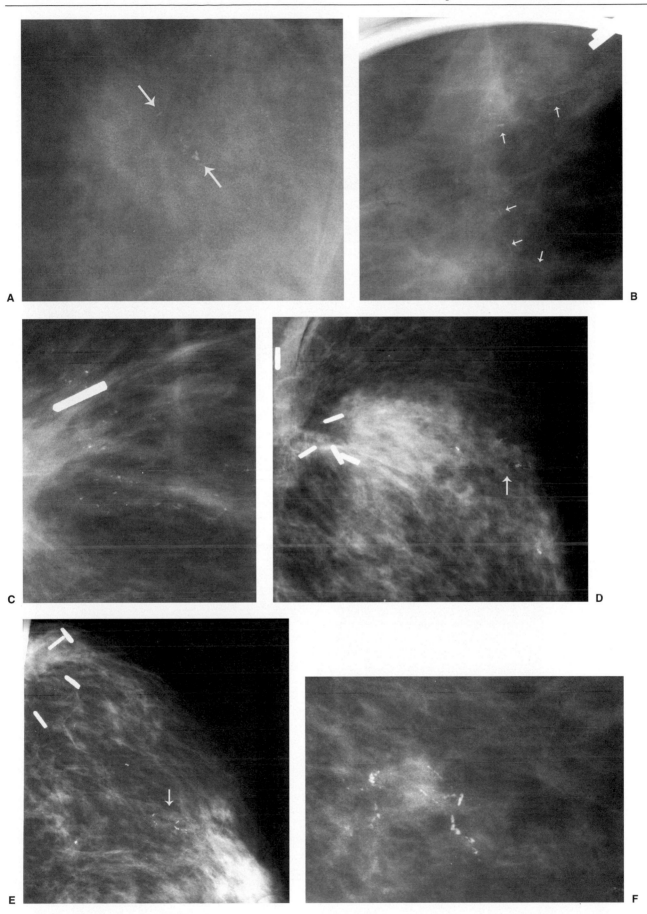

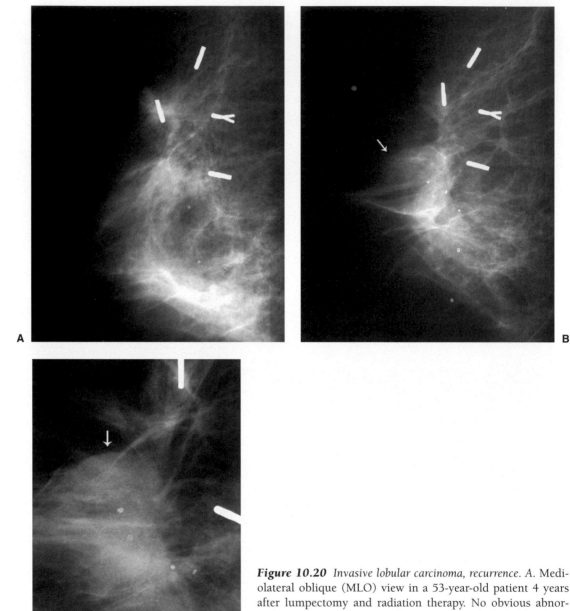

Figure 10.20 *Invasive lobular carcinoma, recurrence. A. Mediolateral oblique (MLO) view in a 53-year-old patient 4 years after lumpectomy and radiation therapy. No obvious abnormality is seen. B. One year later (5 years after lumpectomy), MLO view demonstrating increase in density and nodularity (arrow) that was also apparent on the craniocaudal view (not shown). C. Spot compression view confirms rounded contour consistent with a new mass at a prior lumpectomy site. Invasive lobular carcinoma is diagnosed on excisional biopsy.*

MASTECTOMY SITE

After the breast is removed, palpation of the chest wall is easier. There is little tissue interposed between the examining fingers and the chest wall. Consequently, in patients after mastectomy, recurrences developing at the mastectomy site are usually palpable on a thorough physical examination. Imaging of the mastectomy site probably adds little to the care and management of these patients (2,16). However, some investigators advocate a single mediolateral oblique (MLO) view of the mastectomy side view because some recurrences

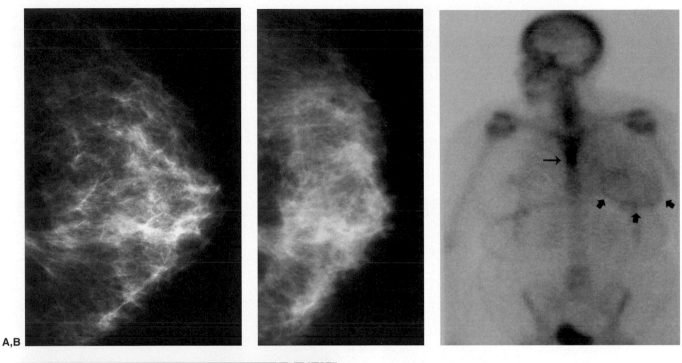

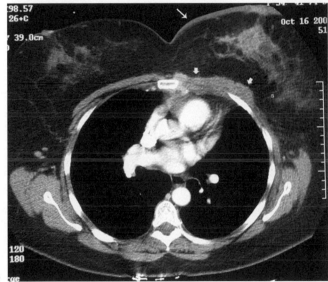

Figure 10.21 *Invasive ductal carcinoma, not otherwise specified, recurrence with diffuse changes and distant metastases.* A. Craniocaudal (CC) view in a 54-year-old patient 2 years after lumpectomy, radiation therapy, and chemotherapy for an invasive ductal carcinoma in the left breast. No obvious abnormality is apparent. *B.* One year after image in part *A* and 3 years following original treatment, CC view demonstrates a diffuse increase in the overall density of the parenchyma, and the breast appears significantly smaller than previously (shrinking). *C.* Bone scan done at this time demonstrates diffuse uptake in the left breast (*thick arrows*) as well as increased uptake by the inferior portion of the sternum (*thin arrow*). *D.* One level of chest computed tomography scan demonstrates skin thickening (*thin arrow*) medially on the left and thickening and irregularity of the pectoral muscle (*thick arrows*). Although not shown, a lytic lesion could be seen with bone windows involving the inferior-most portion of the sternum. Diffuse involvement of the breast is diagnosed on excisional biopsy.

(e.g., ductal carcinoma *in situ*) may be imaged before they become clinically detectable (17). Unless the patient has a large pannus at the mastectomy site, we do not routinely image the mastectomy site.

RECONSTRUCTION

Reconstruction after mastectomy can be done at the time of the lumpectomy (immediate), or it can be delayed. Implants or autologous tissue transplantation are used for reconstruction. We do not routinely image the affected side, when an implant has been used for reconstruction. However, if an autologous tissue transplantation is done, we do a single MLO view of the reconstruction. The goal is to identify recurrences at the chest wall, deep to the reconstruction (18). Patients with autologous tissue transplantation now have tissue interposed between the examining fingers and the chest wall, thereby limiting the physical examination. Additionally, if fat necrosis involves the flap, this hardens the tissue, further limiting physical examination.

Autologous tissue reconstructions are done most commonly using a transverse rectus abdominis myocutaneous (TRAM) flap. The latissimus dorsi muscle is sometimes used. Predominantly fatty tissue is imaged mammographically after construction of a TRAM flap. Areas of increased density are routinely seen superiorly and inferiorly (Figure 10.22). The rectus muscle is usually seen as a round or triangular density posteriorly (19). On follow-up studies, the superior and inferior areas of increased density decrease in size, and

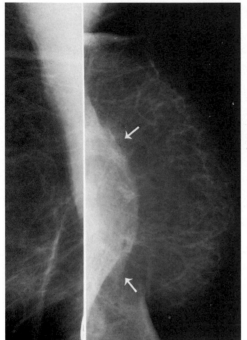

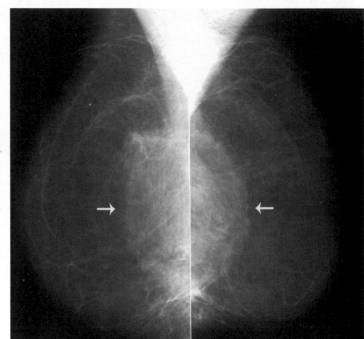

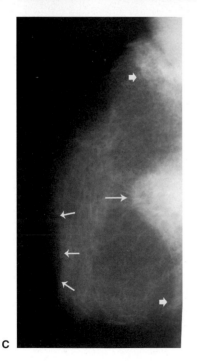

Figure 10.22 *Transverse rectus abdominis myocutaneous (TRAM) flap. A.* TRAM flap on the left after mastectomy. Density posteriorly (*arrows*) represents the rectus muscle. Fatty tissue is seen anterior to muscle. Recurrences close to the chest wall can be detected on this view before they are clinically apparent. *B.* Different patient; bilateral TRAM flaps. Density posterior (*arrows*) represents rectus muscle. Fatty tissue is seen anterior to muscle. *C.* Different patient; TRAM flap demonstrating common densities superiorly and inferiorly (*thick arrows*) to rectus muscle (*long, thin arrow*). A curvilinear contour and density anteriorly (*short, thin arrows*) can be seen in some of these patients and reflects the incisions made to circumvent the umbilicus.

many patients develop oil cysts or more commonly dystrophic calcifications. These calcifications may be curvilinear, coarse, bubbly, or lacelike (Figure 10.23). As described elsewhere, when calcifications begin to develop in areas of fat necrosis, they may be linear and resemble some of the calcifications that develop in association with ductal carcinoma *in situ* with central necrosis (Figure 10.23E).

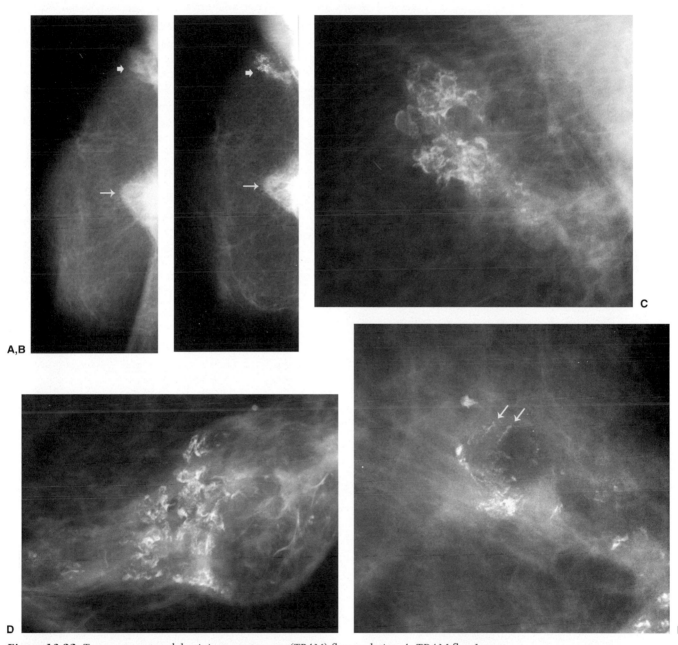

Figure 10.23 *Transverse rectus abdominis myocutaneous (TRAM) flap; evolution.* A. TRAM flap 1 year after surgery. Superior density (*thick arrow*) and rectus muscle (*thin arrow*) are seen posteriorly. B. One year after image in part A, superior density has decreased in size, and calcifications have developed. C. Close-up view of the calcifications demonstrates coarse, curvilinear morphology (bubbly appearance), a common appearance of calcifications developing in areas of fat necrosis. D. Different patient; TRAM flap. Calcifications are developing in inferior density. Coarse, curvilinear calcifications (bubbly appearance) are developing in an area of fat necrosis. E. Early in the development of calcifications related to fat necrosis, linear forms (*arrows*) may be seen. These are associated with an oil cyst and adjacent coarse calcifications.

REDUCTION MAMMOPLASTY

Breast hypertrophy can lead to significant medical issues for affected women. These include respiratory compromise secondary to increases in chest wall weight; alterations in posture; back, thoracic, and breast pain; shoulder grooving; intertrigal infections at the inframammary fold; and psychosocial issues. If the hypertrophy is asymmetric, unilateral reduction is indicated to achieve symmetry.

Several surgical procedures are now available for breast reduction. These usually involve the creation of lateral and medial flaps and a flap for the nipple–areolar complex. A periareolar incision, alone or in combination with a vertical scar to the inframammary fold and a horizontal scar along the inframammary fold are used to either reposition breast tissue or excise tissue and reposition the breast on the chest wall (20).

Potential complications of reduction mammoplasty include nipple necrosis and loss in up to 5% of patients (20). Patients who are smokers or have diabetes or hypertension and are obese have an increased incidence of this complication. Flap necrosis usually involving the lateral flap may occur. Some patients experience periareolar sensory deficits; these often resolve with time. Hypertrophic scarring, postoperative fluid collections, fat necrosis with subsequent oil cyst formation, loss of lactation, cosmetic disappointments (nipple position, asymmetry, breast shape, underreduction or overreduction), regrowth, and recurrent hypertrophy are also potential complications (20).

Common mammographic findings after reduction mammoplasty are variable but distinctive (21) and include the following:

- Nonanatomic distribution of glandular tissue (Figure 10.24)
- Swirling pattern of tissue inferiorly on MLO views (Figure 10.25)
- Fibrotic bands in the subareolar area on CC views (Figure 10.26)
- Distortion
- Oil cysts (Figure 10.27)
- Dystrophic calcifications (Figure 10.27)

Distortion, oil cysts, and calcifications often evolve and become less prominent on follow-up studies.

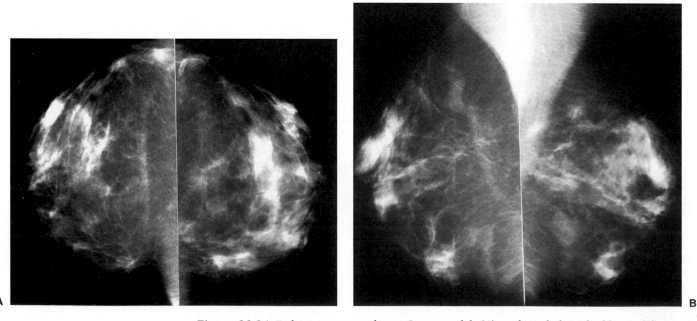

A

B

Figure 10.24 *Reduction mammoplasty.* Craniocaudal (*A*) and mediolateral oblique (*B*) views. Islands of tissue in a nonanatomic distribution.

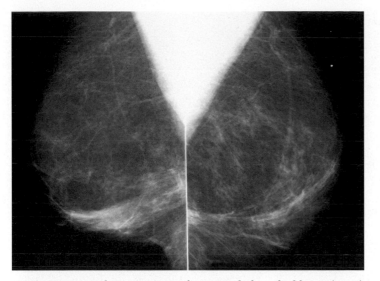

Figure 10.25 *Reduction mammoplasty*. Mediolateral oblique (MLO) views demonstrating tissue swirling inferiorly. Usually, tissue is more common in the upper outer quadrants of the breasts. After reduction mammoplasty, however, the tissue often drops inferiorly and acquires this curvilinear appearance. The nipples on these patients commonly point superiorly secondary to reposition of the nipple–areolar complex; this usually requires use of a bright light to detect.

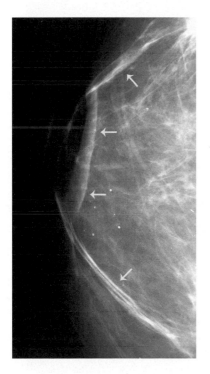

Figure 10.26 *Reduction mammoplasty*. Craniocaudal view demonstrating fibrotic bands (*arrows*) seen in some of these patients. These fibrotic bands are sometimes only seen in the subareolar area.

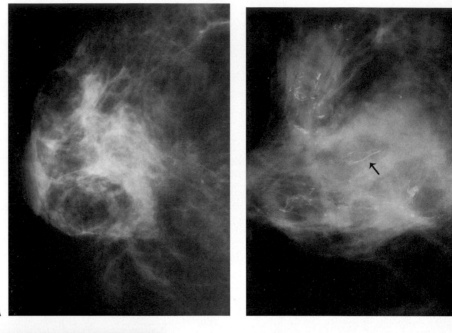

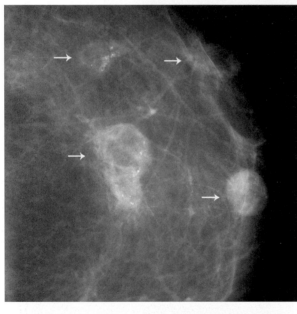

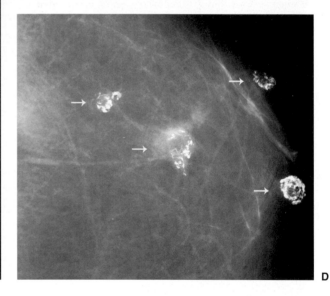

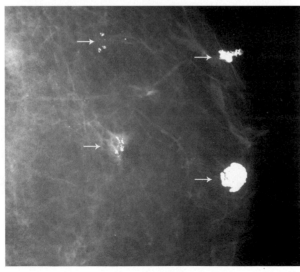

Figure 10.27 Reduction mammoplasty. A. One year after surgery, a mixed-density lesion seen in the right subareolar area is consistent with fat necrosis. *B.* Two years after surgery, the mixed-density lesion is again noted. Dystrophic calcifications are now developing. Some of these are linear (*arrow*). No intervention or short-term follow-up is indicated. This is the normal evolution of fat necrosis. *C.* Different patient, 1 year after reduction mammoplasty. Three mixed-density masses and one (closest to the nipple) seemingly of water density (*arrows*) are seen. Low-density calcifications are starting to develop. *D.* Two years after surgery, the masses (*arrows*) have almost resolved, and all that is seen are dense, coarse calcifications. *E.* Three years after surgery, calcifications are now also resolving (*arrows*).

AUGMENTATION

As an attempt to improve on nature, breast augmentation has been beset with controversy from its earliest days when, in some instances, the women themselves used paraffin and then silicone injections. The development of hard breast masses, draining sinuses, inflammatory reactions, tissue necrosis, and pulmonary and cerebral emboli are just some of the complications encountered in many of these patients. Although paraffin and silicone injections have never been approved in the United States, we see women in whom the long-term sequelae of these procedures in the breast hamper our ability to detect early, potentially curable breast cancer (Figure 10.28). In the 1950s, polyvinyl alcohol sponges (Ivalon) were introduced and used for augmentation with good results, initially. With time, however, contracture, distortion, and hardness of the breasts developed in most patients. High rates of infection and extrusion were reported when other sponges (Etheron, Polystan, polyurethane, Teflon) were used.

Following the first reports describing the use of silicone implants in 1963, a revolution took place that came to a grinding halt in April of 1992. After this date, the U.S. Food and Drug Administration (FDA) imposed a ban on the use of silicone prostheses for the purposes of aesthetic augmentation. As with other augmentation methods, complications were reported as experience accrued with silicone implants. Complications unique to women with breast implants include capsular contracture, gel bleed, rupture, and the potential association with autoimmune disorders. Although the FDA used reports of a potential link between silicone implants and autoimmune disorders to withdraw silicone implants from the market, this remains controversial. No definitive proof has been forthcoming establishing a cause-and-effect relationship.

As foreign bodies, all implants incite a reaction that is characterized by the deposition of an avascular and acellular matrix of continuous bands of fibrous tissue. These fibrous capsules can remain soft and pliable such that the breast has a natural feel and look. In many patients, however, the capsule contracts, "strangulating" the implant. This contrac-

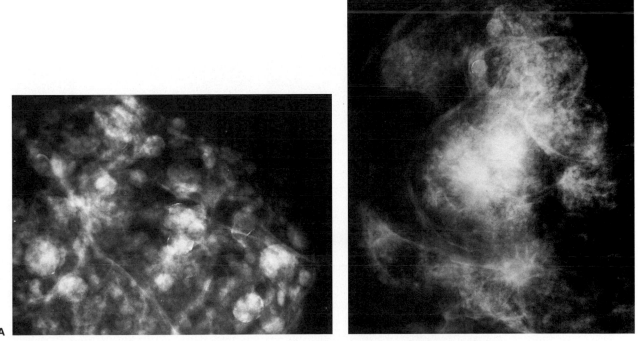

Figure 10.28 *Augmentation, subcutaneous silicone injections. A. A myriad of dense masses are seen, some with curvilinear calcifications consistent with silicone granulomas. B. Slightly different pattern for subcutaneous silicone injections, showing areas of high density and significant distortion. Our ability to detect early breast cancer in these patients is significantly limited.*

ture results in a hard, palpable, visible, and relatively immobile, noncompressible implant. Usually a bilateral process, capsular contraction has been reported in as many as 74% of women with smooth-walled implants (21). In some patients, the capsule can calcify, contributing to the hardness of the implant. Unless the capsule is calcified, it is not usually visible mammographically (Figure 10.29). Many causes for capsular contraction have been suggested, including bleeding, subclinical infections, and inflammatory reactions; however, no definite etiologic factor has been identified.

Treatment approaches for encapsulation include closed and open capsulotomies (20). A closed capsulotomy involves manual circumferential compression of the implant to "pop" the capsule. This releases and helps soften the feel of the implant. Potential complications associated with this procedure include bleeding, implant rupture, and an asymmetric capsular tear distorting the appearance of the breast. Gamekeeper's thumb, resulting from an injury to the ulnar collateral ligament has been reported as a potential complication for the plastic surgeons doing closed capsulotomies. An open capsulotomy is the surgical alternative for releasing the implant from the capsule. The type of implant and placement (subglandular versus subpectoral) can be changed at the time of the capsulotomy, in an attempt to minimize the likelihood of recurring capsular contraction.

During open capsulotomies, silicone is often seen on the surface of intact implants and is found microscopically in the capsule around the implant. This reflects the slow egress of silicone fluid through the semipermeable implant shell, a process commonly referred to as "gel bleed." As pointed out by Middleton and McNamara, however, this phenomenon is more appropriately referred to as "silicone fluid bleed" because it is silicone fluid that egresses from the implant, not the cross-linked silicone gel on the inside of the implant (22,23). All implants have an elastomer shell made of cross-linked silicone that creates a semipermeable barrier for the gel contents of the implant. The extent of the cross-

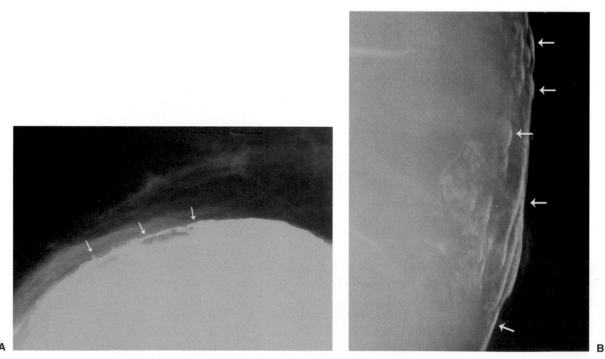

Figure 10.29 *Capsular calcification.* A. Subglandular, silicone implant. All patients develop a fibrous capsule around the implants. This capsule is not apparent, unless it calcifies (*arrows*). When capsular calcifications are present, there is usually significant encapsulation, limiting our ability to do implant-displaced views. B. Saline implant. Capsular calcifications (*arrows*) are seen as plaque-like areas of increased density, when in tangent to the x-ray beam. These calcifications develop in the fibrous capsule, not on the surface of the implant.

linking on the shell determines the rate of silicone fluid bleed as low or high. From the day implants are put in, silicone fluid bleeds out. The cross-linked silicone gel inside the implants escapes only after implant rupture.

Implant rupture can be the result of direct trauma, closed capsulotomies, or aging of the implant with decomposition of the implant shell. Intracapsular rupture refers to the disruption of the implant shell with containment of the implant contents by the capsule. The presence of this type of rupture is best evaluated with magnetic resonance imaging (23) (Figure 10.30). Fragments of the implant shell are imaged floating in the implant contents contained by an intact capsule. Extracapsular rupture results in the extrusion of implant contents outside of the capsule (Figure 10.31). When this is silicone, a high-density, amorphous material or high-density droplets can be seen surrounding the implant (24,25). If long-standing, silicone is seen extending to the axilla and in association with axillary lymph nodes (Figure 10.32). Ultrasonographically, extravasated silicone may be seen as high specular echoes deep to an echogenic line (snowstorm appearance) or as a hypoechoic mass (26–28).

Inframammary, periareolar, and transaxillary surgical approaches are used to place implants in subglandular or subpectoral locations. The subglandular position (Figure 10.33) is more commonly used, reported in 77% to 87% of patients with implants (29). Subpectoral placement (Figure 10.34) may be associated with lower incidence of capsular contraction, possibly related to the massaging of the implant by the overlying muscle. Subpectoral placement facilitates mammographic imaging. Projection of the implant may, however, be limited when subpectoral in location.

The type of implant and its position can often be determined mammographically. On close inspection, textured implants are characterized by subtle undulations of the surface. Saline implants are less radiopaque than silicone implants, so that wrinkles and valves are usually visible (Figure 10.35). Rarely, calcifications can develop on the valve of the implant. These calcifications may be round, punctate, and pleomorphic, simulating the type of calcifications seen in ductal carcinoma *in situ*. As different projections are obtained, these calcifications are always associated with the valve of the implant (Figure 10.36). In other patients, the valvular calcifications are dense and coarse (Figure 10.37). Different densities, constituting the different components of the implants, characterize double-

> Magnetic resonance imaging is the study of choice in evaluating implant integrity.

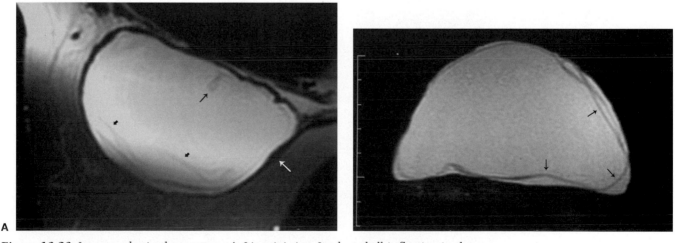

A   B

Figure 10.30 *Intracapsular implant rupture.* A. Linguini sign. Implant shell is floating in the contents of the implant (*thick, black arrows*). The capsule is seen as a signal void surrounding the implant (*white arrow*). Posteriorly, a keyhole shape (*thin, black arrow*) is seen. Note that silicone (bright signal) is seen in the keyhole. When this is seen in isolation (e.g., implant is otherwise intact), it is thought possibly to reflect silicone fluid bleed. B. Linguini sign. Implant shell is floating in the contents of the implant (*arrows*).

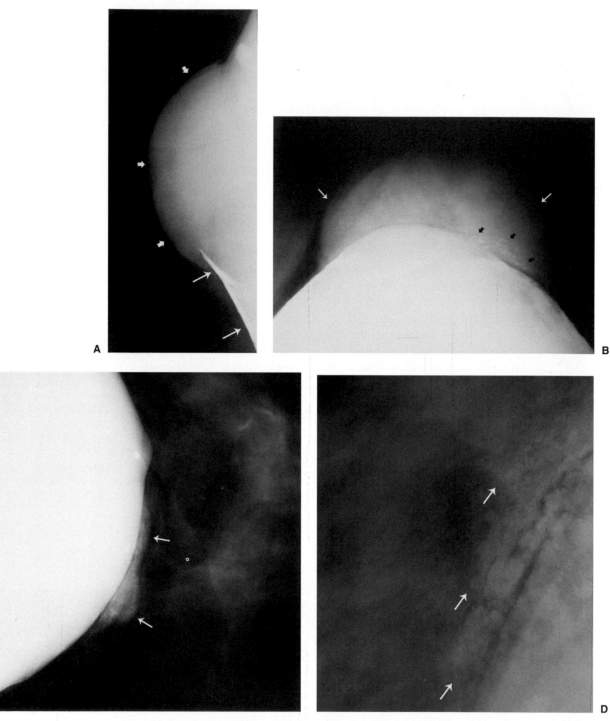

Figure 10.31 *Extracapsular implant rupture. A.* Silicone (*thick arrows*) is seen extending beyond capsular calcifications (*thin arrows*), consistent with extracapsular rupture of the implant. A bulge or herniation of the implant through a capsular tear is an alternative explanation, particularly given the well-circumscribed margins of the protruded material. Localized rupture and bulges or herniations of the implant, through a capsular tear, can be difficult to distinguish from an extracapsular rupture mammographically. *B.* Different patient. Silicone (*white arrows*) extends superiorly to implant, anterior to the pectoral muscle. Some capsular calcifications are also noted (*black arrows*). *C.* Different patient. Small amount of silicone is seen surrounding the medial portion of the implant (*arrows*). Notice the irregular, amorphous margins. This is extravasate silicone. *D.* Different patient; slightly different pattern. Silicone (*arrows*) is external to implant and migrating toward the axilla.

(continued on next page)

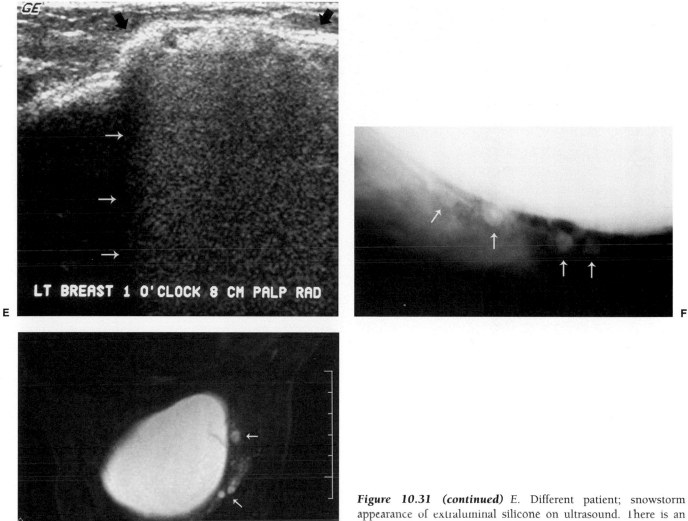

LT BREAST 1 O'CLOCK 8 CM PALP RAD

Figure 10.31 (continued) E. Different patient; snowstorm appearance of extraluminal silicone on ultrasound. There is an echogenic, irregular line (*black arrows*), below which high specular echoes are seen (*white arrows*). *F.* Different patient. Rounded areas of increased density (*arrows*) are consistent with extruded silicone surrounding a portion of the implant in a patient after a motor vehicle crash. *G.* Extraluminal silicone is easily seen on magnetic resonance imaging (*arrows*).

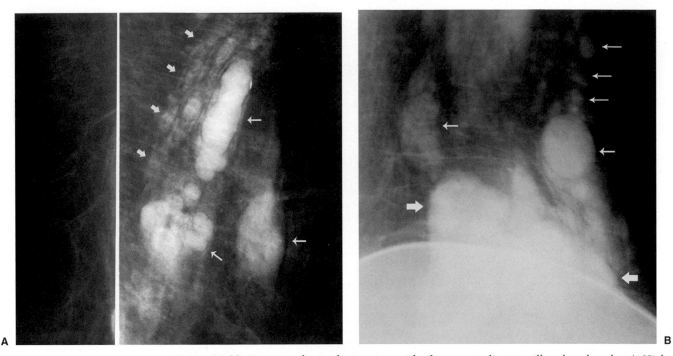

Figure 10.32 *Extracapsular implant rupture with silicone extending to axillary lymph nodes. A.* High-density material is seen, increasing the density of several axillary lymph nodes (*thin arrows*). Silicone is also seen in beaded, linear-like tracks (*thick arrows*); this may represent silicone in lymphatic channels. This appearance is not seen acutely after extracapsular rupture. This represent a long-standing extracapsular rupture. *B.* Different patient. Silicone is seen surrounding the implant (*thick arrows*) consistent with extracapsular rupture. Additionally, silicone is seen extending to axillary lymph nodes (*short, thin arrows*) and beyond the lymph nodes in beaded, linear-like tracks (*long, thin arrows*).

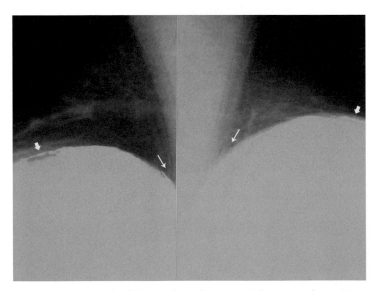

Figure 10.33 *Subglandular implant placement.* Silicone implants. Note the high density of implant contents. Pectoral muscle is seen "diving" down posterior to implants (*thin arrows*). Capsular calcification (*thick arrows*) is present bilaterally.

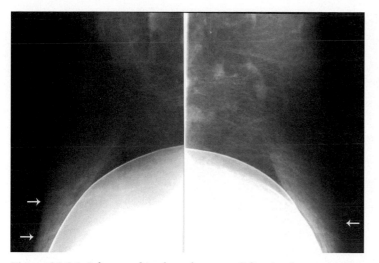

Figure 10.34 *Subpectoral implant placement*. Saline implants; note low density compared with silicone implants. A strip of pectoral muscle (*arrows*) is seen anterior to implants. In some patients, a bright light is needed to visualize adequately the strip of muscle anterior to the implants.

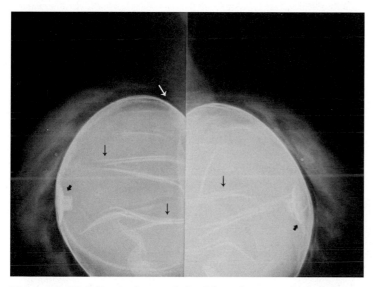

Figure 10.35 *Saline implants, subglandular in location*. The low density of the saline enables visualization of wrinkles involving the implants (*thin, black arrows*) and the valves associated with some of the saline implants (*thick, black arrows*). The pectoral muscle is seen posterior to the implants (*white arrow*).

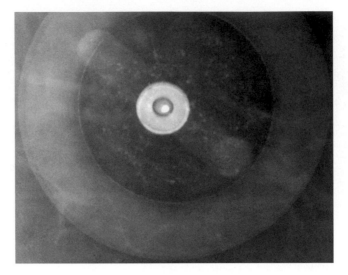

Figure 10.36 Calcifications associated with valve, saline implant. Pleomorphic calcifications involving the valve of this type of saline implant. In all projections obtained, these are associated with the valve on the implant. This is not commonly seen.

lumen implants (Figure 10.38). With subglandular placement, the pectoral muscle can be seen angling acutely posterior to the implant (Figure 10.35). A strip of muscle of varying thickness is usually seen covering the upper portion of the implant when subpectoral in location (Figure 10.34).

Contour deformities, surface undulations, bulges or herniations (Figure 10.39), capsular calcifications, and extracapsular silicone can all be seen mammographically. Intra-

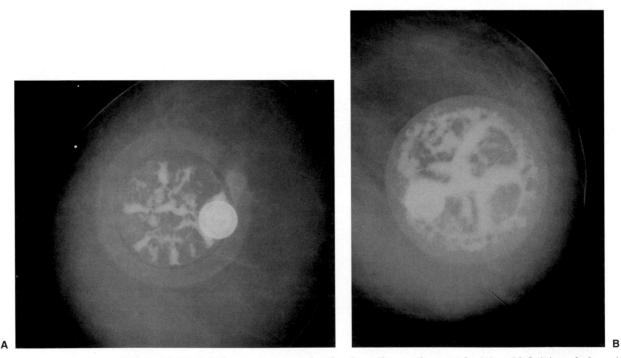

A   B

Figure 10.37 *Calcifications associated with valve, saline implants. Right (A) and left (B) mediolateral oblique views. Dense, coarse calcifications developing on the valve of this type of saline implant. This type of valvular calcification is probably even less common than that shown in Figure 10.36.*

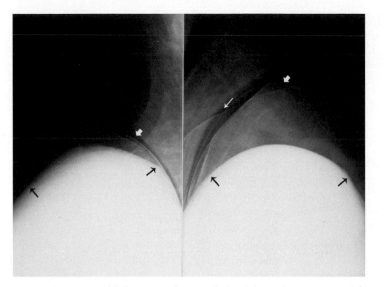

Figure 10.38 *Double lumen implants, subglandular in location.* Two different densities are seen associated with these implants. In this patient, the low-density saline component is on the outside (*thick, white arrows*). Silicone is the inner component (*black arrows*). The pectoral muscle (*thin, white arrow*) is seen posterior to the implants.

capsular ruptures and gel bleed are not seen mammographically but can be seen on magnetic resonance imaging (27). When implants are removed, unilateral or bilateral fluid collections may develop posteriorly at the site occupied by the implants, presumably forming within the preexisting capsule. Alternatively, portions of the capsule may be seen as curvilinear densities of variable thickness posteriorly. These may have, or develop, associated dystrophic calcifications (Figure 10.40).

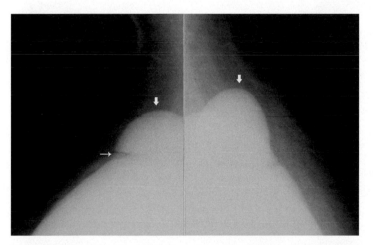

Figure 10.39 *Bulges or herniations.* In some patients, round or oval contour deformities (*thick arrows*) can be seen with areas of constriction (*thin arrow*). The protrusions are well marginated, likely representing a bulge or herniation of an intact implant through tears in the capsule.

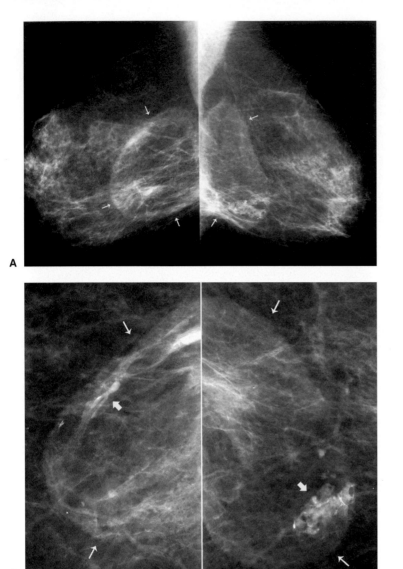

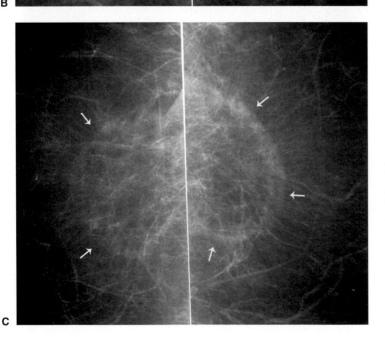

Figure 10.40 *After removal of subglandular implants. A.* Mediolateral oblique views demonstrate a curvilinear density posteriorly (*arrows*) after removal of implants. This is presumably a retained capsule. In some women, a water-density mass appearance is seen consistent with a fluid collection. *B.* Close-up, craniocaudal projection demonstrates curvilinear density (*thin arrows*). Coarse, dense dystrophic calcifications (*thick arrows*) are noted involving portions of the residual capsule. *C.* Different patient; more subtle findings. Curvilinear density (*arrows*) is more prominent on the left than the right, in this patient after implant removal.

ESTROGEN EFFECT

Natural and premature, (surgically or chemically induced) menopause is associated with a variety of signs and symptoms, some of which have significant health implications for the patient while others affect quality of life. Hormone replacement therapy (HRT) is used to treat some of the signs and symptoms associated with menopause. In women who have had a hysterectomy, estrogen replacement is given alone. For patients who have not had a hysterectomy, the risk for uterine cancer is increased if estrogen is given continuously or unopposed; in these patients, estrogen needs to be stopped for a specified amount of time during the month, or progesterone needs to be given.

Postmenopausal women burn less calories at rest, compared with premenopausal women; hence, estrogen levels decrease, and women gain weight. Vasomotor symptoms, including hot flashes and night sweats, affect 85% of women undergoing natural menopause. These symptoms may be exasperated in women undergoing premature, surgically or chemically induced, menopause. These symptoms are significantly improved or relieved in a large number of women using HRT. Bone mineral density, leading to osteoporosis and the increased risk for hip or wrist fractures, decrease rapidly during the first 5 years after menopause. HRT is effective in preventing the decreases in bone mineral density seen postmenopausally, and in some women, HRT actually leads to increases in bone mineral density (30).

The issue of coronary artery disease and of the potential preventive effect of HRT is controversial. Early studies suggest a protective effect for women taking HRT, whereas more recent studies suggest there may be no protective benefit. The potential role of HRT in breast cancer development also remains unclear. It would appear that, at least for the first 10 years of therapy, there might be no significant increase in breast cancer among women taking HRT. Additional studies are needed to elucidate the nature of the relationship, if any, between HRT and the development or stimulation of breast cancer. It is a particularly difficult and controversial issue to address in young women with surgically or chemically induced menopausal symptoms who have a personal history of breast cancer (30).

Mammographically, no change is seen in the appearance of the breast parenchyma in 63% of patients taking HRT. Diffuse density increase (Figure 10.41) or cyst formation is reported in up to 24% of women taking HRT. In about 12% of patients, breast density decreases slightly after therapy is instituted (31,32).

Tamoxifen is an antiestrogenic medication currently used in the treatment and prevention of breast cancer. Decreases in the density of the breast parenchyma can be seen mammographically in a small number of women taking tamoxifen (33). Conversely, increases in the density of the parenchyma can be seen when tamoxifen therapy is stopped. This "rebound" in the tissue should not be mistaken for a recurrence presenting with diffuse changes.

> Increases in the density of the parenchyma or the development of cysts is seen in about 24% of women taking HRT.

MISCELLANEOUS

WEIGHT CHANGES

Alterations in breast size, differences in the glandular-to-fatty tissue ratio, centimeters of compression, and technical factors needed to obtain an optimal image can be noted after significant changes in body weight. Weight loss can result in perceptible decreases in breast size and compression required to obtain an optimal image. Tissue density seemingly increases as the amount of fatty tissue is reduced, and glandular tissue aggregates become denser in some women (Figure 10.42). Conversely, significant increases in weight lead to increases in breast size and dispersal of glandular tissue by increasing amounts of fatty tissue.

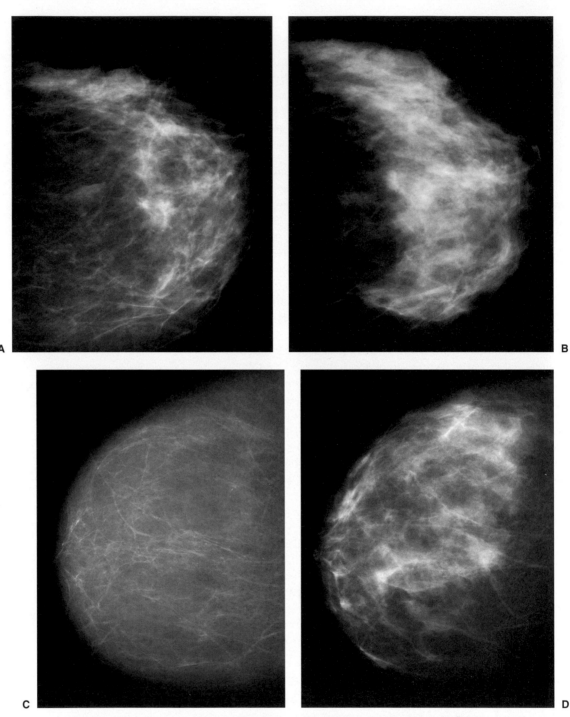

Figure 10.41 *Estrogen effect. A.* Craniocaudal view showing glandular tissue. *B.* Increase in the amount and density of the tissue 1 year after starting hormone replacement therapy (HRT). *C.* Different patient; craniocaudal view showing fatty tissue. *D.* Development of glandular tissue 1 year after HRT started. These patients often describe associated breast engorgement and pain, which can be significant. Cysts are sometimes also seen to develop or enlarge after HRT therapy is started.

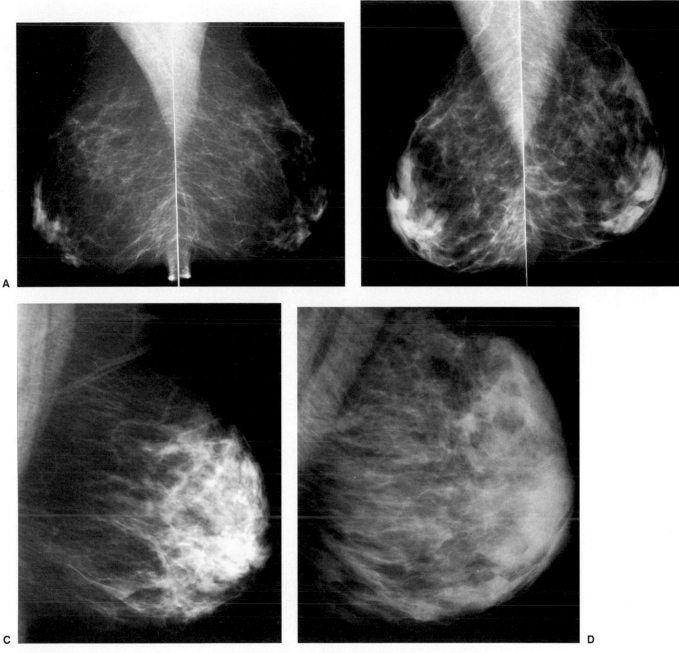

Figure 10.42 *Effect of weight changes. A.* Mediolateral oblique (MLO) views. *B.* Screening mammogram after 60-lb weight loss. The amount of fatty tissue is reduced, and glandular tissue has seemingly increased in amount and density. *C.* Different patient; left MLO view. *D.* Left MLO view after 150-lb weight loss. Amount of fatty tissue is reduced significantly, and the tissue appears increased in amount and density. The amount of compression applied and technical factors used for exposure need to be adjusted.

FOREIGN BODIES

In some patients, foreign bodies may be localized to the breast. Most patients are not aware of their presence and rarely recall the traumatic event. These include, but are not limited to, lead pencil tips, needle or needle fragments, bullets, metallic BBs, or shrapnel. The shape and density of these foreign bodies are usually distinctive enough for their characterization (Figure 10.43). With shrapnel, high-density particles can be seen detailing the track followed by the bullet in the breast (Figure 5.49 in Chapter 5). In some women, nipple rings may be present (Figure 2.40 in Chapter 2). After preoperative wire localizations, wire fragments (Figure 10.4A) are rarely noted on follow-up mammograms, indicating that the localization wire was inadvertently transected during the excisional biopsy.

DACRON CENTRAL LINE CUFF

A 4- to 6-inch subcutaneous tunnel in the medial aspect of the chest is made for Hickman catheter placement. A Dacron cuff is used to anchor the catheter to the subcutaneous tissue midway between the skin and venous entry points. These cuffs may be palpable and are more commonly seen on the right in the upper inner quadrant of the breast. When the catheter is pulled out, the Dacron cuff remains in place and may be seen on the MLO view and less commonly on the CC view (34) (Figure 10.44). Abscess formation around the cuff has been reported and should be suspected when an irregular mass that may contain air is seen associated with the cuff (35).

PORTABLE CATHETERS

Portable catheters (e.g., port-a-cath) are surgically placed on the chest wall, often the upper inner quadrant of either breast. They provide convenient venous access for patients receiving chemotherapy. While in place, they can be seen as a round area of increased density on the MLO view and less commonly medially on the CC view. In a small number of women, a fluid collection (Figure 10.45), area of spiculation (Figure 10.46), or calcifica-

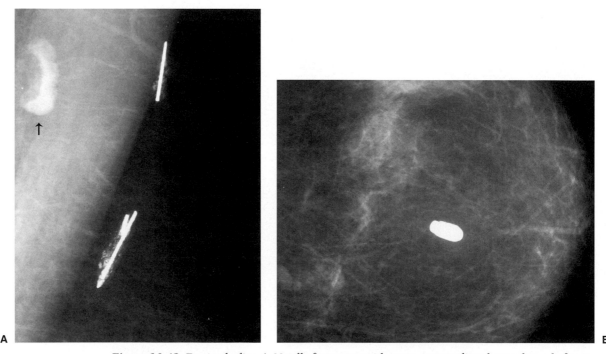

A   **B**

Figure 10.43 *Foreign bodies. A.* Needle fragments with some surrounding dystrophic calcifications. Axillary lymph node (*arrow*). *B.* Different patient showing bullet.

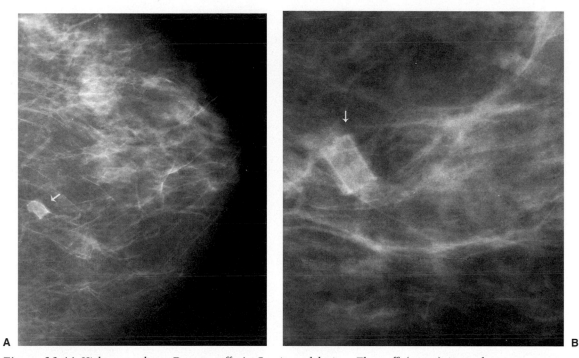

A   B

Figure 10.44 *Hickman catheter Dacron cuff.* A. Craniocaudal view. The cuff (*arrow*) is used to anchor the central line in the medial aspect of the left breast. On mediolateral oblique views (not shown), this is seen superimposed on the pectoral muscle. B. Different patient; close-up of the cuff (*arrow*). When present for a long time, the edges of the cuff can become frayed and indistinct.

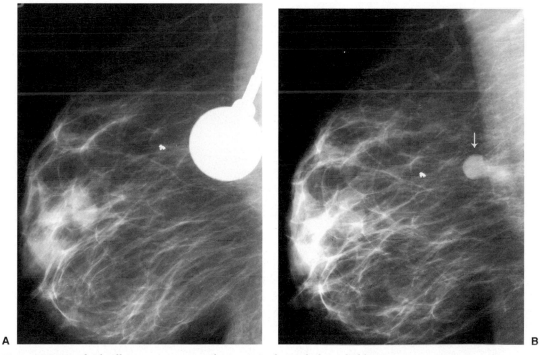

A   B

Figure 10.45 *Fluid collection at port-a-cath site.* A. Right mediolateral oblique view in a patient with a port-a-cath in place for chemotherapy. The catheter could also be seen medially on the craniocaudal (CC) view (not shown). B. A mass (*arrow*) with partially indistinct margins is seen corresponding to the site of the port-a-cath on orthogonal views (CC view not shown).

(*continued on next page*)

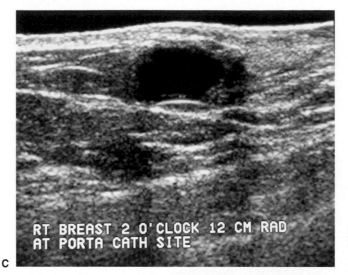

Figure 10.45 (continued) *C.* Ultrasound demonstrates a fluid collection.

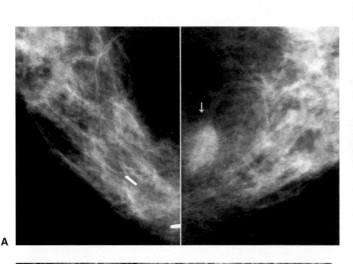

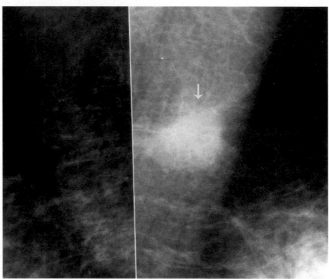

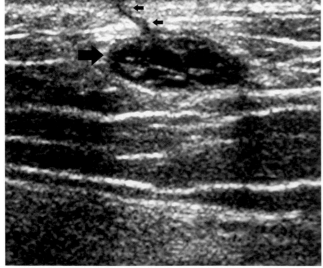

Figure 10.46 *Fluid collection at port-a-cath site.* Craniocaudal (CC) (*A*) and mediolateral oblique (*B*) views show an ill-defined mass (*arrows*) in the upper inner quadrant of the left breast in a patient after lumpectomy, radiation treatment, and chemotherapy for right breast cancer (clips seen on right CC view). *C.* Complex cystic mass (*large arrow*) with posterior acoustic enhancement and track to skin (*small arrows*) corresponding to the mammographic abnormality in the left breast and the site occupied by the port-a-cath used to administer chemotherapy; consistent with fluid collection. In our experience, findings at port-a-cath sites are common and range from round to spiculated masses to, less commonly, dystrophic calcifications. These changes usually resolve on follow-up studies.

tions can be seen developing after removal of the catheter. These changes usually resolve on subsequent mammograms but can simulate a malignancy initially. If the findings are directly correlated to the port-a-cath site, a conservative approach is appropriate.

PACEMAKERS

Pacemakers may be partially or completely seen on MLO views superimposed on the pectoral muscle. If the pacemaker is removed, pacemaker wires may remain, and coarse calcifications may develop in the cavity left by the pacemaker. Depending on the location and size of the pacemaker, positioning on the MLO view may be compromised, and breast or axillary tissue may be excluded from view.

REFERENCES

1. Sickles EA, Herzog KA. Mammography of the postsurgical breast. *AJR Am J Roentgenol* 1981; 136:585–588.
2. Mendelson EB. Evaluation of the postoperative breast. *Radiol Clin North Am* 1992;30:107–138.
3. Stigers KB, King JG, Darvey DD, et al. Abnormalities of the breast caused by biopsy: spectrum of mammographic findings. *AJR Am J Roentgenol* 1991;156:287–291.
4. Burbank F, Forcier N. Tissue marking clip for stereotactic breast biopsy: initial placement accuracy, long-term stability and usefulness as a guide for wire localization. *Radiology* 1997;205: 407–415.
5. Burnside ES, Sohlich RE, Sickles EA. Movement of a biopsy-site marker after completion of stereotactic directional vacuum-assisted breast biopsy: case report. *Radiology* 2001;221: 504–507.
6. DiPiro PJ, Meyer JE, Frenna TH, et al. Seat beat injuries of the breast: findings on mammography and sonography. *AJR Am J Roentgenol* 1995;164:317–320.
7. Harris KM, Costa-Greco MA, Baratz AB, et al. The mammographic features of the postlumpectomy, postirradiation breast. *Radiographics* 1989;9:253–268.
8. Hassell PR, Olivotto IA, Mueller HA, et al. Early breast cancer: detection of recurrence after conservative surgery and radiation therapy. *Radiology* 1990;176:731–735.
9. Bassett LW, Jackson VP, Jahan R, et al. *Diagnosis of disease of the breast.* Philadelphia: WB Saunders, 1997.
10. Brenner RJ, Pfaff JM. Mammographic features after conservative therapy for malignant breast disease: serial findings standardized by regression analysis. *AJR Am J Roentgenol* 1996;171–178.
11. Dershaw DD. Mammography in patients with breast cancer treated by breast conservation (lumpectomy with or without radiation). *AJR Am J Roentgenol* 1995;164:309–316.
12. Krishnamurthy R, Whitman GJ, Stelling CB, et al. Mammographic findings after breast conservation therapy. *Radiographics* 1999;19:S53–S62.
13. Liberman L, Van Zee KJ, Dershaw DD, et al. Mammographic features of local recurrence in women who have undergone breast-conserving therapy for ductal carcinoma in situ. *AJR Am J Roentgenol* 1997;489–493.
14. Philpotts LE, Lee CH, Haffty BG, et al. Mammographic findings of recurrent breast cancer after lumpectomy and radiation therapy: comparison with primary tumor. *Radiology* 1996;201: 767–771.
15. Rissanen TJ, Makarainen HP, Mattila SI, et al. Breast cancer recurrence after mastectomy: diagnosis with mammography and US. *Radiology* 1993;188:463–467.
16. Fajardo LL, Roberts CC, Hunt KR. Mammographic surveillance of breast cancer patients: should the mastectomy site be imaged? *AJR Am J Roentgenol* 1993;161:953–955.
17. Tabar L. *Personal communication,* 1995.
18. Helvie MA, Wilson TE, Roubidoux MA, et al. Mammographic appearance of recurrent breast carcinoma in six patients with TRAM flap breast reconstructions. *Radiology* 1998;209:711–715.
19. Hogge JP, Zuurbier RA, S de Paredes E. Mammography of autologous myocutaneous flaps. *Radiographics* 1999;19:S63–S72.
20. Georgiade NG, Georgiade GS, Riefkohl R. *Aesthetic surgery of the breast.* Philadelphia: WB Saunders, 1990.
21. Miller CL, Feig SA, Fox JW. Mammographic changes after reduction mammoplasty. *AJR Am J Roentgenol* 1987;149:35–38.

22. Hester TR. The polyurethane covered mammary prosthesis: facts and fiction. *Perspect Plastic Surg* 1988;2:135–169.
23. Middleton MS, McNamara MP. *Breast implant imaging.* Philadelphia: Lippincott Williams & Wilkins, 2003.
24. Mund DF, Farria DM, Gorczyca DP, et al. MR imaging of the breast in patients with silicone-gel implants: spectrum of findings. *AJR Am J Roentgenol* 1993;161:773–778.
25. Everson LI, Parantainen H, Detlie T, et al. Diagnosis of breast implant rupture: imaging findings and relative efficacies of imaging techniques. *AJR Am J Roentgenol* 1994;163:57–60.
26. Harris KM, Ganott MA, Shestak KC, et al. Silicone implant rupture: detection with US. *Radiology* 1993;187:761–768.
27. Ganott MA, Harris KM, Ilkanipour ZS, et al. Augmentation mammoplasty: normal and abnormal findings with mammography and US. *Radiographics* 1992;12:281–295.
28. Rosculet KA, Ikeda DM, Forrest ME, et al. Ruptured gel-filled silicone breast implants: sonographic findings in 19 cases. *AJR Am J Roentgenol* 1992;159:711–716.
29. Destouet JM, Monsees BS, Oser RF, et al. Screening mammography in 350 women with breast implants: prevalence and findings of implant complications. *AJR Am J Roentgenol* 1992;159:973–978.
30. Harris JR, Lippman ME, Morrow M, et al., eds. *Disease of the breast,* 2nd ed. Philadelphia: Lippincott Williams & Wilkins, 2000.
31. Stomper PC, Van Voorhis BJ, Ravnikar VA, et al. Mammographic changes associated with postmenopausal hormone replacement therapy: a longitudinal study. *Radiology* 1990;174:487–490.
32. Berkowitz JE, Gatewood OMB, Goldblum LE, et al. Hormonal replacement therapy: mammographic manifestations. *Radiology* 1990;174:199–201.
33. Cardenosa G, Eklund GW. Breast parenchymal change following treatment with tamoxifen [letter to the editor]. *Breast Dis* 1992;5:55–58.
34. Beyer GA, Thorsen MK, Shaffer KA, et al. Mammographic appearance of the retained Dacron cuff of a Hickman catheter. *AJR Am J Roentgenol* 1990;155:1204.
35. Ellis RL, Dempsey PJ, Rubin E, et al. Mammography of breasts in which catheter cuffs have been retained: normal, infected and postoperative appearances. *AJR Am J Roentgenol* 1997;169:713–715.

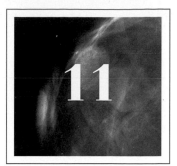

INTERVENTIONAL PROCEDURES

DUCTOGRAPHY

The evaluation and management of patients presenting with nipple discharge is variable among clinicians. Commonly, a prolactin level is checked, and some of the discharge is submitted for cytologic evaluation; if these tests are normal, the patient usually undergoes no further workup unless the discharge is bloody. Patients with bloody nipple discharge are referred to a surgeon and may undergo a subareolar duct excision. Inherent assumptions in these approaches that need to be challenged are outlined in Table 11.1.

Although ductography is not a perfect test, it can help address some of these issues. The presence, location, and extent of a lesion can be demonstrated in many patients with spontaneous nipple discharge. The location of the duct containing the lesion and its distribution in the breast can be established preoperatively. When findings consistent with duct ectasia or fibrocystic changes are diagnosed, surgery may be averted. Finally, if preoperative ductograms are done using a methylene blue–contrast combination (1:1), the contrast allows us to verify that we cannulated the abnormal duct; the methylene blue stains the duct so that it is easy to identify intraoperatively by the surgeon intraoperatively and by the pathologist at the time the specimen is processed. This helps ensure that the lesion is localized, excised, and evaluated histologically.

Clinically, patients with intraductal lesions may present describing nipple discharge. When asked how they notice the discharge, patients invariably provide one of three histories. They notice dark spots on their bra cups or spots on their nightclothes, or after taking a hot bath or shower, they notice that their nipple is dripping. If the discharge is only expressed after vigorous manipulation of the breast and nipple, the likelihood of finding an intraductal lesion is low, and ductography is not indicated.

Ductography is a safe, easy, and simple contrast evaluation of a lactiferous duct (1–4). The only relative contraindication to ductography is the presence of mastitis, and no significant complications have been described with the water-soluble contrast agents currently in use. Ductography is used to evaluate women presenting with spontaneous nipple discharge, regardless of the character of the discharge (Figure 11.1). Adequate lighting and magnification of the nipple are helpful in identifying the secreting duct opening. Full-strength iodinated contrast material is drawn into a 3-mL Luer-Lok syringe. A 30-gauge blunt-tip sialography needle with attached tubing is screwed onto the Luer-Lok syringe,

Ductography is used to evaluate women presenting with spontaneous nipple discharge, regardless of the character of the discharge.

Table 11.1: Common Assumptions in Women with Nipple Discharge

Assumption	Fact
1. Negative cytology results reliably exclude pathology.	Negative cytology does not reliably exclude significant pathology.
2. Only bloody nipple discharge is significant.	Ductal carcinoma *in situ* can present with serous or clear, heme occult–negative nipple discharge.[a]
3. The location and extent of a lesion in the duct can be reliably identified intraoperatively so that the dissection is extended as needed to include, but not transect, the lesion.	Not all papillomas are close to the subareolar area and when cancer is present if this is often extensive and not subareolar in location.
4. The pathologist can reliably identify the location of the lesion in the specimen for histologic evaluation.	Staining of the duct with methylene blue facilitates intraoperative identification of the duct for the surgeon and during processing of the specimen for the pathologist.

[a]How a patient notices the discharge is more important than the character of the discharge. Expressed nipple discharge is usually physiologic. Spontaneous nipple discharge needs to be evaluated regardless of its appearance.

making sure that the connection is tight so that air bubbles are not drawn into the syringe. Contrast material is run through the tubing until all air bubbles are removed from the system. Topical anesthesia and dilators are not needed for this procedure.

The patient is positioned supine with the ipsilateral arm placed above her head. The nipple is inspected for the presence of crusting or a dilated prominent duct opening. Using an alcohol wipe, the nipple is swabbed to remove any keratin plugs that may obstruct the duct opening. Next, the breast is examined. A "trigger point" may be identified in some patients (5). When this trigger point is compressed, nipple discharge is obtained. As you move away from this point, the discharge stops. In some patients with an intraductal lesion, the discharge can be copious and projectile.

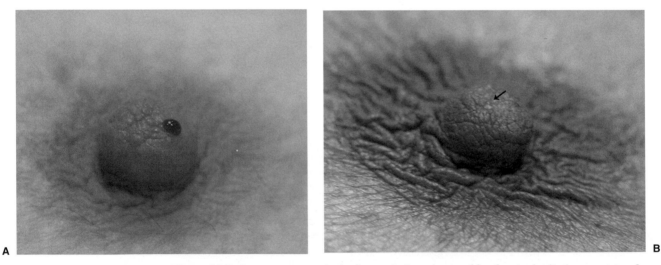

Figure 11.1 *Spontaneous nipple discharge. A.* Spontaneous bloody nipple discharge arising from a single duct opening. *B.* Spontaneous clear nipple discharge (*arrow*) arising from a single duct opening. If the patient presents with spontaneous nipple discharge, the character of the discharge does not dissuade us from evaluating the patient with ductography. Breast cancers can present with clear, or serous, heme occult–negative discharge.

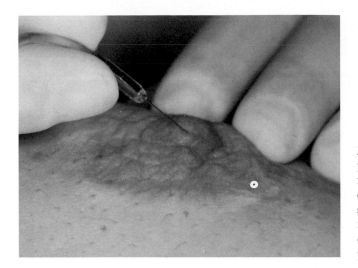

Figure 11.2 *Duct cannulation.* After the duct producing the discharge is identified, the cannula is angled, and the tip is placed in the duct opening. Next, the cannula is gently straightened. In most patients, the cannula falls in the duct to the hub. No pressure is exerted. The patient should experience no pain during cannulation.

If you identify a trigger point, use it to express small amounts of discharge. Elicit just enough to moisten and glisten the opening. If a larger amount of discharge is obtained, other openings are flooded, precluding correct identification of the offending duct. With a clear idea of which opening the discharge is coming from, angle the cannula and place the tip on the duct opening (Figure 11.2). After the cannula is engaged in this manner, straighten it so that the cannula falls into the duct to the level of the hub. After cannulation, take a few seconds to observe the tubing. Because the tubing is now in a closed system with the cannulated duct, duct contents can sometimes be seen refluxing back into the tubing (Figure 11.3). If this is not observed, start to inject contrast and look at the nipple. As intraductal fluid is displaced by contrast, some of the fluid may come out to form a drop around the cannula (Figure 11.4). When either of these observations is made, you have some assurance that you cannulated the potentially abnormal duct.

A small amount of contrast (0.2 to 0.4 mL) is injected initially, and the cannula is taped on the nipple (Figure 11.5). Injecting larger amounts of contrast at the onset may obscure small lesions (Figure 11.6) or those that are close to the nipple. Full-paddle magnification views in the craniocaudal (CC) and 90-degree lateral projections are then obtained. After a review of these initial images, additional contrast can be injected as needed, to opacify the duct proximally.

Little is known about the ductographic appearance of normal ducts. There seems to be considerable variation in length, amount of branching, distribution, and caliber (Fig-

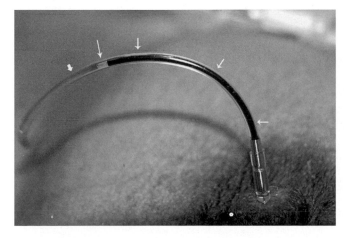

Figure 11.3 *Reflux of duct contents into tubing.* Cannula in the duct to the hub. Immediately after cannulation, observe the tubing for a few seconds before injecting contrast. The tubing is now in a closed system with the cannulated duct such that duct contents can sometimes be seen refluxing into the tubing. If this is seen, it confirms cannulation of the duct producing the discharge. In this patient, the refluxing material is bloody (*short, thin arrows*). An air bubble (*long, thin arrow*) separates the refluxing duct contents from the contrast (*thick arrow*). When the discharge is clear or serous, mixing of the duct contents with the contrast can be seen occurring in the tubing.

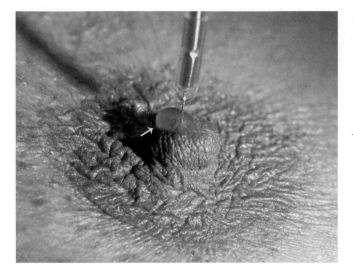

Figure 11.4 Duct contents forming droplet around cannula. If duct contents do not reflux into the tubing, duct contents can sometimes be seen forming a droplet (*arrow*) around the cannula as contrast is injected. The contrast displaces duct contents. When this is seen, it confirms cannulation of the duct producing the discharge.

ure 11.7). Occasionally, a contained contrast blush is seen, the overall appearance of which suggests the possibility of lobular opacification (Figure 11.8). We use the sialography cannula as an internal measure of duct caliber. Arbitrarily, we define normal duct caliber as up to 3 times the width of the cannula.

Solitary papillomas are diagnosed in about half of women presenting with spontaneous nipple discharge (1–7). Papillomas are most commonly found within dilated ducts in a subareolar location. Although the entire duct may be dilated in these patients, the segment of duct between the lesion and the nipple is most commonly involved. Papillomas, however, can occur anywhere in the duct, and duct dilation is not always present (Figure 11.9). Filling defects (Figure 11.10), obstruction of the main duct (Figure 11.9A) or a branch (Figure 11.11), and, less commonly, wall irregularity (Figure 11.12) are ductographic findings in patients with papillomas. In some patients, contrast can be seen pooling irregularly in the interstices of the lesion. The lesions sometimes appear to expand and disrupt the integrity of the duct; however, when excised, the wall of these ducts is intact (Figure 11.13). In patients with fibrocystic changes, the discharge is often green (7). Ductography findings include connection with one or several cysts (Figure 11.14) or diffuse wall irregularities. Thick, white, pasty discharge may be seen in patients with underlying

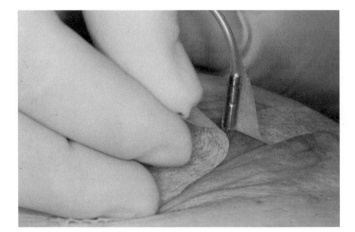

Figure 11.5 Taping cannula in place. After 0.2 to 0.4 mL of contrast is injected, the cannula is taped onto the nipple using two pieces of paper tape. Leaving the cannula in place permits additional injections of contrast as needed to evaluate the duct. The cannula also helps minimize the amount of contrast that is forced out of the duct when compression is applied.

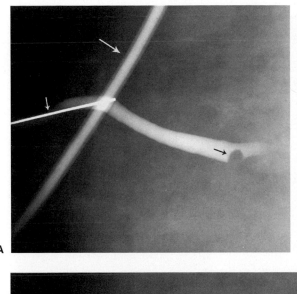

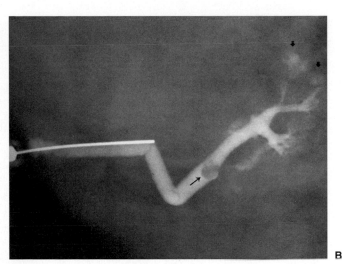

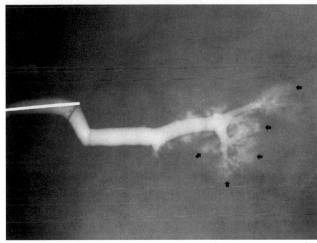

Figure 11.6 *Masking of lesion; lobular blushing; papilloma. A.* Initial films following injection of 0.2 mL of contrast demonstrate a filling defect (*arrow*) in a mildly dilated duct. No proximal opacification is noted. Cannula (*short thin arrow*) is present; tubing with contrast (*long thin arrow*) should be moved out of the field of view by the technologist. *B.* After an additional 0.2 mL of contrast, the filling defect (*thin arrow*) is still seen. Branches of the duct are now filling with contrast, and there is some "blushing" (*thick arrows*), possibly reflecting contrast in the lobular units. *C.* An additional 0.2 mL of contrast is injected. The lesion is no longer seen because of the amount of contrast injected. Increased amount of blushing is noted (*thick arrows*). Small lesions and lesions that are close to the nipple can be obscured if too much contrast is injected initially. A small amount is injected initially. If the cannula is left in place, it is easy to inject additional contrast as needed to evaluate the duct proximally.

duct ectasia as the cause of nipple discharge (7). These ducts are dilated in the subareolar region and often change abruptly in caliber as the duct courses proximally (Figure 11.15).

Finally, breast cancer can present with spontaneous nipple discharge (1–7). Most of the patients with underlying cancer as the cause of the nipple discharge have normal mammograms (Figure 11.16). Ductal carcinoma *in situ* (DCIS) is the most common finding in patients with normal mammograms. These represent about 5% of all patients presenting with spontaneous nipple discharge. A small number of patients present with spontaneous nipple discharge and a finding suggestive of cancer (e.g., malignant-type calcifications, ill-defined or spiculated mass) on their mammograms. In these patients, the discharge is evaluated with a ductogram, and the mammographic finding is evaluated, as needed, based on the finding. Until a relationship is established, these may represent synchronous, yet unrelated, processes (Figure 11.17). The ductographic findings in women with breast cancer overlap with those described for papillomas. Cancer-containing ducts, however, are not usually very dilated, and diffuse wall irregularities with focal areas of dilation and sacculation are more common than discrete filling defects (Figure 11.18). Less common signs of cancer on ductography include contrast extravasation and displacement of the opacified duct (3).

Some potential pitfalls include the masking of small lesions, or those close to the nipple, if too much contrast is injected at the onset (Figure 11.6). Air bubbles may rarely be mistaken for a lesion. Air bubbles, however, are well-defined, round, and lucent, and they

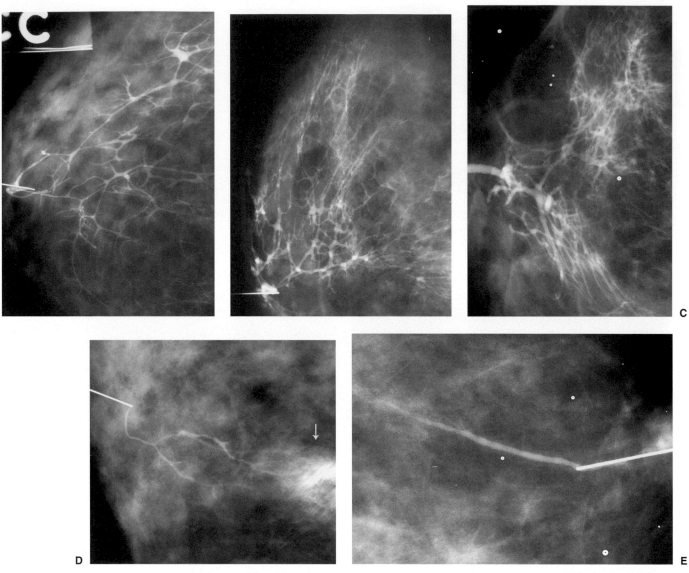

Figure 11.7 *Normal ducts. A.* Using the cannula as an internal measure, this duct is normal in caliber. This duct demonstrates a wide area of drainage with a moderate amount of branching. No focal abnormality is apparent. *B.* Different patient. Normal caliber duct (cannula at nipple) with a wide area of drainage and more branching than seen in the previous patient. *C.* Different patient. The subareolar portion of the duct is at the upper limits for what we define as a normal caliber. Significant branching and a wide distribution in the parenchyma. *D.* Different patient. In contrast to the prior examples, this duct is attenuated with a minimal number of branches and a limited drainage area. In these smaller ducts, proximal extravasation of contrast (*arrow*) is seen as attempts are made to distend the duct further. *E.* Different patient. This duct has no detectable branch points, and its distribution is limited in the breast. Normal caliber.

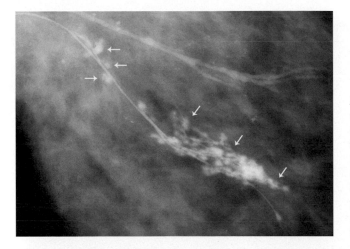

Figure 11.8 *Lobular blush; normal duct.* In some patients, a contained contrast blush is seen in a lobular-like distribution (*arrows*) around the duct. This is often seen in normal-caliber ducts such as those seen in this patient. Scattered benign calcifications are seen in the surrounding tissue.

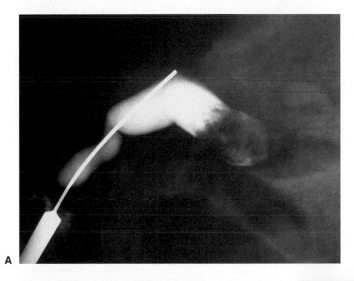

A

Figure 11.9 *Papillomas. A.* A lesion is present obstructing the cannulated duct close to the nipple. The irregular interface at the obstructing site reflects contrast pooling in the interstices of the papilloma. The duct between the lesion and the nipple is dilated (compare to cannula). The subareolar location of this lesion, within a distended duct, is a common presentation for papillomas. *B.* Different patient. The lesion (*arrow*) is obstructing one of the terminal branches in this duct. The duct is normal in caliber, and there is a significant amount of branching and a wide area of drainage. Despite the magnification technique, some of these lesions can be difficult to identify, and close evaluation of all branches is important. Imagine how limited we would be in trying to detect these small lesions without magnification. *C.* Photographic coning to area of lesion. Obstructing lesion and two adjacent filling defects (*arrows*) are evident in this patient. Preoperative ductography is done and then used to direct a wire localization of the lesion.

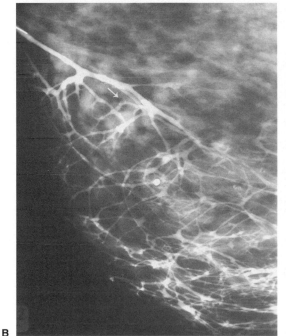

B

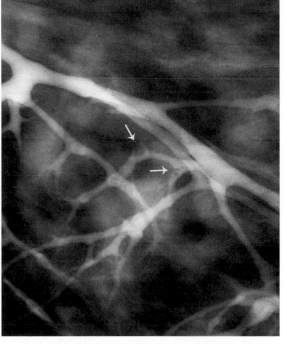

C

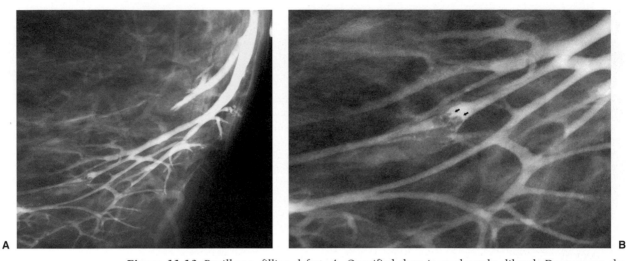

Figure 11.10 *Papilloma, filling defect.* A. Opacified duct is moderately dilated. Do you see the lesion? Despite the magnification technique, some of these lesions can be difficult to identify, and close evaluation of all branches is important. Imagine how limited we would be in trying to detect these lesions without magnification. B. Photographic coning to the area of the lesion demonstrates a filling defect (*arrows*) in the opacified duct. The edges of the lesion are irregular, consistent with contrast pooling in the interstices of the papilloma. Notice the distance from the nipple to the lesion. Although papillomas are often in a subareolar location, not all of them are. Without knowing the location of this lesion preoperatively, do you think the surgeon would extend the dissection to this point? Even if the dissection was extended to this point, can we be sure the pathologist would know where to look for the lesion for complete histological evaluation?

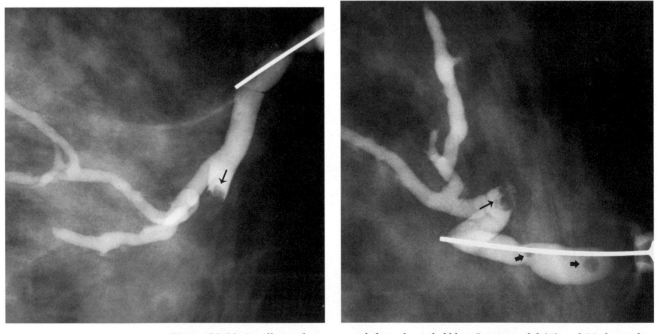

Figure 11.11 *Papilloma obstructing side branch; air bubbles.* Craniocaudal (A) and 90-degree lateral (B) views demonstrating a lesion (*thin arrows*) obstructing one of the branches of the opacified duct. The duct is dilated. Air bubbles (*thick arrows*) are well circumscribed and lucent. They are not seen on the craniocaudal view in this patient.

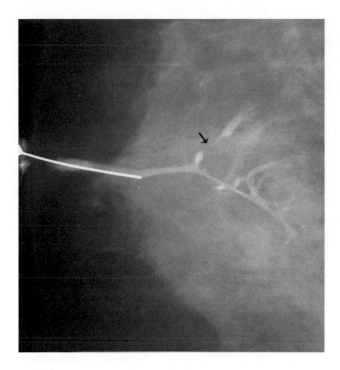

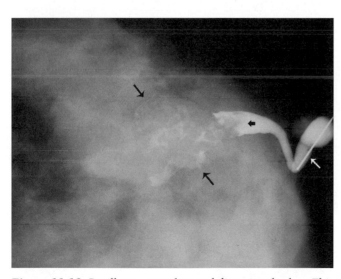

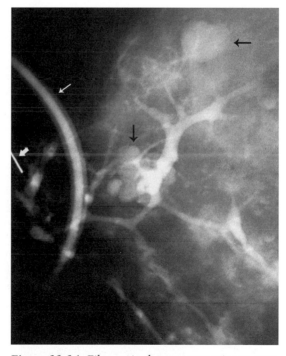

Figure 11.12 *Papilloma, wall irregularity.* Normal-caliber duct with apparent narrowing and irregularity involving a side branch of the duct (*arrow*). Ductographic findings for ductal carcinoma *in situ* and papillomas often overlap, hence the need to recommend biopsy.

Figure 11.13 *Papilloma, expanding and distorting the duct.* This lesion (*thick, black arrow*) is obstructing the duct. Contrast (*thick, black arrow*) is seen seemingly outside the confines of the duct, but this is actually contrast in the interstices of the lesion, and the duct itself is normal. The duct is dilated compared with the cannula (*white arrow*).

Figure 11.14 *Fibrocystic changes, connection to cysts.* Normal-caliber duct with contrast opacifying multiple cysts (*black arrows*). A portion of the contrast-containing tubing (*thin, white arrow*) used for the ductogram is seen superimposed on the breast. Ideally, the technologist moves the tubing away from the field of view. Portion of cannula (*thick, white arrow*) is seen.

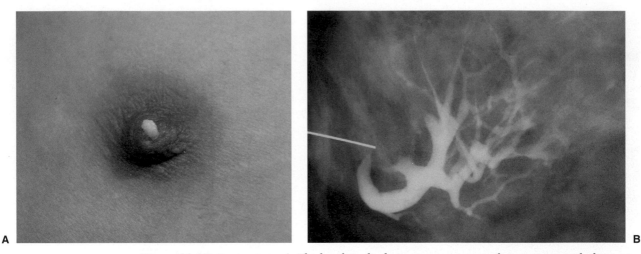

Figure 11.15 *Duct ectasia. A.* Thick, white discharge is seen commonly in women with duct ectasia. *B.* Different patient; dilated duct in its subareolar distribution. The more proximal branches assume a normal caliber. No focal finding is identified.

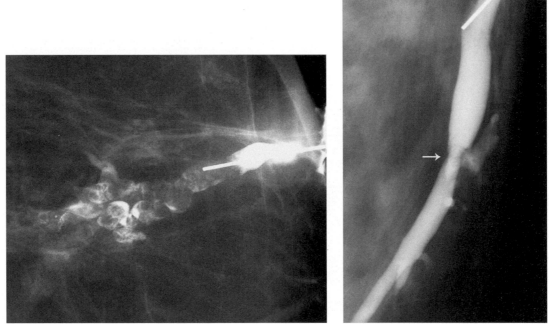

Figure 11.16 *Ductal carcinoma* in situ *(DCIS). A.* Intraductal lesion with interstices outlined by contrast. The duct is dilated between the lesion and the nipple. A papilloma with associated and adjacent DCIS (low to intermediate nuclear grade with no central necrosis) is diagnosed histologically. *B.* Different patient; focal area of narrowing (*arrow*) in opacified duct. The duct is minimally dilated. DCIS is diagnosed histologically.

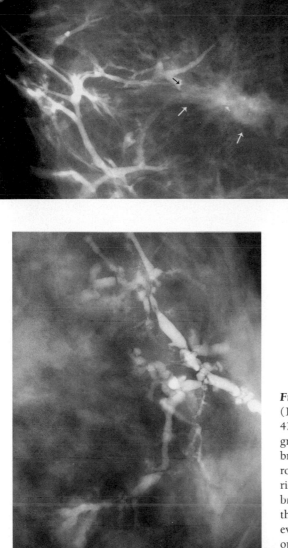

Figure 11.17 *Invasive ductal carcinoma, not otherwise specified.* Patient has a spiculated mass on her mammogram and spontaneous nipple discharge. The opacified duct is borderline dilated. A side branch of the duct is obstructed (*black arrow*), with a meniscus noted at the obstruction site. This corresponds to the area of the spiculated mass (*white arrows*) on orthogonal views (only one view is shown) consistent with an invasive ductal carcinoma presenting with nipple discharge and a mass seen on the mammogram.

Figure 11.18 *Ductal carcinoma* in situ *(DCIS).* *A.* Craniocaudal magnified (1.8×) view of the anterior aspect of the left breast. Diffusely abnormal duct in a 42-year-old patient with spontaneous nipple discharge and a normal mammogram. This duct extends proximally in the upper central portion of the left breast. Multiple areas of narrowing and sacculation are identified, as are abrupt, rounded terminations of the duct. *B.* Mediolateral oblique magnified view posteriorly. Focal areas of sacculation are seen terminating several of the duct branches (*thick arrows*). Clusters of calcifications (*thin arrows*) are also noted on the magnification views, although not very striking on the routine views, however, with magnification, concern in increased. DCIS diffusely involving the opacified duct and surrounding tissue is diagnosed histologically. *C.* Different patient; diffusely abnormal duct with areas of sacculation and narrowing.

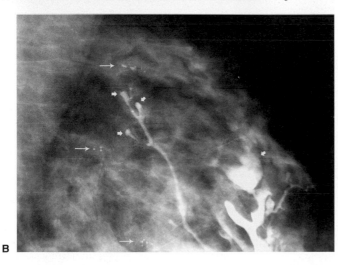

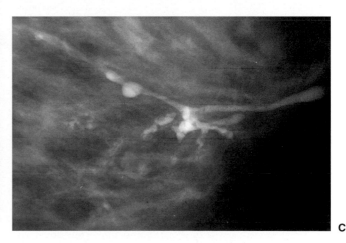

change in position between films (Figure 11.19). Rarely, an extensive amount of air out-lines portions of the ductal system. This is probably not related to the contrast injection, but the cause is not clear (Figure 11.19). Duct perforation with contrast extravasation is uncommon. It is not easy to perforate a normal duct. It requires a certain amount of force and is painful, and the patient describes a burning sensation as soon as you start injecting contrast. In attempting to distend small ducts, contrast extravasation proximally in side branches of the duct and opacification of lymphatic channels can sometimes be seen (Figure 11.20). These patients tolerate the injection initially but describe a burning sensation after a few drops of contrast have been injected.

Rarely, pseudolesions may be seen on ductography. Diffuse wall abnormalities may be seen on the initial ductogram, yet at the time of the preoperative ductogram, the findings are not confirmed (Figure 11.21). Nonspecific fibrocystic changes are diagnosed in these patients. It is unclear why this is seen, but it may represent debris in the lumen of the duct. Finally, false-negative ductography secondary to the cannulation of the wrong duct occurs in about 15% of patients. Duct openings are closely apposed on the surface of the nipple; hence, identifying the one with the discharge can be a challenge. If a patient presents with

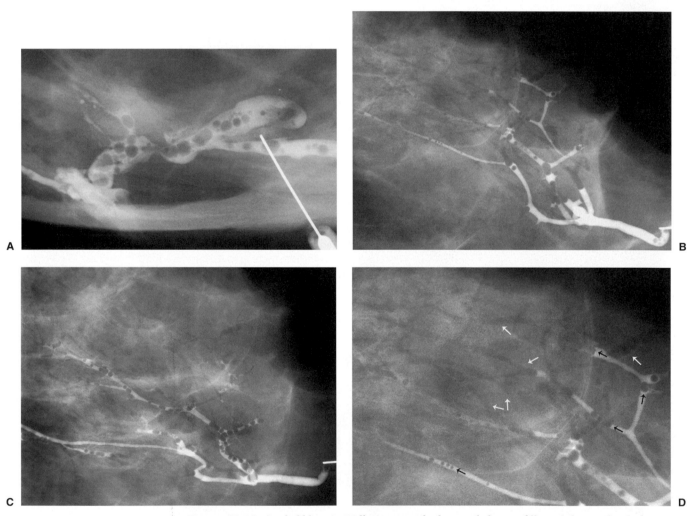

Figure 11.19 *Air bubbles. A.* Well-circumscribed, round, lucent filling defects. These change in position between views. *B.* Different patient. Craniocaudal (CC) and 90-degree lateral (C) views. Photographic cone down, CC projection (*D*). Air bubbles (*black arrows*) are present in the opacified duct, and there is air (*white arrows*) outlining proximal branches of the duct. The source of the air is not clear. Although there is dense tissue, the air is not apparent on the preductogram films, and yet no air was present in the syringe or cannula at the time of the injection.

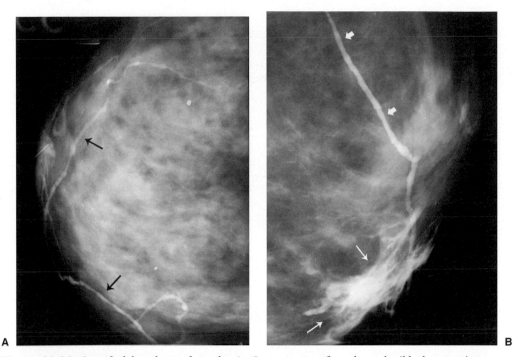

Figure 11.20 *Opacified lymphatic channels. A.* Contrast opacifies channels (*black arrows*) in a nonanatomic distribution for ducts. *B.* Different patient; proximal extravasation (*thin arrows*) resulting from an attempt to opacify the cannulated duct. Burning is described by the patient when the extravasation occurs. Contrast opacifies a channel (*thick arrows*) in a nonanatomic distribution for a duct. Opacification of lymphatics is seen in some patients with proximal contrast extravasation, as in this patient.

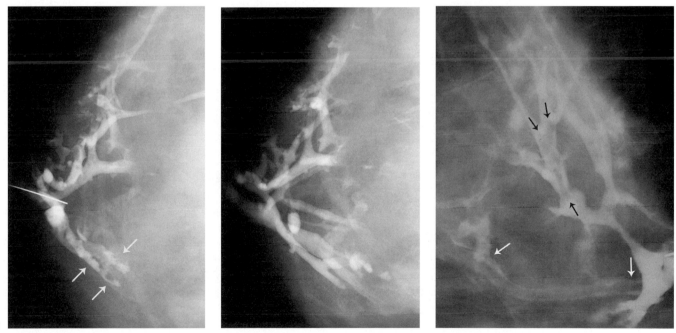

Figure 11.21 *Pseudolesions. A.* Diagnostic ductogram demonstrates a diffusely irregular duct with filling defects and wall irregularities (*white arrows*). Excision is recommended. *B.* Preoperative ductogram demonstrates a normal duct. Previously noted abnormalities are not reproduced. Nonspecific fibrocystic changes are reported histologically. *C.* Different patient; tubular-like filling defects are noted in different portions of this duct (*arrows* demonstrate extent of filling defects). It is unclear whether these represent duct contents.

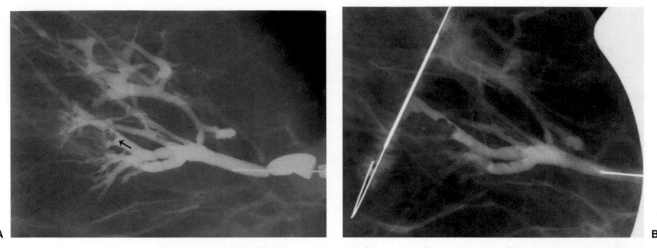

Figure 11.22 *Papilloma. A.* Diagnostic ductogram demonstrating a filling defect (*arrow*) in a side branch of an arborized duct. *B.* On the day of surgery, the ductogram is repeated and used to guide a wire localization. Midportion of reinforced wire segment is just posterior to the intraductal lesion.

a classic history (e.g., dark spots on the bra cup) and physical examination suggestive of an intraductal lesion (focal crusting on the nipple, identifiable trigger point with copious discharge), a normal ductogram is not accepted. The patient is asked to return for a repeat study, and ultrasound is used in an attempt to localize the lesion.

If an intraductal lesion is identified on ductography, excision is usually recommended. A preoperative ductogram with a methylene blue–contrast combination (1:1) can be helpful to the surgeon intraoperatively and ensures that the pathologist will process and evaluate the lesion. Occasionally, in women with lesions that are a distance from the nipple or proximal to multiple branch points in the duct, a wire localization of the lesion is done using the ductogram as a guide (Figure 11.22). In these patients, the ductogram is done with undiluted contrast material (e.g., no methylene blue is injected).

After the study is completed, the cannula is removed, and the nipple is covered with gauze or a nursing pad. This prevents contrast material from leaking out onto the patient's clothes. Many patients describe a significant reduction or complete cessation of the discharge for several weeks after the ductogram. It is unclear why this occurs, but it is usually not a problem for the preoperative ductogram because discharge is still obtained when the nipple is compressed.

CYST ASPIRATION AND PNEUMOCYSTOGRAPHY

Aspiration of cysts is undertaken when there are associated significant symptoms, atypical features on ultrasound, or at the patient's request. Pneumocystography is sometimes undertaken in patients in whom an intracystic or mural abnormality is suspected.

Aspiration of cysts is undertaken in three situations: when there are associated significant symptoms (e.g., tenderness, burning), when there are atypical features on ultrasound, or at the patient's request. As cysts enlarge and tension on the wall and surrounding tissue increases, patients may describe significant discomfort and tenderness. Some investigators have suggested that as cysts enlarge, some of the fluid escapes into the surrounding breast parenchyma, eliciting an aseptic inflammatory response. Aspiration under these circumstances often relieves the symptoms (2,8,9).

We consider aspiration when the ultrasound findings are not diagnostic of a cyst (Figure 11.23). Pneumocystography is sometimes undertaken in patients in whom an intracystic or mural abnormality is suspected. Palpation, ultrasound, or mammography can be used to guide the aspiration. Even with palpable cysts, our preference is to aspirate them using ultrasound guidance. Direct observation with ultrasound expedites needle movements and is helpful in determining the amount of pressure needed to puncture cyst walls that are sometimes thickened and inflamed. After the aspiration, no residual abnormality

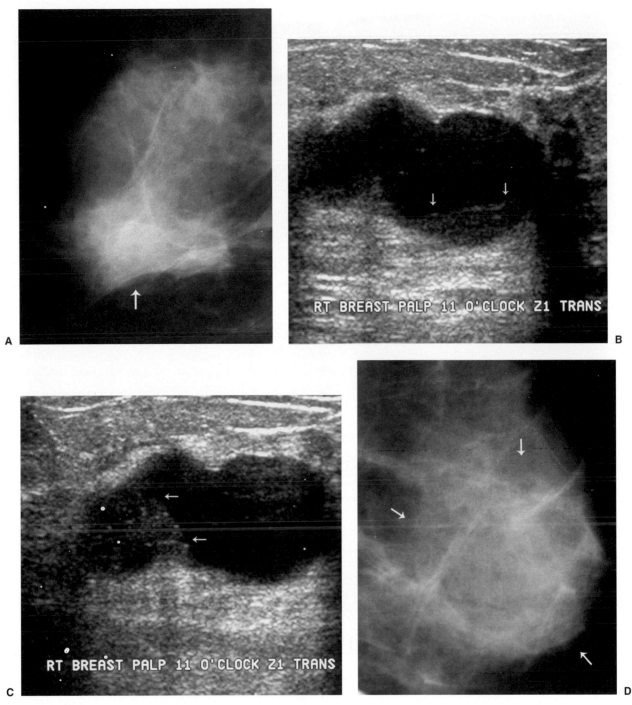

Figure 11.23 *Cysts. A.* Right mediolateral oblique view. A mass with obscured margins (*arrow*) is imaged corresponding to a palpable area. *B.* With the patient in a supine position, ultrasound demonstrates a macrolobulated mass with posterior acoustic enhancement and internal echoes (*arrows*) in the dependent portion of the cyst. *C.* Decubitus position. Internal echoes have now shifted into what is now the dependant portion of the cyst (*arrows*). This shift in the echoes confirms that the finding is a cyst. When we can establish the diagnosis of a cyst, we do not routinely undertake aspiration unless the patient is symptomatic or requests it. *D.* Different patient. A mass with obscured margins (*arrows*) is imaged corresponding to a tender lump.

(continued on next page)

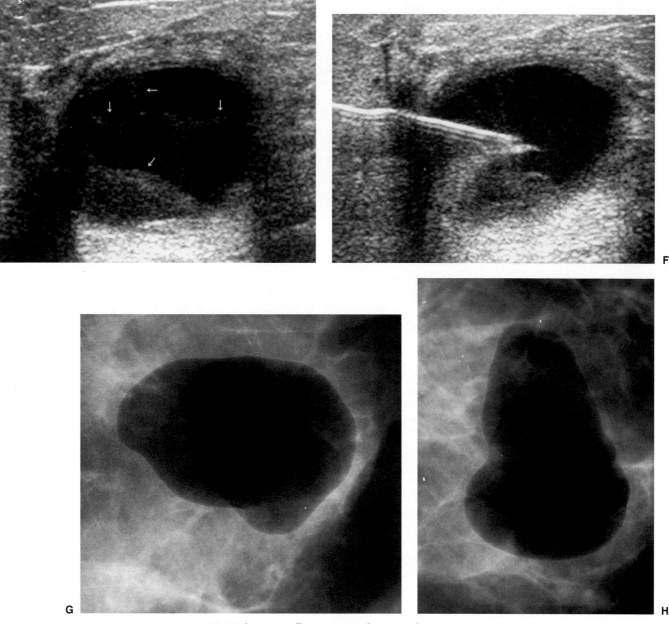

Figure 11.23 (continued) E. A cystic lesion with posterior acoustic enhancement is imaged corresponding to the area of concern to the patient. Internal echoes and apparent septations are noted (*arrows*). The wall is not sharply defined. Aspiration and pneumocystography are undertaken for diagnostic purposes. F. Needle with tip in the center of the cyst. The aspiration is monitored with real time ultrasound, and many of the echoes are seen being aspirated into the needle. The wall of the cyst is not sharp. This is often seen with tender, possibly "aseptically inflamed," cysts. After the contents are aspirated, 50% of the volume of fluid aspirated is replaced with air. Craniocaudal (*G*) and 90-degree lateral (*H*) double spot compression magnification (1.8×) views following the injection of air. A smooth-walled cyst cavity is seen with no intracystic component. There is wall thickening, and the surrounding tissue is normal.

should be seen ultrasonographically (Figure 11.24). If a persistent abnormality is seen, a core biopsy or short-term follow-up ultrasound (6 to 8 weeks) is undertaken (Figure 11.25). When pneumocystography is done, half the amount of aspirated fluid is replaced with air. Spot compression magnification views of the cyst are obtained in orthogonal projections (CC and 90-degree lateral views) to evaluate the cyst wall.

When using ultrasound guidance, we select an approach that enables us to introduce the needle parallel to the chest wall and transducer (see Needle Biopsy section for a more detailed description). The skin is cleaned with povidone-iodine (Betadine) and alcohol. One or 2 mL of lidocaine (2%) is used to slowly raise a skin wheal. Under ultrasound guidance, the anesthesia needle is advanced up to the cyst, and lidocaine is infiltrated along the expected course of the needle. A few minutes are allowed to elapse after the administration of the lidocaine. Using ultrasound guidance, a 20-gauge spinal needle is used to puncture the cyst. With real-time scanning, it is easy to appreciate how much pressure to apply in traversing the cyst wall. With the tip of the needle in the center of the cyst, the inner stylet is removed, and the needle is connected to a 10-mL syringe. Under direct ultrasound visualization, suction is applied until all of the contents are evacuated. There should be no residual abnormality after the aspiration. In patients with cysts having thick contents, an 18-gauge spinal needle may be needed to evacuate the cyst completely. The aspirated fluid is not submitted for cytologic evaluation, unless the aspirate is bloody (or the patient makes the request).

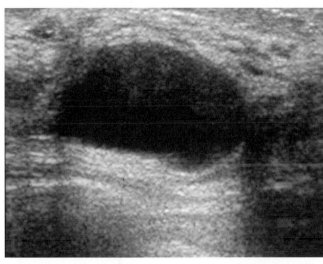

A

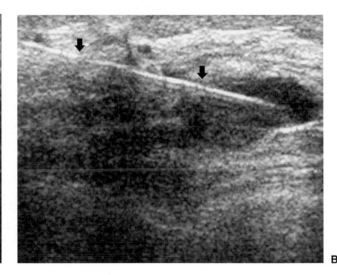

B

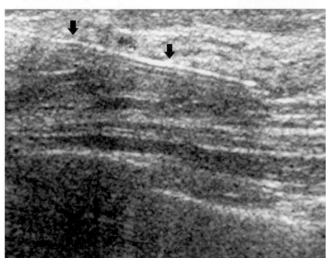

C

Figure 11.24 *Cyst.* A. Nearly anechoic cyst with posterior acoustic enhancement and internal echoes. The distribution of the echoes is such that they may not represent reverberation artifact. B. After puncturing the cyst with a 20-gauge spinal needle (*arrows*), the aspiration is monitored with real time ultrasound. C. No abnormality should be seen at the completion of the aspiration. No area of hypoechogenicity is seen surrounding the tip of the needle (*arrows*).

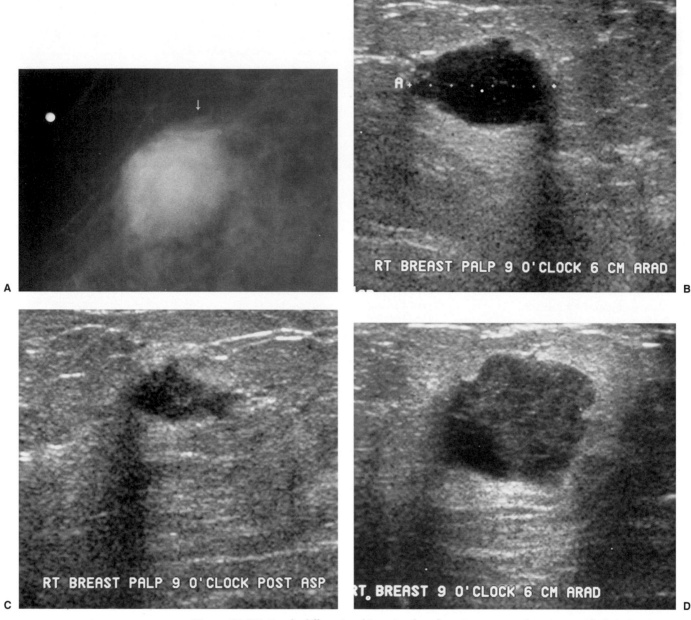

Figure 11.25 *Poorly differentiated invasive ductal carcinoma, not otherwise specified. A.* Spot tangential view in a 36-year-old patient who presents with a tender lump. A round mass with microlobulated and ill-defined margins is seen. *B.* Complex cystic mass with internal echoes and posterior acoustic enhancement. Closely evaluate the margins and note irregular microlobulations. Aspiration is undertaken. *C.* Residual irregular abnormality is seen after aspiration. The fluid is submitted for cytology. Necrosis, inflammatory cells, and viable cells with atypia are reported. A trial of antibiotics is recommended with a follow-up ultrasound in 4 weeks. *D.* Five weeks later, a round mass with a heterogeneous echotexture and posterior acoustic enhancement is imaged at the prior aspiration site. Ultrasound-guided core biopsy is done to establish the diagnosis.

Air can be injected into the cyst cavity. Some investigators have suggested that inject-ing air may have a therapeutic benefit by reducing the likelihood of cyst recurrence (2,8,9). In these patients, no mammographic images are obtained after the air is injected. Alternatively, a pneumocystogram (2,8,9) can be done, for diagnostic purposes, to evalu-ate potential intracystic (Figure 11.26) or mural lesions (Figure 11.27). After the cyst is drained, the needle is stabilized, and the fluid-filled syringe is replaced with a syringe con-taining air. Fifty percent of the aspirated fluid is replaced with air. The needle and syringe are then removed. Ultrasonographically, an irregular echogenic line is seen after air is injected (Figure 11.28). Spot compression magnification views of the cyst are obtained to

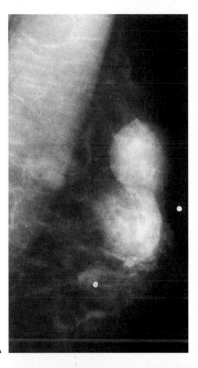

A

Figure 11.26 *Papilloma. A.* A 60-year-old patient presents with a lump. Two masses are apparent mammographically. One of these is palpable (metallic BB). *B.* On ultrasound, one of these two masses is a classic cyst (not shown). The second shown here is a complex cys-tic mass that is predominantly cystic with a solid component. Aspiration and pneumocys-tography are undertaken. The fluid is serous in appearance. "Findings consistent with cyst contents" are reported cytologically (the pathologist is aware that a papillary lesion is sus-pected). *C.* Pneumocystogram image demonstrates intracystic lesion (*arrow*). The remain-der of the cyst cavity has a smooth wall. Excisional biopsy following ultrasound-guided wire localization is undertaken (Figure 11.46).

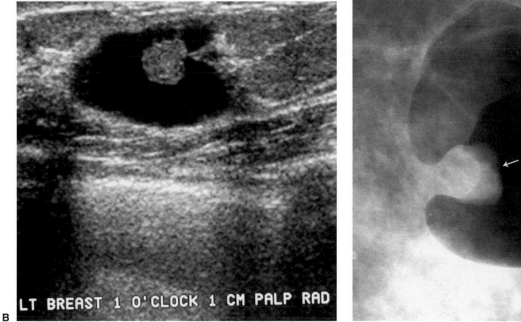

LT BREAST 1 O'CLOCK 1 CM PALP RAD

B

C

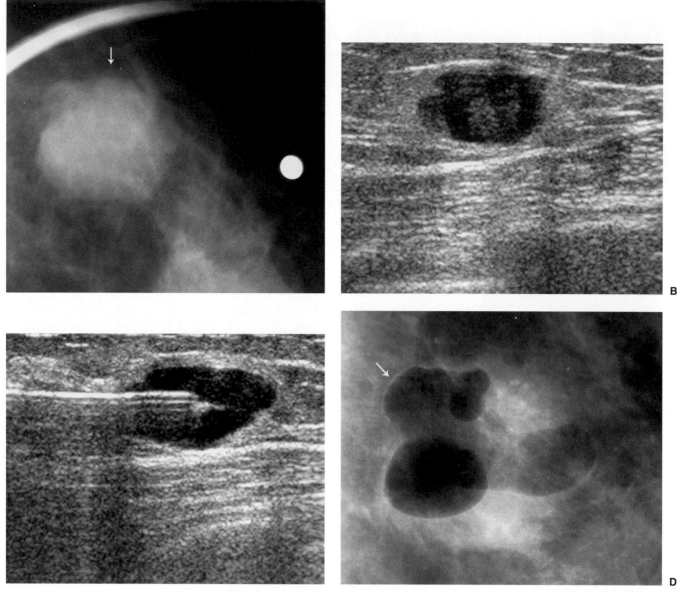

Figure 11.27 *Poorly differentiated, multicentric invasive ductal carcinoma, not otherwise specified; associated with extensive high-nuclear-grade ductal carcinoma* in situ. *A. Spot tangential view in a 71-year-old patient who presents with a lump. A round, macrolobulated mass (arrow) corresponds to palpable area. No other abnormalities are apparent mammographically. B. An oval complex cystic mass corresponds to the palpable area. Aspiration is undertaken. C. Needle tip in center of mass. Aspiration is monitored using real-time ultrasound. Malignant cells are described cytologically. D. Pneumocystogram demonstrates an irregular mass (arrow) with thickened walls and surrounding soft tissue abnormality. Unsuspected multicentric disease is diagnosed after mastectomy. No axillary lymph node involvement is reported (0 of 10 lymph nodes).*

evaluate the wall of the cyst and the appearance of the surrounding tissue (Figures 11.26 and 11.27).

In women with small lesions, or when the lesion is deep in a larger breast or far posteriorly, cyst aspirations can be done using mammographic guidance (see Preoperative Wire Localization section). A fenestrated paddle is used to establish the coordinates for the lesion. With the patient still in compression, a 20-gauge spinal needle is advanced slowly at the coordinates for the lesion as suction is applied. When fluid is obtained, the needle

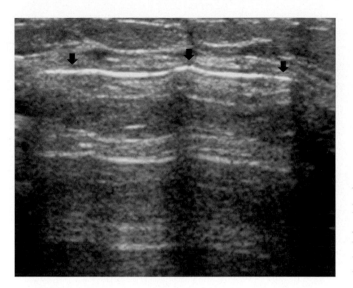

Figure 11.28 Air. An echogenic line (*arrows*) is seen after injection of air into a cyst cavity. Although not evident in this patient, shadowing may be seen in some patients deep to the injected air.

is stabilized until all of the fluid is aspirated. The needle is left in place, and follow-up orthogonal images are obtained to document resolution of the lesion.

FINE-NEEDLE ASPIRATION

Fine-needle aspiration (FNA) of breast lesions is advocated by some as a quick, reliable method of accurately establishing a diagnosis (10,11). Others contend that inadequate specimens (reported in as many as 47% of patients) and false-negative rates (sensitivity range of 65% to 99%; specificity of 64% to 100%; and accuracy of 81% to 98%) are unacceptably high (10,11). FNA can be successfully used in evaluating patients with palpable and mammographically detected lesions. As with anything, however, good technique and experience are invaluable in maximizing the usefulness of the method. Also, having a trained cytopathologist, who is comfortable with breast aspirates, is critical; the pathologist needs to be comfortable in making definitive statements regarding the adequacy of the sample and the presence of malignancy. Ideally, the cytopathologist is available while the aspiration is done so that the adequacy of the specimen can be determined immediately. If additional material is needed, more samples can be obtained.

For nonpalpable lesions, fenestrated paddles, stereotactic devices, or ultrasonography can be used to localize the lesion accurately. At this time, we are almost exclusively using ultrasound guidance for FNA. We reserve the use of FNA for lesions that may otherwise be difficult to approach with a core needle biopsy (Figure 11.29). The predetermined skin entry point is wiped with povidone-iodine and alcohol; lidocaine (2%) is used to raise a skin wheal and is infiltrated in the expected course of the needle. For one-handed aspirations, the needle (22 or 25 gauge) can be attached to a syringe in a pistol-grip holder. Alternatively, with the tip of the needle in the center of the lesion, the needle can be attached directly to a syringe. Suction is applied, and the needle is moved within the lesion in short, quick strokes as the angle of the needle is varied. The excursions of the needle within the lesion are monitored under real time ultrasound. Suction is released before the needle is pulled out of the lesion; otherwise, cells may be inadvertently sucked into the syringe. The needle is removed and disconnected from the syringe. A syringe filled with air is attached to the needle so that the cells can be expressed out of the needle and onto a glass slide. The material on the slide is smeared using another clean slide. Fixation can be accomplished by allowing the material to air-dry or by placing the slide in 95% alcohol. The methods to be used in handling the aspirates should be reviewed with the pathologist at your institution because there are variations.

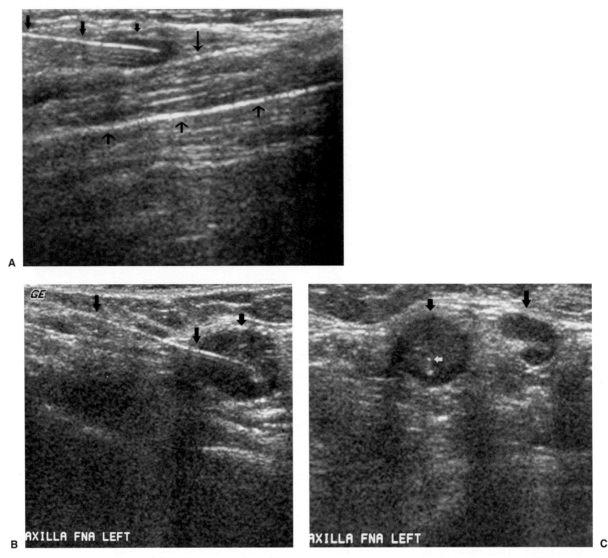

Figure 11.29 *Fine-needle aspiration, lymph node. A.* Oval hypoechoic mass (*short, thick arrow*) in patient with implants (not shown). Although a lymph node was suspected based on palpation and ultrasonographic appearance, the patient specifically requested that we establish the diagnosis. Mass is directly on the deep pectoral fascia (*long, thin arrow*). Pleural reflection is seen as an echogenic line deep to the pectoral muscle (*short, thin arrows*). A 22-gauge spinal needle is advanced parallel to the chest wall with ultrasound guidance. With the tip of the needle in the center of the mass, suction is applied using a syringe. Short, rapid excursions within the mass are monitored ultrasonographically. The cytopathologist determines the presence of sufficient material in samples to establish the diagnosis of a lymph node. *B.* Different patient. Enlarged axillary lymph node (*short arrow*) with bulging cortex and loss of hyperechogenic hilar region suggesting metastatic disease in a patient with a mass and associated calcifications in the breast (Figure 4.39H in Chapter 4 for ultrasound image of breast lesion). Fine-needle aspiration is used to establish the presence of metastatic disease. Using ultrasound guidance, the tip of a 22-gauge spinal needle (*long arrows*) is advanced to the center of the mass. *C.* Ultrasound image in orthogonal plane. Needle is seen in cross section (*white arrow*) in mass (*short, black arrow*). Needle positioning (*white arrow*) is verified on orthogonal planes. A syringe is attached to the needle and small rapid strokes, with slight variations in the angle of the needle, are undertaken and monitored with ultrasound. Suction is released, and the needle is pulled out. The cytopathologist determines the presence of sufficient material in samples to establish the diagnosis of metastatic disease. A second adjacent lymph node (*long, black arrow*) is noted.

NEEDLE BIOPSY

First described by Parker and associates, stereotactically, and then ultrasonographically, guided biopsies of the breast represent a significant advancement in patient care and management. These authors first described the use of a spring-loaded mechanism and a 14-gauge needle and more recently described a vacuum-assisted device that can be used with 14- or 11-gauge needles to increase the amount of tissue obtained (12–16). These techniques revolutionized the practice of breast imaging and are now well established with significant literature to support their routine use (12–22).

At the onset of this discussion, it is important to emphasize that the availability of these relatively simple techniques should not be used to replace or undermine complete mammographic workups. If, after evaluation, a lesion fits the criteria for a probably benign lesion (Chapter 12), we recommend short-interval follow-up. However, the findings and all available options, including imaging-guided and excisional biopsies, are discussed with the patient. If the patient requests an imaging-guided biopsy, it is done. The other important concept related to these procedures is the need for radiologic and pathologic concordance and follow-through. At the time you make the biopsy recommendation, ask yourself what you are willing to accept as a diagnosis for this finding and, given the diagnostic considerations, what will be your next step? If the pathology results do not correlate with the imaging features of the lesion, you need to be prepared to repeat the biopsy or refer the patient for an excisional biopsy (Figure 11.30).

Commonly used sampling methods include automated gun-needle devices and directional vacuum-assisted biopsy probes. The automated gun-needle devices are spring

> Ask yourself: "What will I accept as a diagnosis for this finding?" Radiologic and pathologic concordance is critical after imaging-guided FNA and needle biopsy.

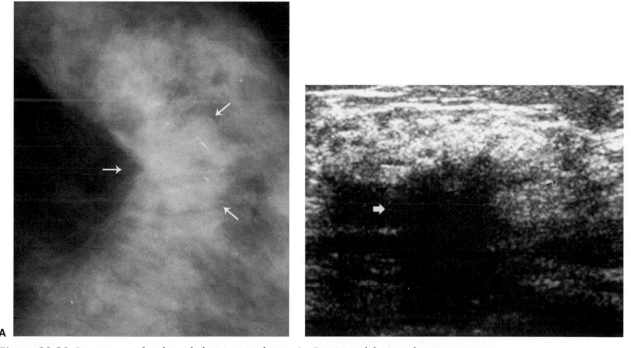

Figure 11.30 *Importance of radiopathologic concordance.* A. Craniocaudal view demonstrates an irregular mass (*arrows*) drawing tissue in at the fat–glandular tissue interface ("tent sign") associated with scattered linear calcifications. B. Ultrasound demonstrates irregular mass with significant shadowing (*arrow*). Appropriately, a biopsy is recommended. What are you willing to accept as a diagnosis for this lesion? Benign fibrocystic changes are reported histologically. What is your next step? This lesion is malignant until proved otherwise. Benign fibrocystic changes are not concordant results for a lesion with the imaging features shown. Excisional biopsy (or repeat imaging biopsy) is recommended. It is critical that there be radiopathologic concordance after imaging-guided biopsy.

loaded to move the two components making up the devices. The inner sampling needle has a 4- to 5-mm needle tip followed by a tissue trough that is either 10 to 15 mm (short throw) or 21 to 25 mm (long throw) in length. The larger trough is preferred because more tissue is obtained. The second component is the outer cutting cannula. When the gun is fired, the inner sampling needle moves forward, followed almost instantaneously by the outer cutting cannula, which in effect cuts the tissue securing a sample in the tissue trough. The needle is pulled out after each firing so that the tissue can be removed. These guns have a cocking mechanism. The first position in the mechanism exposes the tissue trough; the second position prepares the gun for another firing by withdrawing the sampling needle back into the outer cannula. The guns have a safety device to prevent premature firing during needle positioning and a trigger to set the needle mechanism in motion. Reusable and disposable guns are available; the reusable guns are more cost effective and appear to have more force in propelling the needle forward and cutting through dense fibrous tissue. Needle lengths include a 10-cm long needle used primarily for ultrasound-guided biopsies and a 16-cm long needle used for stereotactically guided procedures. It is helpful to have the patient hear the "pop" the gun makes when it is fired before starting the procedure so that during the procedure she is not startled by the sound.

Different needle gauges (e.g., 14 and 11 gauge) can be used with the directional vacuum-assisted biopsy probes. A needle with a tissue trough attached to a vacuum device is advanced into the lesion, and a cutter is advanced over this sampling needle. The tissue sample is withdrawn (sucked) into a chamber outside of the breast from where it is retrieved. The position of the sampling needle can be turned in small increments, and each time, the cutter is advanced over the sampling needle. The tissue is sampled circumferentially (360 degrees) around the needle without having to take the needle out of the breast between samples; the tissue is retrieved from the needle using the vacuum device. Larger amounts of tissue are consistently obtained with these devices and as such are preferred for sampling calcifications; targeting of individual calcifications at the onset is not as critical with this system. Small masses and tight clusters of calcifications can be removed piecemeal such that placement of a clip is required to mark the site of the lesion. If cancer is diagnosed, it is possible to excise the tumor bed widely. When a clip is deployed, CC and 90-degree lateral views are obtained to document the location of the clip at the end of the procedure (Figure 11.31).

We perform about 90% of our biopsies using ultrasound guidance and the spring-loaded 14-gauge core biopsy needles. This includes some patients with calcifications. Our general rule is that if we can see it with ultrasound, we prefer to do the biopsy using ultrasound guidance. We perform stereotactically guided biopsies using a spring-loaded 14-gauge core biopsy needle, or the 11-gauge vacuum-assisted needle for some patients with calcifications and small masses. Two groups of patients undergo stereotactically guided biopsies: (a) those in whom the lesion cannot be seen ultrasonographically with enough confidence to do the biopsy (mainly patients with calcifications, but also a small number of patients who have predominantly fatty tissue and an isoechoic mass on ultrasound); and (b) patients with large breasts and a centrally or posteriorly located small lesion. In these patients, immobilization of the breast and lesion with compression facilitates and expedites the biopsy procedure.

Ultrasound-guided biopsies are quick, easy on the patient, require no compression, and use no radiation. The prone position and the turning of the head and neck, required for stereotactic biopsies, are not well tolerated by some patients. The ability to achieve orthogonal views of the needle and establish its relationship to the lesion during ultrasound-guided procedures is helpful in determining the accuracy of the biopsy. This, in conjunction with the appearance of the cores and their behavior when placed in the formalin, helps us determine the number of samples we obtain to establish a diagnosis. If the core is yellow, floats, and has fat locules dispersing from its edges onto the surface of the formalin, additional core samples are obtained. If the core is stiff, predominantly white, and sinks or dips as soon as it is put in the formalin, it is likely diagnostic, particularly if the needle is seen through the lesion on orthogonal images (Figure 11.32A). Core samples of mucinous carcinomas are often gelatinous and glisten (Figure 11.32B).

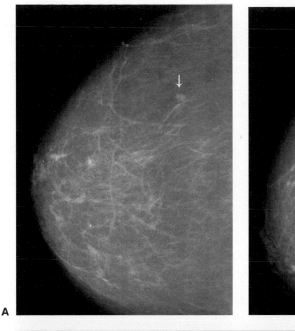

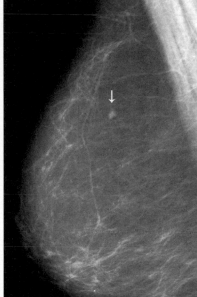

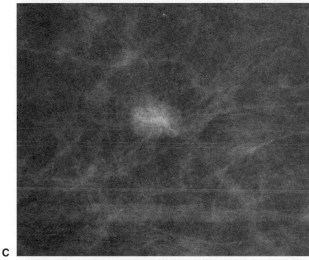

Figure 11.31 *Well-differentiated invasive ductal carcinoma, not otherwise specified; clip placement after biopsy.* Craniocaudal (*A*), mediolateral oblique (*B*), and spot compression (*C*) views demonstrate a mass with minimally ill-defined margins (*arrows*) in a 72-year-old woman that is new compared with prior studies. Biopsy is indicated. Directional vacuum-assisted biopsy is done with an 11-gauge needle. Two clips are deployed at completion of study (it was not clear that the first clip had deployed, so a second was placed). Craniocaudal (*D*) and mediolateral oblique (*E*) views obtained at the completion of the biopsy procedure demonstrate position of metallic clips. The clips (*thin arrows*) are used to localize the area of the tumor at the time of the lumpectomy. A small air locule is seen (*thick arrows*).

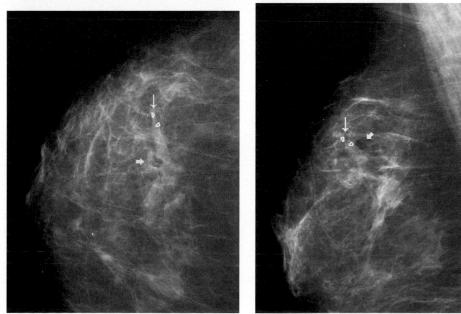

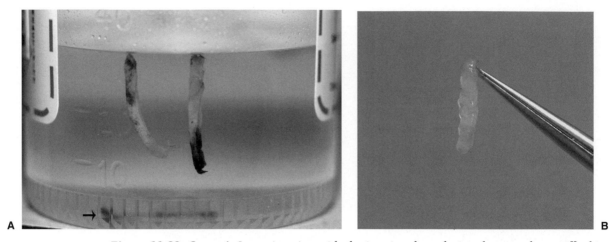

Figure 11.32 *Cores. A.* In conjunction with the imaging done during the procedure, stiff white cores that "dip" or "sink" (*arrow*) are suggestive of adequate sampling. We routinely examine our core samples carefully to help determine the number of cores needed to establish a diagnosis. *B.* Cores obtained from mucinous carcinomas often have a distinctive appearance. They glisten and appear gelatinous. When placed in the formalin, small water droplets form along the edges.

Relative contraindications to these procedures include warfarin sodium (Coumadin) and aspirin therapy. For biopsies done using a 14-gauge needle, we do not routinely stop these medications. In these patients, we take some extra time to tamponade between passes and at the end of the procedure (in our experience, aspirin use appears to be associated with a greater likelihood of bleeding compared with warfarin sodium). For patients undergoing vacuum-assisted 11-gauge biopsy, we prefer to stop these medications for several days before the biopsy. Lesions that are close to the chest wall or far laterally may not be approachable stereotactically. If the patient is unable to lie prone for 30 to 60 minutes or if the breast compresses to less than 2 cm ("pancake breast"), stereotactic guidance may not be a reasonable option.

ULTRASOUND GUIDANCE

For ultrasound-guided biopsies of mammographically detected abnormalities, ask yourself: "does the lesion I am seeing with ultrasound correlate with the lesion detected mammographically?"

Before undertaking an ultrasound-guided biopsy of a mammographically detected lesion, it is important to review mammographic and ultrasonographic images to make sure the lesion seen ultrasonographically correlates with the mammographic finding (see triangulation discussion in Chapter 3). If there is ever a question about the correlation, confirmation is sought before undertaking the biopsy. In these patients, all of the preliminary steps (e.g., povidone-iodine and alcohol wipes, lidocaine) for an ultrasound-guided core biopsy are taken. The needle used to inject the lidocaine is advanced to the lesion and left in place so that a mammographic image can be obtained. This helps to determine the relationship of the needle to the lesion seen mammographically (Figure 11.33). If correlation is established between mammographic and ultrasonographic findings, the patient is returned to the ultrasound room, and the biopsy is completed. As more experience is acquired with ultrasound and mammographic correlation, the need to take this extra step decreases significantly.

For ultrasound-guided procedures, the lesion is localized, and an approach is selected. We make every effort to select an approach that allows us to biopsy the lesion with the needle parallel to the transducer and chest wall. When the needle is parallel to the transducer, it is seen in its entirety. If the needle is angled, it becomes more difficult to localize the tip of the needle (Figure 11.34). The possibility of a pneumothorax is virtually eliminated, when the needle is moved parallel to the chest wall. As a routine, we hold the gun upside down. If the gun is held upright, it is difficult in some situations to advance the

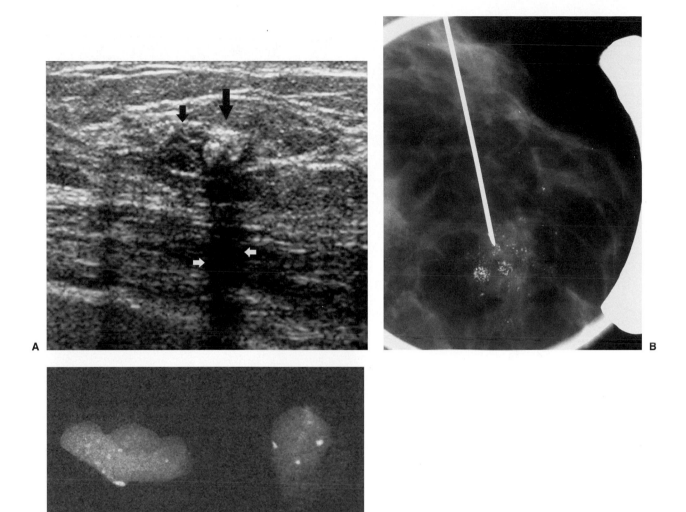

Figure 11.33 *Ductal carcinoma* in situ, *with central necrosis and areas of associated invasive ductal carcinoma. Correlating ultrasonographic and mammographic findings. A.* Ultrasound study demonstrates an irregular area of hypoechogenicity (*short, thick black arrow*) and focal hyperechogenicity (*long, thick black arrow*) associated with shadowing (*white arrows*). *B.* Spot compression view of the left breast demonstrates the needle used to inject the lidocaine in the area of the calcifications. Whenever we are not sure that mammographic and ultrasonographic findings correlate, we advance the needle used for the lidocaine up to the suspected lesion under ultrasound guidance and obtain a follow-up mammogram to document correlation. The biopsy is completed under ultrasound guidance using a 14-gauge needle. *C.* Core specimen radiograph demonstrates calcifications associated with the two cores obtained.

needle without some angulation (Figure 11.35). The skin entry site, using this method, is usually a distance from the transducer so that contamination of the biopsy site is minimized and the likelihood of getting blood on the transducer is reduced. Sterile technique and lidocaine (2%) are used. With ultrasound, lidocaine (2%) does not obscure the lesion; we use about 10 mL of lidocaine on the skin and along the expected needle track. We infuse the lidocaine under real time ultrasound to ensure that lidocaine is deposited up to the margin of the lesion (Figure 11.36). This also provides a good estimate of the trajectory that needs to be taken and helps establish a plane through the tissue. A small skin nick is made with a No. 11 surgical blade.

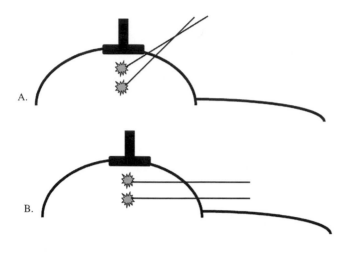

Figure 11.34 *Ultrasound approach to a lesion. A.* When the needle is angled, it may be difficult to see and difficult to determine the position of the tip. Because the needle is going to move forward in the breast almost instantaneously when the gun is fired, it is important to know the relationship of the tip of the needle to the lesion and chest wall. *B.* When the needle is kept parallel to the transducer, it is clearly seen. The position of the tip and its relationship to the lesion are established easily. Using this approach, the needle is parallel to the chest wall. Consequently, the likelihood of a pneumothorax is almost completely eliminated. When using this approach, the skin entry site is an adequate distance from the location of the transducer, minimizing the likelihood that the needle or skin entry site is contaminated or getting blood on the transducer.

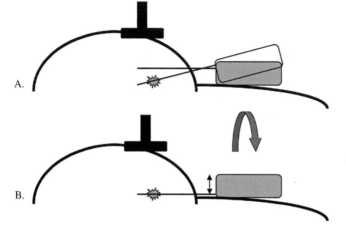

Figure 11.35 *Position of gun in approaching deep lesions. A.* When doing a biopsy of a lesion that is deep in the breast or in a small-breasted patient or a patient with a protuberant abdomen, consider how you hold the "gun." Because the needle comes out of the gun barrel close to the top, there is some dead space between the needle and the bottom of the gun. This causes you to angle the needle down as you try to approach the lesion. *B.* With the gun flipped upside down, the needle can be seen in its entirety, the tip of the needle can be identified without difficulty, and the lesion is approached with the needle parallel to the chest wall. The likelihood of a pneumothorax is almost completely eliminated.

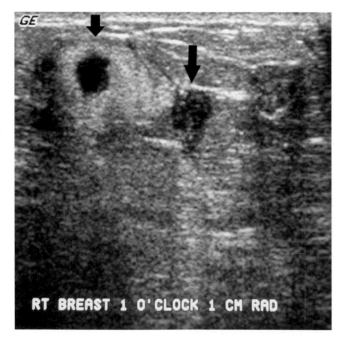

Figure 11.36 *Lidocaine injection along needle track.* Using a 25-gauge needle, lidocaine (2%) is used to raise a skin wheal. Lidocaine is also injected in the breast along the expected course of the needle. Under ultrasound guidance, the needle is advanced up to the lesion (*long arrow*), and lidocaine is injected (*short, thick arrow*) at the lesion and as the needle is withdrawn. As shown here, the injected lidocaine is imaged as round areas of hyperechogenicity with associated central areas that are anechoic. A total of about 10 mL of lidocaine is used; there is no reason that these procedures should be the least bit uncomfortable for patients. This process also seems to help create a track to the lesion.

Although some advocate having a technologist hold the transducer over the lesion as the radiologist advances the needle, this is probably more awkward and difficult for the radiologist (it has been likened to two people trying to drive a stick-shift car together: one manipulating the clutch, the other the stick-shift). The movements of the transducer are useful in knowing how to make fine adjustments to the position of the needle. Consequently, at our facility, the radiologist doing the procedure manipulates the transducer with one hand (nondominant hand) and the gun-needle device with the other (dominant mass). With this approach, one hand is moved at a time. At the onset, with the lesion centered on the screen, the needle is advanced to the expected location of the lesion in one movement. Firm pressure is applied over the lesion with the transducer to minimize any tissue movement as the needle approaches the lesion. In many cases, the needle is seen as it is advanced toward the lesion. If the needle is not seen, the gun-needle device is stabilized, and the transducer is rocked minimally from one side to other looking for the needle (Figure 11.37). If it is not found with these maneuvers, the skin entry point is approached with the transducer to localize the needle so that it can be followed back toward the lesion. The movement made with the transducer, in going from the needle to the lesion, defines the movement that has to be made with the needle. If the transducer is moved to the right in going from the needle to the lesion, the needle needs to be backed up slightly and readjusted slightly toward the right. These are fine, delicate movements (the lesion is approached in small increments) that are made until the needle is brought in line with the lesion. Prefire images are obtained to document the relationship of the needle to the lesion (Figure 11.38). The patient is warned that she is going to hear a "pop" in the room before the gun is fired. Postfire images are obtained, demonstrating the relationship of the needle to the lesion with orthogonal images (Figure 11.38). The needle is taken out of the breast, and the specimen is teased off the trough and placed in 10% formalin. If additional cores are obtained, air tracks

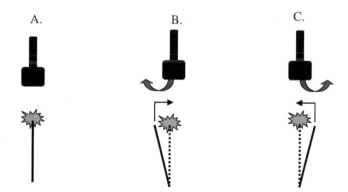

A. B. C.

Figure 11.37 *Using transducer movements to determine needed needle adjustments in approaching a lesion.* A. With the transducer over the lesion, advance the needle to the expected location of the lesion in one movement. With experience, you will frequently see the needle moving to the lesion (it's amazing, but your right hand usually knows where your left hand is!). B. If you advance the needle to the expected location of the lesion and you do not see it coming into the field of view (e.g., the lesion), *STOP* moving the needle. Gently rock the transducer to the left and right of the lesion to localize the needle. In this case, you find the needle to the left of the lesion. As you go from the needle back to the lesion, the movement of the transducer tells you what you need to do with the needle. The needle is withdrawn slightly and moved minimally to the right. Using fine, delicate, slow movements of the needle, walk the needle to the lesion. As you make the adjustments, remember to move only one hand at a time. If you are moving the needle, keep the transducer over the lesion. If you are moving the transducer to find the needle, do not also move the gun-needle mechanism. C. In this case, you find the needle to the right of the lesion. In going from the needle back to the lesion, the transducer is moved to the left. The needle is withdrawn slightly and moved to the left in small increments until the needle is seen lined up with a portion of the lesion.

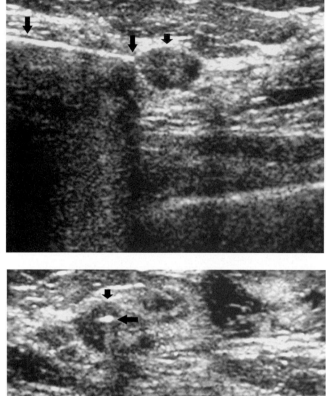

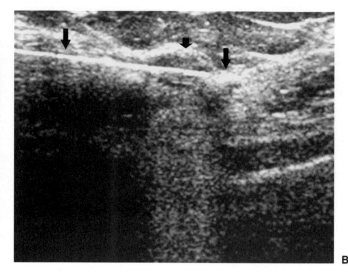

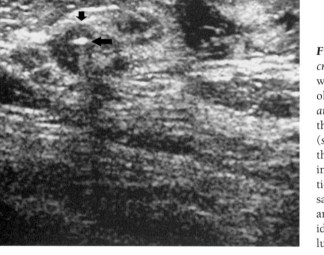

Figure 11.38 *Well-differentiated invasive ductal carcinoma (0.7 cm), not otherwise specified. Ultrasound-guided biopsy. A.* This oval, well-circumscribed, hypoechoic mass (*short arrow*) in a 72-year-old patient is a new finding. The needle is in prefire position (*long arrows*). *B.* Postfire image demonstrates the needle (*long arrows*) through the lesion (*short arrow*). *C.* Orthogonal view of the mass (*short arrow*) demonstrates the needle (*long arrow*) in cross section through the center of the mass. We use the appearance of the cores, in conjunction with orthogonal images demonstrating the relationship of the needle to the lesion, to individualize the number of samples taken. Our goal is to make a diagnosis with the least amount of intervention. In this patient, micrometastatic disease is identified in the sentinel lymph node biopsy done at the time of the lumpectomy.

may be seen in the lesion and should not be mistaken for the needle (Figure 11.39). Air often has a beaded appearance, and if the transducer is held over the lesion for a few seconds, the bubbles will shift in position. Depending on the images and the appearance of the cores, the number of passes is individualized for each patient. Core radiography is obtained when calcifications are the target (Figure 11.33).

In a patient with a lesion deep in the breast, a couple of maneuvers can be used to facilitate approaching the lesion with the needle parallel to the chest wall (Figure 11.40). The one we use most commonly involves "diving" the needle down in a controlled manner at the skin entry point to the expected depth of the lesion. The gun is then leveraged down so that the needle can be advanced in a more horizontal plane. Alternatively, the tip of the needle can be wedged into the lesion and the gun again leveraged down so that the needle and lesion are raised upward. The third approach available is to deposit and create a pool of saline deep to the lesion that helps raise the lesion. We have not found this method very helpful because, after the first pass, the fluid collection generally dissipates, precluding a second pass without more saline being deposited.

Associated complications with these procedures are uncommon. Cellulitis or, less commonly, mastitis may develop in some patients. Bleeding with hematoma formation

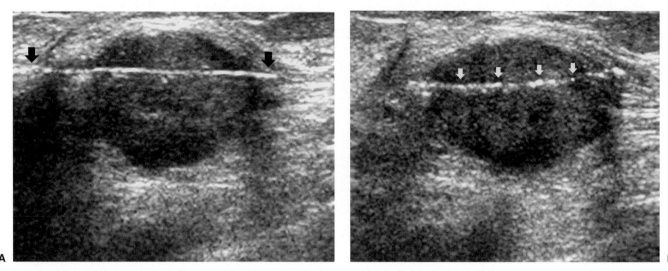

A   B

Figure 11.39 *Poorly differentiated, invasive ductal carcinoma, not otherwise specified. Air in needle track. A.* Round mass with posterior acoustic enhancement in a 73-year-old patient. A 14-gauge needle is through the mass (*arrows*). *B.* After the first pass, air (*arrows*) could be seen moving back and forth along the needle track. Air has a beaded appearance, as noted here, and if observed during real time ultrasound, the bubbles shift in position as the mass is compressed. Be careful not to mistake this for your needle.

is rare but can be seen in some patients. This sometimes occurs during the procedure (Figure 11.41). It is important to stop and tamponade the bleeding before proceeding. Finally, pneumothoraces can occur; however, if an approach that is parallel to the chest wall is taken and needle movements are monitored using ultrasound, this is unlikely.

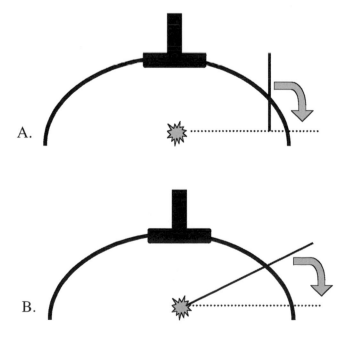

Figure 11.40 *Maneuvers to reach deep lesions and approach them parallel to the chest wall. A.* The needle is advanced down carefully and in a controlled manner to the expected depth of the lesion. The gun-needle mechanism is levered down, so that the needle is now horizontal. *B.* The tip of the needle is wedged into the lesion, and the gun-needle mechanism is levered down, raising the needle and with it the lesion at the tip.

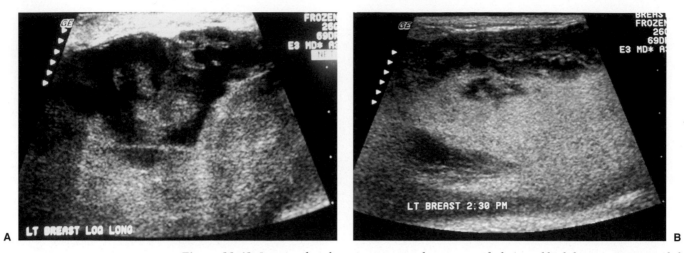

Figure 11.41 *Invasive ductal carcinoma, not otherwise specified. Acute bleed during imaging-guided biopsy. A.* Complex cystic mass. Ultrasound-guided biopsy using a 14-gauge needle is undertaken. The patient is taking no medications. When the needle was removed from the breast after the first pass, blood actively squirted out through the skin nick. Pressure with ice packs was kept on area for 20 minutes until bleeding stopped. *B.* Ultrasound image about 40 minutes after first pass demonstrates hyperechogenic material in the mass consistent with blood. Immediately after the first pass, the echogenic material (blood) could be seen on real time, swirling in the mass and increasing in amount. No surgical intervention is required.

STEREOTACTIC GUIDANCE

Dedicated prone tabletops and add-on devices attached to mammography units are available. In determining the approach, the shortest distance from the skin to the lesion is desirable. This is established by reviewing CC and 90-degree lateral views. If it is determined that the shortest distance to the lesion is by taking a mediolateral approach (e.g., the lesion is closest to the medial aspect of the breast on the CC view), the patient is positioned on the table so that the compression is applied on the medial aspect of the breast in a 90-degree lateral projection. A scout is taken to document that the lesion is imaged in the fenestrated portion of the paddle. If the lesion is seen, stereo-pair images are obtained by moving the x-ray tube 15 degrees to the right and 15 degrees to the left. On this stereo pair, multiple targets are selected if the 14-gauge gun-needle device is to be used, or one point is selected in the center of the area of interest for the vacuum-assisted devices (Figure 11.42). Using reference points on the images, the computer calculates horizontal (X), vertical (Y), and depth (Z) coordinates for the lesion. Lidocaine is used to raise a skin wheal; for stereotactic procedures, care needs to be exercised in the amount of lidocaine used. Lidocaine can sometimes obscure the lesion and can spread calcifications in a cluster apart. A skin nick is made big enough to accommodate whichever needle you are using. The needle is advanced into the breast at the predetermined coordinates. For the automated gun-needle device, the 14-gauge needle is advanced to within 5 mm of the Z value; for the directional vacuum-assisted biopsy probe, the 11-gauge needle is advanced to within 2 mm of the Z value, and prefire films are obtained (Figure 11.42). If the needle is lined up with respect to the lesion, the gun is fired, and postfire images are obtained (Figure 11.42). If using the 14-gauge gun-needle device, the needle is taken out of the breast, and the specimen is teased off the trough. If using the vacuum-assisted device, samples are obtained at the discretion of the radiologist at various points circumferentially around the needle. The specimens are withdrawn using suction so that the needle is not withdrawn after each sample is procured. As mentioned earlier, if there is a possibility that the entire lesion can be removed during biopsy, a metallic clip is deployed through the needle, and stereo images can be taken (Figure 11.42). Follow-up orthogonal images are obtained

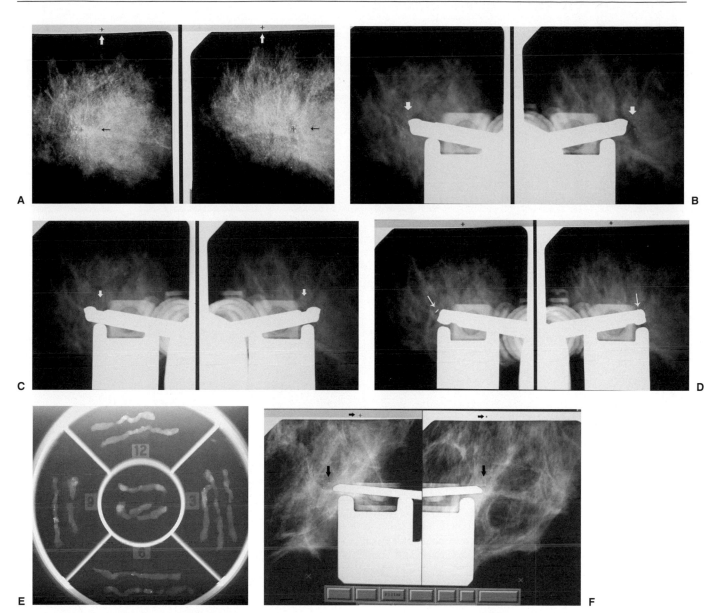

Figure 11.42 *Stereotactically guided breast biopsies. A.* Stereo scout images in a patient with calcifications for directional vacuum-assisted biopsy with an 11-gauge needle. Cluster of calcifications is seen in both images (*black arrows*). Reference cursors are appropriately positioned (*white arrow*). A point in calcification cluster is selected (*black hatch mark*) for targeting. The unit calculates X, Y, and Z coordinates for the area of interest. Coordinates determined by the unit are dialed in, and the needle is advanced to within 2 mm of the Z value. *B.* Prefire images. The calcifications are just beyond the tip of the needle (*arrows*). The patient is warned that she will hear a "pop," and the gun is fired. *C.* Postfire, prebiopsy images. The calcifications now surround the needle notch (*arrows*). Biopsies are taken circumferentially within the cluster. *D.* Stereo pair after deployment of the clip. The clip (*arrows*) is seen well in one of the two stereo pairs, and only a small portion is seen on the right-hand image. Craniocaudal and 90-degree lateral views are also obtained (not shown) to document clip positioning. *E.* Core, specimen radiograph. Calcifications are present in several of the cores. Ductal carcinoma *in situ* is diagnosed. *F.* Prefire stereo images in a different patient. Calcifications (*long arrows*) are targeted for biopsy with an automated gun-needle device using a 14-gauge needle. Reference points in each stereo image are appropriately positioned (*short arrows*) at the top of the images. In this patient, multiple targets are selected for sampling. When using this system, targeting is critical. To the extent possible, try to select the same calcification (or point) in both stereo pairs; otherwise, the sampling will be off. With this setup, the needle is advanced to within 5 mm of the Z value calculated by the unit. The patient is warned of the "pop" she will hear, and the gun is fired.

(continued on next page)

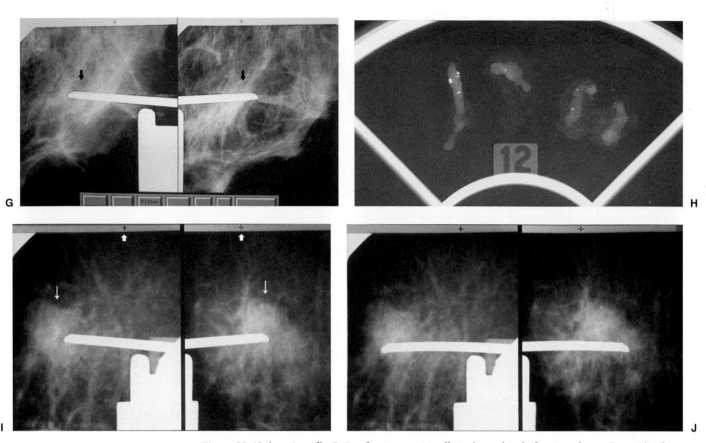

Figure 11.42 (continued) *G.* Postfire images. Needle is through calcification cluster (*arrows*). The needle is taken out of the breast to retrieve tissue and repositioned for subsequent pass. *H.* Core radiograph. Calcifications present in several of the cores. Compare with part *E* relative to size of cores. Ductal carcinoma *in situ* is diagnosed. *I.* Prefire images in a different patient with a mass (*thin arrows*). Several targets are selected in the mass. Coordinates are calculated by the unit in conjunction with reference points (*thick arrows*) in each stereo pair. The needle is advanced to within 5 mm of the Z value calculated by the unit. Patient is warned of the "pop" she will hear, and the gun is fired. *J.* Postfire stereo images. Needle is through a portion of the mass. Invasive ductal carcinoma is diagnosed.

mammographically to document clip placement (Figures 11.31 and 11.43). Core radiography is done if the target is calcifications (Figure 11.33).

Patients with a diagnosis of invasive carcinoma or DCIS are referred to a surgeon. Patients with benign findings that are radiologically and pathologically congruent (e.g., fibroadenoma) are returned to screening. With a diagnosis of atypical ductal hyperplasia, excision is recommended; 20% to 56% and 0% to 38% of cases of atypical ductal hyperplasia diagnosed using 14-gauge automated systems or directed vacuum-assisted devices,

Figure 11.43 *Mucinous carcinoma; tubular hematoma. A.* Craniocaudal view from a screening study in a 65-year-old woman showing a new mass (*thin arrow*). Intramammary lymph nodes (*thick arrows*) have been stable for years. *B.* Spot compression view showing mass with ill-defined margins. Arterial calcification is noted. Biopsy with directional vacuum-assisted biopsy probe and 11-gauge needle is done to establish diagnosis. Clip is deployed after biopsy. *C.* Craniocaudal view immediately after biopsy (mediolateral oblique view not shown). Clip (*short, thin arrows*) is seen adjacent to air locule (*thick arrow*). Intramammary lymph nodes (*long, thin arrows*) are again noted. *D.* A 90-degree lateral view is done when the patient presents for preoperative wire localization of clip 9 days after imaging-guided biopsy. Tubular density is noted along the biopsy needle track. Clip (*thick arrow*) is seen at inferior-most extent of hematoma. *E.* Craniocaudal view obtained after localization wire is deployed demonstrates hematoma end-on as dense, round mass (*thin arrow*). Reinforced segment of localization wire is seen adjacent to clip (*thick arrow*).

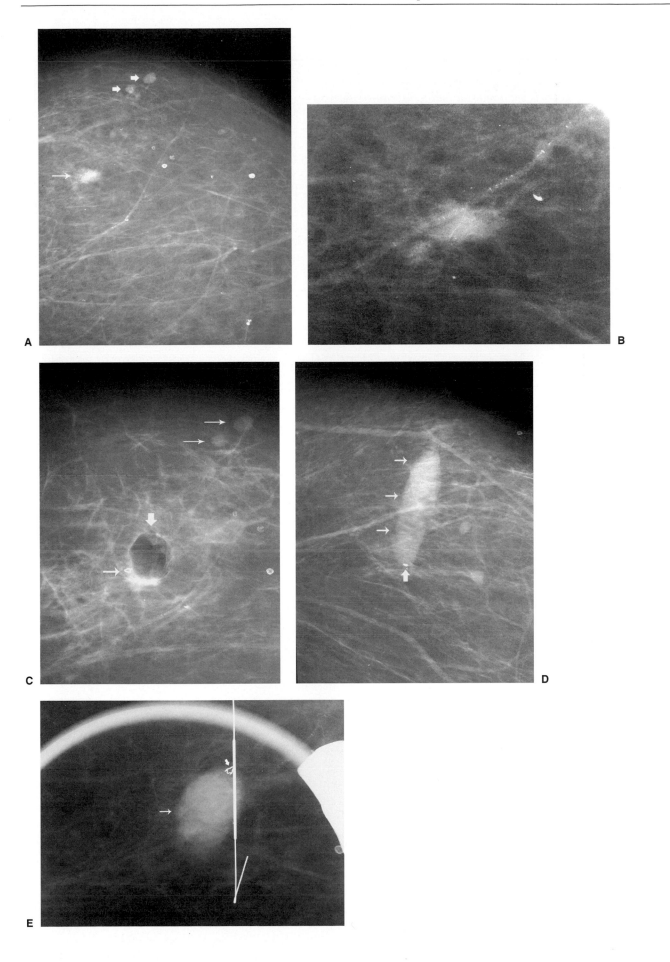

respectively, are upstaged to malignancy on excision (23–26). Excisional biopsy may also be recommended for patients with "cellular" fibroadenomas, if the pathologist is concerned the lesion could represent a phyllodes tumor. Controversy surrounds the appropriate management of lobular neoplasia (e.g., atypical lobular hyperplasia and lobular carcinoma *in situ*), complex sclerosing lesions, and papillary lesions diagnosed on imaging-guided biopsies (25–28). Following a discussion with the pathologist and surgeon, a decision is made about the need for excision that takes into consideration pertinent history and clinical, imaging, and histologic findings.

Radiography of the core samples is indicated if the biopsy is being done for calcifications.

After the procedure, the biopsy site (needle track) is compressed for at least 10 minutes. The patient is provided a small ice pack that fits in her bra to minimize any bruising or discomfort. There are no restrictions after the biopsy. The patient is asked to return the next afternoon for an evaluation of the biopsy site and a discussion of the results. When the patient returns, surgical consultation can be scheduled, if appropriate, or the patient is provided with follow-up recommendations. For all biopsies with positive results, the referring physician is contacted directly with the findings, and surgical referral is discussed with the physician before scheduling the patient.

CLIP PLACEMENT TO MARK TUMOR LOCATION

Neoadjuvant therapy is used in some patients who desire conservative treatment to downstage the tumor. These patients present with a large lesion or with an average-sized lesion in a small breast that might otherwise preclude conservative therapy. An imaging-guided biopsy of the breast, primary tumor is done to establish the diagnosis and determine the status of estrogen and progesterone receptors and HER-2/neu. If a potentially abnormal lymph node is imaged in the ipsilateral axilla, FNA or core biopsy is done to establish the presence of disease in the axilla.

As patients are treated, some tumors shrink dramatically after the first two or three courses of chemotherapy. In these patients, a metallic clip is placed in the tumor under ultrasound guidance (Figure 11.44) to mark its location. Orthogonal, images are obtained after clip placement to document the final position of the clip. If the tumor shrinks so that it is no longer palpable or resolves completely after completion of the chemotherapy, the clip is used to guide preoperative wire localization of the original tumor location (29).

PREOPERATIVE WIRE LOCALIZATION

As the number of imaging-guided biopsies that are performed increases, the number of preoperative wire localizations decreases. At this time, we perform preoperative wire localizations almost exclusively in patients who have already had an imaging-guided biopsy and have a diagnosis of breast cancer or a lesion such as atypical ductal hyperplasia that requires excisional biopsy. Rarely, in patients who, for technical reasons, cannot undergo imaging-guided biopsy, we perform preoperative wire localization for diagnostic purposes. As with core biopsies, the number of localizations done under ultrasound guidance has increased significantly in the past several years, and only a few are now done using mammographic guidance.

Basically, if we can see the lesion with ultrasound (and this includes some patients with calcifications), we perform the localization using ultrasound guidance. Ultrasound-guided procedures are much easier for patients because the patient remains supine, and no compression or radiation is used. Consequently, vasovagal reactions are almost completely eliminated. Ultrasound-guided localizations also facilitate the surgical approach. Unlike mammographically guided localizations, during which the patient is sitting up with her breast pulled out and compressed, the patient lies supine for ultrasound-guided localizations, simulating her position in the operating room. In conjunction with the placement of the wire, the skin overlying the lesion is marked with an X, and the distance from the

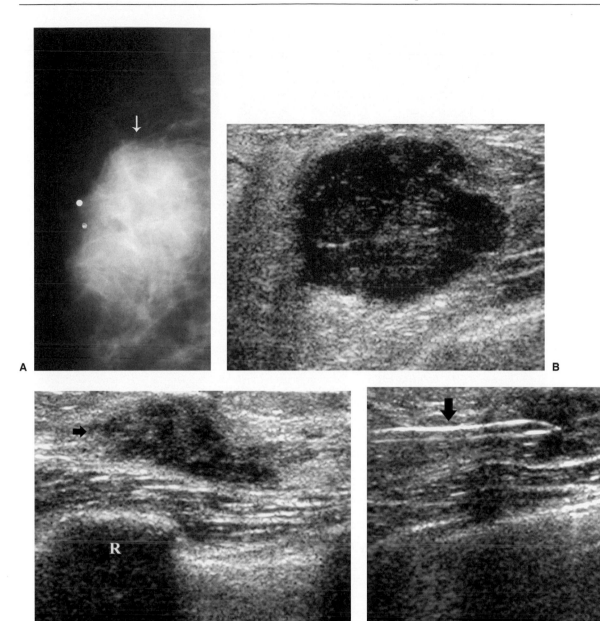

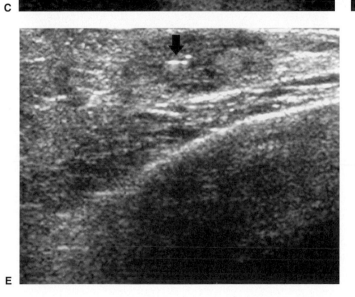

Figure 11.44 *Poorly differentiated invasive ductal carcinoma, not otherwise specified, with metastasis to at least one ipsilateral axillary lymph node. Neoadjuvant therapy. A. Oval mass (arrow) in a 57-year-old patient. Screening mammogram 9 months previously, even in retrospect, is normal. B. Round mass with irregular margins and posterior acoustic enhancement. Enlarged lymph node in ipsilateral axilla is identified. Diagnosis is established with core biopsies of the breast lesion and axillary lymph node (not shown). Patient received two courses of chemotherapy with significant response. She now presents for clip placement to localize tumor bed. C. Ultrasound 2 months after image in part B. Mass (arrow) is still seen but now smaller. Rib (R) is seen. D. Needle (arrow) is used for clip placement. The tip of the needle is in the center of the mass; the clip is deployed E. Clip (arrow) is seen in the mass after the needle is removed.*

(continued on next page)

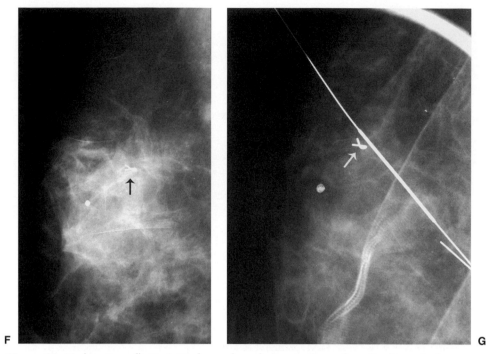

F   G

Figure 11.44 (continued) *F.* A 90-degree lateral view is done after clip (*arrow*) placement. Craniocaudal view is also done (not shown). *G.* Film from preoperative wire localization demonstrates that reinforced wire segment is adjacent to clip (*arrow*). Four months after initial presentation (after four courses of chemotherapy), 2 months after clip placement, the patient presents for preoperative wire localization. At this time, no abnormality is identified ultrasonographically. Localization of the clip is undertaken using mammographic guidance. No residual tumor is identified histologically in the lumpectomy specimen or in the removed axillary lymph nodes. Neoadjuvant therapy is given to reduce tumor size, which enables patients who otherwise might not be candidates to undergo conservative treatment.

skin to the lesion is provided to facilitate the excision of the lesion. The incision can be made to intercept the wire, rather than dissecting along the wire, as many surgeons do after mammographically guided localization.

A variety of needle-wire systems are available, including spring hookwire (30), modified spring hookwire (31–33), J wire (34), and "barbed" wire systems. These come in various lengths, including 3, 5, 7, 9, 11, and 15 cm. We usually use the modified spring hookwire; however, any of these systems accomplishes the goal of the localization procedure, which is to provide a guide or "road map" for the surgeon in removing the lesion in question while sparing much of the surrounding normal tissue. The modified spring hookwire has a hook at the end that helps anchor the wire in place and a 2-cm long reinforced segment that is 1 cm from the tip of the hook. The reinforced segment adds stiffness to that portion of the wire, minimizing the likelihood that the wire is inadvertently transected. Additionally, it provides a reference point for describing the location of the lesion to the surgeon. We aim to place the reinforced wire segment within or in close proximity to the lesion. Although the hook anchors the wire, it is important that the wire not be used as a retractor, particularly in predominantly fatty breast tissue; otherwise, the wire can be inadvertently dislodged.

If ultrasound guidance is used, the patient is supine or in a slight oblique position (Figure 11.45). A skin entry point is selected that will allow the needle to be advanced parallel to the chest wall and transducer (as described for needle biopsies). Lidocaine (2%) is used to raise a skin wheal, and a small amount is used along the expected course of the needle to the lesion. A needle that is long enough to go beyond the lesion by at least 1 cm is selected. With the tip of the needle 1 cm beyond the lesion, the reinforced wire segment

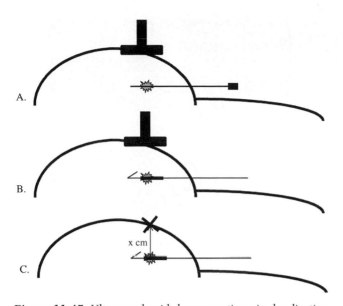

Figure 11.45 *Ultrasound-guided preoperative wire localization.*
A. With the transducer over the lesion, the localization needle
is advanced through the lesion. Orthogonal images of the needle are obtained when localizing small lesions. If the needle is
through the lesion on the orthogonal ultrasound images, the
wire is deployed, and the needle is pulled out of the breast. *B.*
As long as the wire is parallel to the transducer, it is seen beau-
tifully, even though it is thin. Its position through the lesion is
documented in orthogonal planes. *C.* The distance from the
skin to the lesion and wire is measured, and an X is placed on
the skin directly over the lesion. This assists the surgeon in
intersecting the wire rather than following it in from the skin
entry point.

will be in close proximity to the lesion. The wire is removed from the needle and set aside
to prevent inadvertent deployment or contamination of the wire. Under ultrasound guidance, the needle is advanced through the lesion and beyond it by 1 cm. If the lesion is
small, an orthogonal view of the needle is done to document the relationship of the needle to the lesion (Figure 11.46). With the needle through the lesion, the wire is passed
through the needle so that the burnish mark on the wire is at the hub of the needle. The
needle is then pulled out of the breast, making sure that the wire is not inadvertently
advanced into the breast or pulled out with the needle. Ultrasound images of the wire and
its relationship to the lesion are taken in orthogonal planes. The distance from the skin to
the lesion is determined, and an X is marked on the skin directly over the lesion. A single
mammographic image with compression applied parallel to the course of the wire is
obtained (Figure 11.46). After the hookwire is deployed, we never compress the breast
perpendicular to the wire. This can result in uncontrolled repositioning of the wire,
including having the wire pull out from the lesion completely (accordion effect) (Figure
11.47).

Safe, precise localizations can also be accomplished by using mammographic guidance (30–38). CC and 90-degree lateral views are reviewed to determine the shortest distance from the skin to the lesion (Figure 11.48). Needle length is determined by measuring from the skin to the lesion and selecting a needle that is long enough to go beyond the
lesion by at least 1 cm.

Several compression paddles are available for these localization procedures. The most
commonly used has a single fenestration with radiopaque markers along two sides for ease
of coordinate mapping and needle placement. The second type contains multiple perfora-

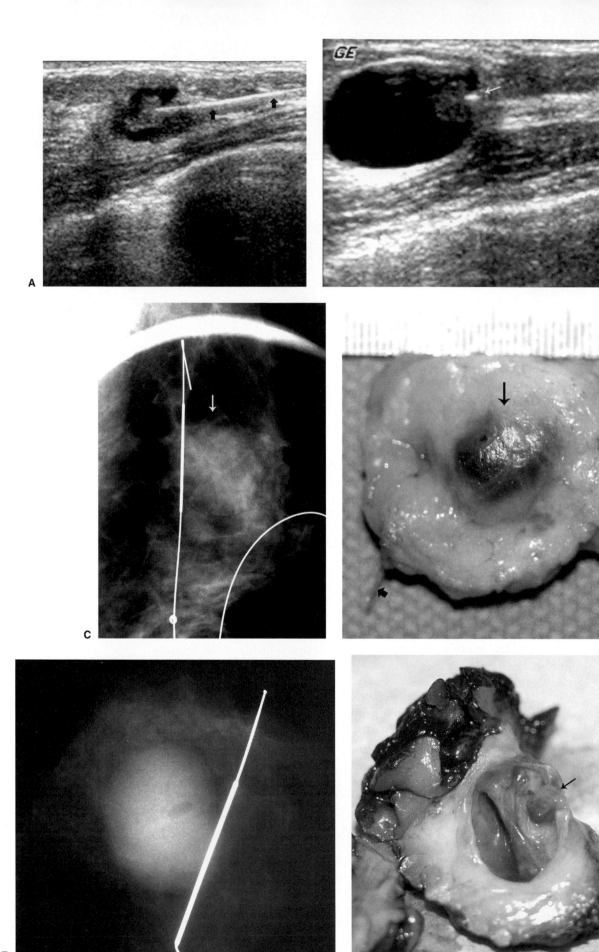

A

B

C

D

E

F

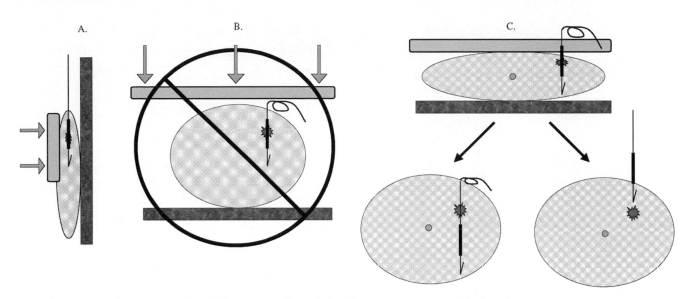

Figure 11.47 *Localization wires should be compressed parallel to their course, not perpendicular. A.* After the wire is in position, we compress the breast parallel to the wire without any difficulty. *B.* We do not, however, compress the breast perpendicular to the wire. *C.* If the breast is compressed perpendicular to the course of the wire, the wire can be inadvertently advanced further into the breast or pulled out of the lesion.

tions arranged at set intervals. With this type of paddle, the perforations need to be large enough to allow passage of the needle hub so that the compression paddle can be released when the gantry is repositioned for the orthogonal view. A relatively minor disadvantage of these multiple-perforation paddles is that repositioning of the breast may be required if the lesion does not project directly below one of the perforations. These types of paddles come in two sizes: full compression paddles (the size of those used for routine screening views) and smaller paddles (the size of a spot compression paddle). The small paddles are particularly useful in women with small breasts and in patients with posterior, axillary, or subareolar lesions (Figure 11.49). In these situations, optimal compression and breast immobilization are difficult to accomplish with a full-sized compression paddle.

Let us consider a patient with a cluster of calcifications (Figure 5.40C in Chapter 5 for CC magnification view) and a diagnosis of DCIS after imaging-guided biopsy. The patient now presents for preoperative wire localization of the calcifications. CC and 90-degree lateral views demonstrate that the calcifications are closest to the lateral skin surface on the CC view. Consequently, a 90-degree lateromedial (LM) view, using the fenestrated compression paddle, will be the starting view in this patient. Firm compression is applied to prevent inadvertent patient motion. Ideally, the technologist marks the corners of the fenestration on the patient's skin so that it is easy to determine whether she moves

Figure 11.46 *Papilloma; preoperative ultrasound-guided wire localization. A.* Needle (*arrows*) through intracystic lesion. Note that the needle is parallel to deep pectoral fascia. (Diagnostic films for this patient are shown in Figure 11.26.) *B.* Orthogonal ultrasound image demonstrates localization needle in cross section (*arrow*) through the stalk of the intracystic lesion. *C.* Single mammogram film obtained, compressing parallel to wire demonstrates the relationship of the localization wire to the mass (*arrow*). As desired, the reinforced wire segment is through the posterior portion of the mass (*arrow*). *D.* Image of specimen. Localized mass is grossly apparent (*thin arrow*) as a blue-domed cyst. Although not in focus on this image, the localization wire is seen extending beyond the specimen (*thick arrow*). *E.* With sectioning of the lesion, fluid is released. *F.* The papilloma (*arrow*) is attached to otherwise smooth cyst wall. A residual amount of fluid is seen in the dependant portion of the cyst.

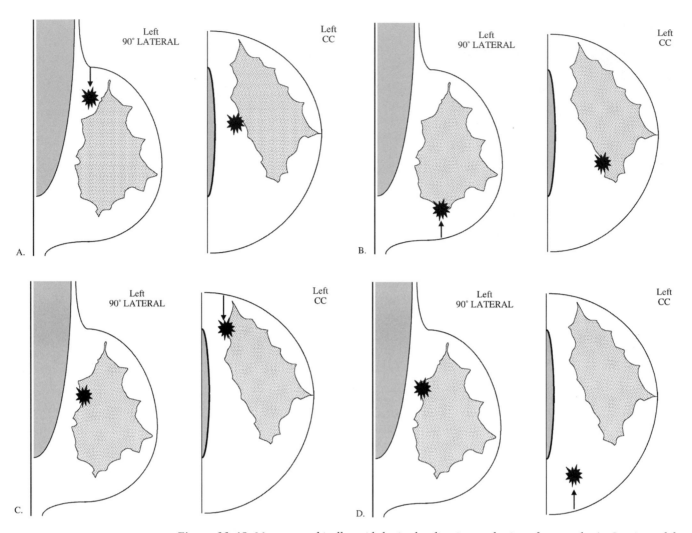

Figure 11.48 *Mammographically guided wire localizations; selection of approach. A. Craniocaudal* (CC) and 90-degree lateral views are reviewed. The shortest distance from the skin to the lesion determines the approach. In this case, the lesion is closest to the superior skin surface on the 90-degree lateral view (*arrow*). The starting position for the localization is a CC view: the superior skin surface is compressed with the fenestrated compression paddle. *B.* In this example, the lesion is closest to the inferior surface of the breast on the 90-degree lateral view (*arrow*). The starting position for the localization is a from-below (FB) view: the inferior skin surface is compressed using the fenestrated compression paddle. *C.* In this case, the lesion is closest to the lateral skin surface on the CC view (*arrow*). The starting position for the localization is a 90-degree lateromedial view. The lateral aspect of the breast is compressed using the fenestrated compression paddle. *D.* In this case, the lesion is closest to the medial skin surface on the CC view (*arrow*). The starting position for the localization is a 90-degree mediolateral view. With this view, the medial aspect of the breast is compressed using the fenestrated compression paddle.

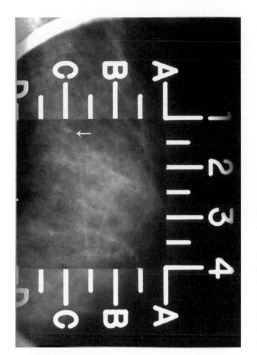

Figure 11.49 *Small localization compression paddle.* Cluster of calcifications (*arrow*) for wire localization is seen far posterolaterally in the patient. Location of calcifications and breast compression to 1.5 cm preclude stereotactically guided biopsy. This small compression paddle with a fenestration and alphanumeric grid is particularly helpful in patients with a small breast or in localizing lesions that are located far posteriorly, high in the axilla or in the subareolar area. These areas are hard to access and compress adequately with the standard-sized compression paddle.

between the time it takes to obtain this first image, and when the needle is put in. The film is obtained, and the coordinates for the lesion are plotted on this film (Figure 11.50). The collimator crosshairs or laser lights are aligned to the appropriate coordinate settings. With the centering light of the mammographic unit, a shadow of the crosshairs marking the lesion's coordinates is cast onto the patient's compressed breast. The skin is cleaned with povidone-iodine and alcohol. Lidocaine (2%) is used to raise a skin wheal. A 5-cm needle is selected, and the wire is removed from the needle and set aside before starting; this prevents inadvertent deployment or contamination of the wire. The tip of the needle is placed at the intersecting point of the coordinates, and the needle is aligned, using the centering light of the mammographic unit, so that the shadow of the needle hub is cast on the skin entry site (if the hub of the needle is held with the thumb and index fingers, and the rest of fingers are splayed away, the radiologist's hand will not interfere with the ability to see the shadow of the coordinates and needle hub). The needle is advanced in one motion, perpendicular to the skin and parallel to the chest wall, as far as possible. Another 90-degree LM view is obtained with the needle in place (Figure 11.50). Because the wire is placed through the needle, this film serves to describe the eventual relationship between lesion and wire in this plane (e.g., this projection need not, and should not, be repeated after the wire is deployed; it would require that compression be applied perpendicular to the wire). Compression is released slowly, allowing breast tissue to reexpand around the needle so that the hub is flush with the skin surface. At this point, the patient, who has remained stationary, is encouraged to sit back and relax while the x-ray tube is rotated 90 degrees.

The patient's breast is repositioned with the needle now parallel to the film; in this patient, it is a CC view. Compression for this orthogonal image is best done with the spot compression paddle. Use of the spot paddle at this point allows us to determine the position of the tip of needle and its relationship to the lesion while permitting easy access to the hub of the needle for adjustments in needle positioning. If the full compression paddle is used, the space between the film holder and the compression paddle may limit access for needle repositioning and deployment of the wire (Figure 11.51). The spot CC view in our example is obtained and processed while the patient's breast remains in compression (Figure 11.50). Before the wire is deployed, the relationship of the needle to the lesion is determined on the orthogonal view. On the initial film (in this case, the 90-degree LM view), the hub and tip of the needle should be superimposed on the lesion. If a long

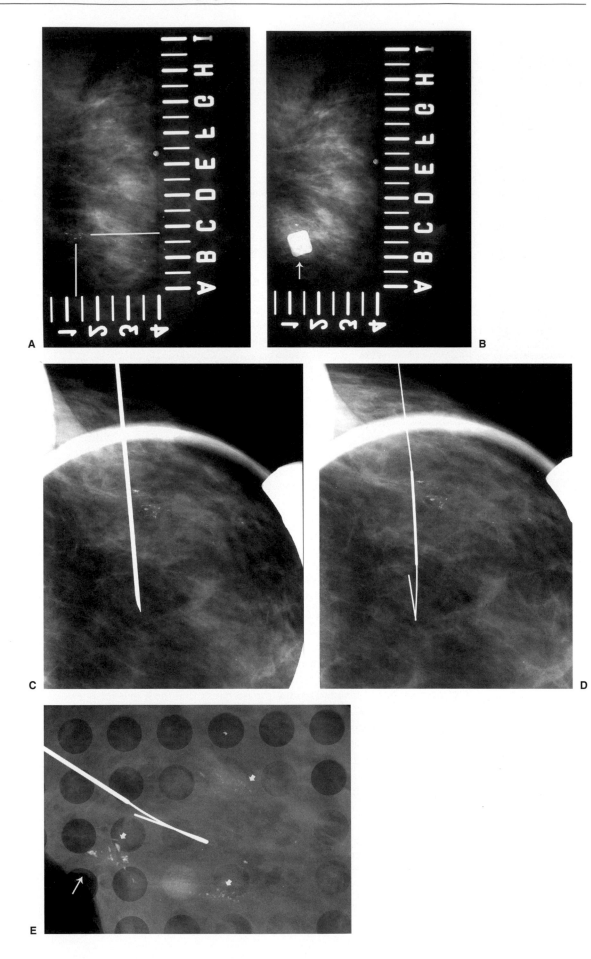

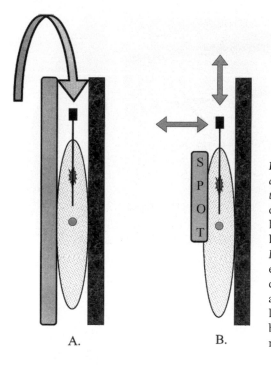

A.   **B.**

Figure 11.51 *Use of spot compression paddle during mammographically guided wire localization.* A. When obtaining the orthogonal view to document the relationship of the needle to the lesion, access to the hub of the needle may be limited if the large compression paddle is used. B. If the spot compression paddle is used, however, there is easy access to the hub of the needle. The needle can be pulled out slightly and in a controlled manner if the tip is beyond the lesion by more than 1 cm. It is also easy to stabilize the wire so that there is no inadvertent motion of the wire as the needle is pulled out.

enough needle was selected, the lesion is skewered. On the second film (in this case, a CC view), the location of the lesion along the course of the needle is determined. If the needle is more than 1 cm beyond the lesion, it is pulled out enough so that the tip is about 1 cm beyond the lesion. With this needle positioning, the reinforced wire segment will be in close proximity to the lesion. If the needle is in a satisfactory position, the wire is advanced through the needle until the burnish mark on the wire is at the hub of the needle. The wire is then held in place as the needle is withdrawn; care is needed to make sure that the wire is not inadvertently advanced into the breast or pulled out with the needle (Figure 11.52). A repeat CC view is obtained at this point to document the position of the wire. Compression is released, and the external portion of the wire is secured to the skin. A theoretical localization using a CC approach and an actual localization using a 90-degree mediolateral approach are presented for review (Figures 11.53 and 11.54). In patients with multiple lesions or an extensive area of calcifications not undergoing mastectomy, multiple wires are used to localize each mass or bracket the area of calcifications (Figure 11.55).

Figure 11.50 *Mammographically guided preoperative wire localization.* A. A 90-degree lateromedial (LM) view in a patient with a cluster of calcifications closest to the lateral skin surface on the craniocaudal (CC) view. A 90-degree LM view is the starting point using the standard-sized fenestrated compression paddle. The coordinates for the cluster of calcifications is determined (*white lines*). Collimator crosshairs are positioned so that a shadow is cast on the woman's breast at these coordinates. The needle is advanced in one movement to the hub, and a repeat 90-degree LM view is obtained. B. A 90-degree LM view. Hub of needle (*arrow*) is superimposed on calcification cluster. If a long enough needle has been selected, the calcifications will be found along the course of the needle. This view defines the positioning of the wire (wire is passed through needle) and thus does not need to be repeated after the wire is deployed. Compression is released, and a CC view is obtained to determine where the calcifications are found along the course of the needle. C. CC view using the spot compression paddle. Patient remains in compression after this view is done until after the wire is deployed. Needle is through the posterior edge of the calcification cluster. D. Repeat CC view after wire is deployed. Superficial portion of reinforced wire segment is at the posterior edge of the calcification cluster. E. Specimen radiograph (3× magnification). Localized calcifications have been excised. Wire with hook has been excised. Proximity to one of the margins (*arrow*) is discussed with surgeon. Although the specimen radiograph is a two-dimensional representation of a three-dimensional structure, proximity to the margins can sometimes be suggested based on the image. Coordinates for the three areas of calcifications (*thick arrows*) are indicated for the pathologist.

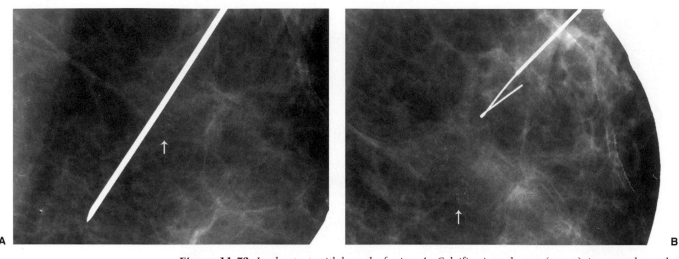

A   **B**

Figure 11.52 *Inadvertent withdrawal of wire.* A. Calcification cluster (*arrow*) is seen along the course of the needle. The wire is deployed. As the needle is pulled out, the wire needs to be stabilized (much as is done with a catheter exchange). Care must be exercised not to advance the wire as the needle is pulled out, nor to withdraw the wire with the needle. B. On the final image taken to document the relationship of the wire to the lesion, it is clear that the wire was inadvertently pulled out with the needle. The hook and reinforced segment of the wire are short of the cluster of calcifications (*arrow*). When the wire is short of the lesion, as in this patient, a second wire needs to be deployed; otherwise, it becomes very difficult for the surgeon to excise the area of concern.

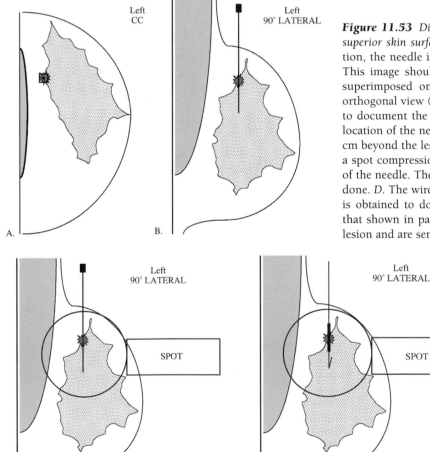

Figure 11.53 *Diagrams, wire localization of a lesion closest to the superior skin surface.* A. With the patient in a craniocaudal position, the needle is advanced in the breast all the way to the hub. This image should show the hub of the needle and the needle superimposed on the lesion. Compression is released. B. The orthogonal view (in this case a 90-degree lateral view) is obtained to document the relationship of the needle to the lesion and the location of the needle tip. The tip of the needle should be about 1 cm beyond the lesion. C. The 90-degree lateral view is done using a spot compression paddle so that there is easy access to the hub of the needle. The patient is kept in compression after this view is done. D. The wire is deployed, and a repeat 90-degree lateral view is obtained to document final wire positioning. This image and that shown in part A describe the relationship of the wire to the lesion and are sent to the surgeon for use during the biopsy.

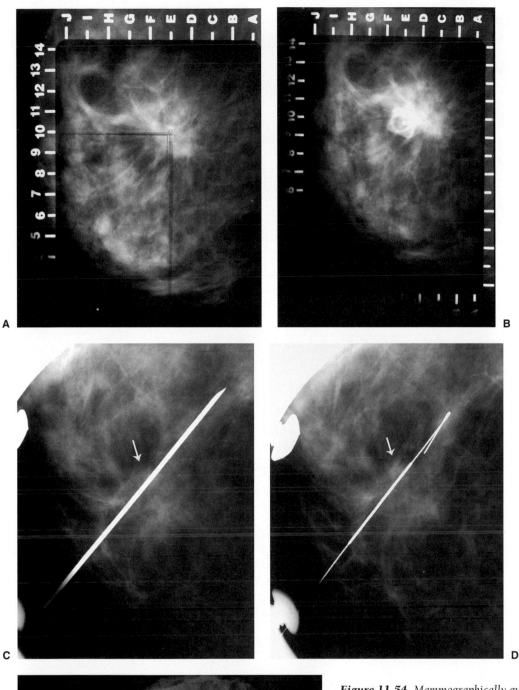

Figure 11.54 *Mammographically guided wire localization, 90-degree mediolateral approach. A. A 90-degree mediolateral view with fenestrated compression paddle. Coordinates for the spiculated mass are determined. The needle tip is placed at the intersection of the coordinates and advanced to the hub. B. A 90-degree mediolateral view after needle placement. The hub of the needle is superimposed on the lesion. If a long enough needle is selected, the lesion will be skewered. At this point, compression is released, and the orthogonal view is obtained; in this patient, it is a craniocaudal view. C. Craniocaudal view done using a spot compression paddle. This view demonstrates where the mass (arrow) is located along the course of the needle. D. The wire is deployed, and the needle is taken out, making sure the wire is not moved inadvertently as the needle is manipulated. Final image taken demonstrates that the reinforced wire segment is through the spiculated mass (arrow). E. Specimen radiograph confirms excision of the spiculated mass and wire.*

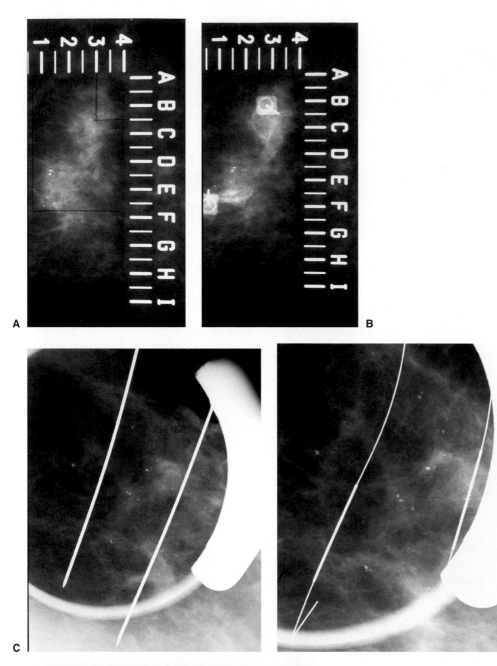

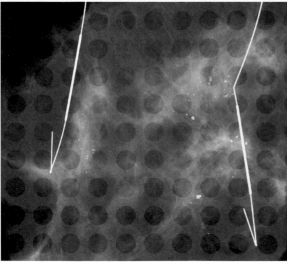

Figure 11.55 *Bracketing of extensive lesions.* A. A 90-degree latero-medial (LM) view. Fenestrated compression paddle with alphanumeric grid is used to compress the lateral aspect of the breast. Coordinates for the calcification clusters are determined as shown on the film. Needles are advanced at the two sets of coordinates. B. A 90-degree LM view. After needles are placed, a repeat LM view is done to document the relationship of the needles and the calcification clusters in this plane. C. Craniocaudal (CC) view done using spot compression paddle. Calcifications are seen surrounding both needles. D. Repeat CC view after deployment of the wires. Although the patient has moved slightly, the relationship of the wires to the calcifications can be determined. E. Specimen radiograph demonstrates wide area of calcifications in the specimen bracketed by the wires. Ductal carcinoma *in situ* is diagnosed. In women with extensive areas of calcification or multiple lesions, multiple wires are used to bracket the area of concern for the surgeon.

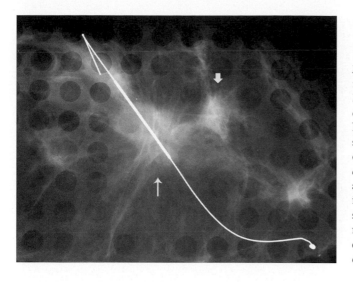

Figure 11.56 *Specimen radiography, detection of unsuspected lesions.* Specimen radiograph confirms excision of a spiculated mass (*thin arrow*). Wire is seen through this mass. A second unsuspected mass (*thick arrow*) is seen in the radiograph and confirmed to be a second invasive ductal carcinoma. In some patients, additional masses or calcifications may be detected on the specimen radiograph.

SPECIMEN RADIOGRAPHY

After imaging-guided localization, surgical specimens are radiographed (39,40) or, in some situations, imaged using ultrasound.

This serves several purposes:

Following imaging-guided wire localizations, a specimen radiograph or ultrasound is indicated to document excision of the localized lesion.

- Documents excision of the localized lesion (Figures 11.50 and 11.54)
- Documents removal of the localization wire
- Is used to mark the location of the lesion for the pathologist
- Detects unsuspected lesions (Figure 11.56)
- Can suggest proximity of lesion to margins

The specimen is placed in a container that has an alphanumeric grid that can be used to compress the specimen. Based on the radiograph, a pin is put through the lesion, or four pins can be used to bracket the area of concern (Figure 11.57). What is marked and how it is marked are indicated for the pathologist. Specimen radiography is done with compression of the specimen and magnification technique. The radiograph can be obtained on a mammography unit; alternatively, dedicated specimen radiography units are available.

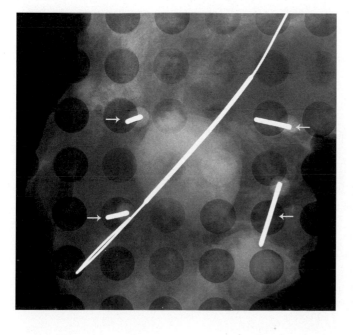

Figure 11.57 *Marking location of lesion for pathologist on specimen radiograph.* Based on the specimen radiograph, the location of the lesion is marked for the pathologist using four pins (*arrows*) to ensure that the lesion of interest is evaluated histologically.

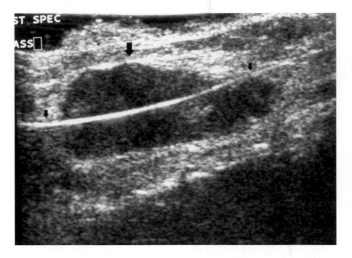

Figure 11.58 Specimen sonogram. If the lesion is visible on ultrasound, ultrasonography can also be used to document excision of the lesion and wire. In patients in whom the lesion is not seen mammographically, ultrasound of the specimen is required. The mass (*large arrow*) is readily seen in the specimen with the wire still through it (*small arrows*).

Magnification factors of up to 3.8 times can be obtained with some of the radiography units available. As a routine, we obtain two specimen radiographs. One remains in the patient's jacket, and the second is submitted to pathology with the specimen. After the radiograph is obtained and verification of lesion removal is established, the surgeon is notified with the results; if there are concerns about proximity to a margin, this is discussed at this time also.

With lesions that are not apparent mammographically and are localized using ultrasonography, the specimen is imaged using ultrasound. A protective sheath is put on the transducer, and a small amount of gel is applied to the specimen. The transducer is manipulated over the specimen in a systematic manner to determine the location of the lesion (Figure 11.58). When the lesion is identified, a pin or needle can be put through it to mark the area for the pathologist.

PARAFFIN BLOCK RADIOGRAPHY

When a biopsy is done for calcifications and the calcifications are not identifiable on the microscopic slides, we can assist the pathologist by obtaining a radiographic image of the paraffin blocks (41,42). Magnified images of the blocks are obtained using the lowest pos-

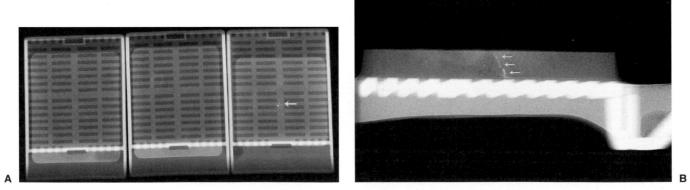

A   B

Figure 11.59 Paraffin block radiography. A. After excision of calcifications, the pathologist occasionally requests assistance in locating the calcifications. The paraffin blocks are radiographed (if there is any unsectioned tissue, this can also be evaluated). The block containing the calcifications (*arrow*) is identified. B. Orthogonal view of the block. This is obtained to determine the depth of the calcifications (*arrows*) in the block.

sible kilovoltage peak, with a milliamperage of 5 to 6. The block with calcifications is identified, and an orthogonal view of the block is obtained to establish the depth of the calcifications in the block (Figure 11.59).

REFERENCES

1. Cardenosa G, Doudna C, Eklund GW. Ductography of the breast: technique and findings. *AJR Am J Roentgenol* 1994;162:1081–1087.
2. Fajardo LL, Jackson VP, Hunter TB. Interventional procedures in diseases of the breast: needle biopsy, pneumocystography and galactography. *AJR Am J Roentgenol* 1992;158:1231–1238.
3. Leborgne R. Estudio radiologico del sistema canalicular de la glandula mamaria normal y patologica. Montevideo, Uruguay, Impresora Uruguaya S.A. *Juncal* 1943:1511.
4. Tabar L, Dean PB, Zoltan P. Galactography: the diagnostic procedure of choice for nipple discharge. *Radiology* 1983;149:31–38.
5. Haagensen CD. Disease of the breast. 3rd ed., Philadelphia, Saunders, 1986:136–175.
6. Woods ER, Helvie MA, Ikeda DM, et al. Solitary breast papilloma: comparison of mammographic, galactographic and pathologic findings. *AJR Am J Roentgenol* 1992;159:487–491.
7. Leis HP, Cammarata A, LaRaja RD. Nipple discharge: significance and treatment. *Breast* 1985; 11:6–12.
8. Tabar L, Pentek Z, Dean PB. The diagnostic and therapeutic value of breast cyst puncture and pneumocystography. *Radiology* 1981;141:659–663.
9. Ikeda DM, Helvie MA, Adler DD, et al. The role of fine-needle aspiration and pneumocystography in the treatment of impalpable breast cysts. *AJR Am J Roentgenol* 1992;158:1239–1241.
10. Azavedo E, Svane G, Auer G. Stereotactic fine needle biopsy in 2594 mammographically detected non-palpable lesions. *Lancet* 1989;1:1033–1035.
11. Jackson VP. The status of mammographically guided fine needle aspiration biopsy of nonpalpable breast lesions. *Radiol Clin North Am* 1992;30:155–166.
12. Parker SH, Lovin JD, Jobe WE, et al. Stereotactic breast biopsy with a biopsy gun. *Radiology* 1990;176:741–747.
13. Parker SH, Lovin JD, Jobe WE, et al. Nonpalpable breast lesions: stereotactic automated large-core biopsies. *Radiology* 1991;180:403–407.
14. Parker SH, Jobe WE, eds. *Percutaneous breast biopsy*. New York: Raven Press, 1993.
15. Parker SH, Burbank F, Jackman RJ, et al. Percutaneous large-core breast biopsy: a multi-institutional study. *Radiology* 1994;193:359–364.
16. Parker SH, Klaus AJ, McWey PJ, et al. Sonographically guided directional vacuum-assisted breast biopsy using a handheld device. *AJR Am J Roentgenol* 2001;177:405–408.
17. Liberman L. Percutaneous imaging-guided core breast biopsy: state of the art at the millennium. *AJR Am J Roentgenol* 2000;174:1191–1199.
18. Liberman L, Fahs MC, Dershaw DD, et al. Impact of stereotaxic core biopsy on cost of diagnosis. *Radiology* 1995;195:633–637.
19. Liberman L, Feng TL, Dershaw DD, et al. US-guided core breast biopsy: use and cost effectiveness. *Radiology* 1998;208:717–723.
20. Meyer JE. Value of large-core biopsy of occult breast lesions. *AJR Am J Roentgenol* 1992;158: 991–992.
21. Perez-Fuentes JA, Longobardi IR, Acosta VF, et al. Sonographically guided directional vacuum assisted breast biopsy: preliminary experience in Venezuela. *AJR Am J Roentgenol* 2001;177: 1459–1463.
22. Fornage BD, Coan JD, David CL. Ultrasound-guided needle biopsy of the breast and other interventional procedures. *Radiol Clin North Am* 1992;30:167–185.
23. Liberman L, Cohen MA, Dershaw DD, et al. Atypical ductal hyperplasia diagnosed at stereotaxic core biopsy of breast lesions: an indication for surgical biopsy. *AJR Am J Roentgenol* 1995;164: 1111–1113.
24. Jackman RJ, Birdwell RL, Ikeda DM. Atypical ductal hyperplasia: can some lesions be defined as probably benign after stereotactic 11-gauge vacuum assisted biopsy, eliminating the recommendations for surgical excision? *Radiology* 2002;224:548–554.
25. Philphotts LE, Shaheen NA, Jain KS, et al. Uncommon high risk lesions of the breast diagnosed at stereotactic core needle biopsy: clinical importance. *Radiology* 2000;216:831–837.
26. Reynolds HE. Core needle biopsy of challenging benign breast conditions: a comprehensive literature review. *AJR Am J Roentgenol* 2000;174:1245–1250.

27. Liberman L, Sama M, Susnik B, et al. Lobular carcinoma in situ at percutaneous breast biopsy: surgical biopsy findings. *AJR Am J Roentgenol* 1999;173:291–299.
28. Berg WA, Mrose HE, Ioffe OB. Atypical lobular hyperplasia or lobular carcinoma in situ at core needle breast biopsy. *Radiology* 2001;218:503–509.
29. Edeiken BS, Fornage BD, Bedi DG, et al. US-guided implantation of metallic markers for permanent localization of the tumor bed in patients with breast cancer who undergo preoperative chemotherapy. *Radiology* 1999;213:895–900.
30. Kopans DB, Meyer J. Versatile spring hookwire breast lesion localizer. *AJR Am J Roentgenol* 1982; 138:586–587.
31. Kopans DB, Deluca S. A modified needle-hookwire breast lesion localizer. *AJR Am J Roentgenol* 1982;138:586–587.
32. Kopans DB, Lindfors K, McCarthy KA, et al. Spring hookwire breast lesion localizer: use of rigid-compression mammographic systems. *Radiology* 1985;157:537–538.
33. Kopans DB, Swann CA. Preoperative imaging-guided needle placement and localization of clinically occult breast lesions. *AJR Am J Roentgenol* 1989;152:1–9.
34. Homer MJ. Nonpalpable breast lesion localization using a curved-end retractable wire. *Radiology* 1985;157:259–260.
35. Gisvold JJ, Martin JK. Prebiopsy localization of nonpalpable breast lesions. *AJR Am J Roentgenol* 1984;143:477–481.
36. Hall FM, Frank HA. Preoperative localization of nonpalpable breast lesions. *AJR Am J Roentgenol* 1979;132:101–105.
37. Meyer JE, Kopans DB, Stomper PC, et al. Occult breast abnormalities: percutaneous preoperative needle localization. *Radiology* 1984;150:335–337.
38. Kalisher L. An improved needle for localization of nonpalpable breast lesions. *Radiology* 1978; 128:815–817.
39. Holland R. The role of specimen x-ray in the diagnosis of breast cancer. *Diagn Imaging Clin Med* 1985;54:178–185.
40. Rebner M, Pennes DR, Baker DE, et al. Two view specimen radiography in surgical biopsy of nonpalpable breast masses. *AJR Am J Roentgenol* 1987;149:283–285.
41. Cardenosa G, Eklund GW. Paraffin block radiography following breast biopsies: use of orthogonal views. *Radiology* 1991;180:873–874.
42. Rebner M, Helvie MA, Pennes DR, et al. Paraffin tissue block radiography: adjunct to breast specimen radiography. *Radiology* 1989;173:695–696.

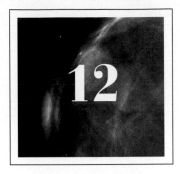

THE MAMMOGRAPHY REPORT AND THE MEDICAL AUDIT

THE MAMMOGRAPHY REPORT

The mammographic report should be concise, accurate, and directive. For screening exams, a report with pertinent negatives is used for normal studies, and a report stating there is a mass, distortion, or calcifications requiring further evaluation is issued for potentially abnormal studies. Description and characterization of findings are relegated to the diagnostic setting. Time and time again, we find that the information available to us on the screening study is limited and may actually be misleading. In our opinion, trying to make definitive statements on a screening study is not optimal. As discussed in Chapter 2, the only assessment categories we use for screening studies are as follows: 1, negative; 2, benign; and 0, incomplete, requiring additional imaging evaluation.

For a diagnostic exam after a screening study, we need to determine whether there is a lesion and, if there is, to characterize it and make a decision about the next appropriate step. For a diagnostic exam in a patient presenting with a sign or symptom related to the breast, we need to correlate imaging findings (if any) with the area of clinical concern. This may require one or two mammographic images or an ultrasound and, in some patients, imaging-guided needle biopsy. The bottom line: Is there a finding that may represent breast cancer? What is the next step? Return to screen? Short-interval follow-up because the lesion is probably benign? Or biopsy? On these studies, all assessment categories are used, although category 0 is not typically used.

Before dictating a report, review films with comparisons (if available), make a decision about what you think is going on, and provide an appropriate recommendation and direction. Focus immediately on the relevant observations. Do not use the report to make up your mind as you go along, describing every inconsequential ("ditzel") and benign finding. If you do not have enough information to make up your mind, then do whatever you need to do to get the information. On clinically occult lesions, the radiologist interpreting the mammogram should provide guidance and a final recommendation.

Read your reports. Do they make sense? Are they logical, or do you jump from one finding to the next or from one breast to the other? Make every effort to issue reports that are helpful to the clinician. Eliminate excessive verbiage that is often confusing and can

Work hard at making your mammography reports concise, accurate, and directive. After complete imaging workups, make up your mind about the significance of any findings.

be misleading. Be precise; instead of saying a mass is small or large, give a measurement. The description of the findings belongs in the body of the report, and the impression should be your decision with a recommendation that is supported and justified by the findings of your workup. The impression should not be a repetition of the findings.

In organizing your mammography reports, provide the information listed in Box 12.1 (1–3).

The "probably benign" category is used in the diagnostic setting. We do not use this category on screening studies because characterization of the lesion is required to justify this designation (4–9). Masses that appear well circumscribed on screening studies may have small spiculations and irregular margins on spot compression and spot compression magnification views. Ultrasound is undertaken because if the mass is a simple cyst, short-interval follow-up is not appropriate. Calcifications that appear benign on screening studies may have pleomorphic features on magnification views, and some that appear linear and of concern are identified as benign with additional evaluation. Finally, some of the lesions are characterized as benign after additional images or ultrasound, and short-interval follow-up is not indicated.

This category should not be used to circumvent complete mammographic workups or decision making. It is probably a designation that is only appropriate in women with no prior studies. If the lesion is present on prior studies with no interval change or a decrease in size, a short-interval follow-up adds no additional information. If the lesion has increased in size compared with prior studies and is solid on ultrasound, a biopsy is indicated (not short-interval follow-up).

Usually, short-interval follow-up refers to one extra study of the affected breast 6 months after the initial study. Rarely, when considering an inflammatory, postsurgical, or traumatic etiology for a finding, is anthing less than 6 months appropriate. The probably benign lesions and the data in support of follow-up are defined for mammographic findings (not ultrasound findings) and include localized or multiple findings (4–9). Included among the localized findings are nonpalpable, noncalcified, solid, round or oval, predominantly well-circumscribed masses, irrespective of the size of the mass or age of the patient; nonpalpable, focal asymmetry with concave margins and interspersed fat; an asymptomatic, single, dilated duct; and a cluster of small, round or oval calcifications. Included among the multiple findings are multiple (three or more) similar findings, distributed randomly and often bilaterally: circumscribed masses and round or oval, small calcifications in tight clusters (or scattered individually throughout the breast).

Box 12.1: Mammography Report Outline

Type of study (e.g., screening, diagnostic, ultrasound)
Reason for study
Comparison studies
Tissue type
Description of findings with pertinent negatives when appropriate
Location of lesion
Impression
Recommendation
Assessment category (required under the Mammography Quality Standards Act for all mammographic studies)
  Category 1: negative
  Category 2: benign findings; negative
  Category 3: probably benign finding; short interval follow-up is recommended
  Category 4: suspicious abnormality, biopsy should be considered
  Category 5: highly suggestive of malignancy; appropriate action should be taken
  Category 0: incomplete, need additional imaging evaluation (or prior studies for comparison)

The likelihood of malignancy for probably benign lesions as reported by Sickles (4–8) is as follows:

- 1.4% for solid circumscribed mass
- 0.6% for focal, asymmetric density
- 0.4% for localized microcalcifications
- 0.3% for multiple solid, circumscribed masses
- 0.2% for generalized microcalcifications

After appropriate workup, the findings and low likelihood of malignancy are discussed with the patient. Although a recommendation for short-interval follow-up is made, options of imaging guided and excisional biopsies are also presented to the patient. A biopsy may be undertaken if the patient is particularly anxious, unlikely to return for follow-up, or pregnant or planning a pregnancy.

PATIENT NOTIFICATION LETTERS

As regulated by the Mammography Quality Standards Act (MQSA), the results of mammographic studies and appropriate recommendations must be communicated directly to patients in writing using lay language. Forms with check-off boxes can be used, and if the studies are interpreted while the patient is still in your department, the notification can be given directly to the patient. If screening studies are batch interpreted, the letters have to be mailed within 30 days of the study.

MEDICAL AUDIT

One of the main purposes of the medical audit is to evaluate the accuracy of mammography and mammographic interpretation (10–13). As discussed in Chapter 1, the goal of mammography is the detection of early, potentially curable breast cancer, ideally lesions smaller than 1 cm. The medical audit aims to determine whether this goal is being accomplished and how much is being done to accomplish it (e.g., recalls, biopsies, 6-month follow-up). It is also an excellent teaching and learning tool. With review and feedback from our own follow-up exams and biopsies, we can improve; hence, the numbers should not be viewed statically but over a period of time.

For the medical audit, raw data that need to be tracked and collected for the medical audit are listed in Box 12.2, and derived data are listed in Table 12.1 (10–13). Please note

In addition to being an excellent learning tool, the medical audit provides invaluable information about the success of your mammography program and feedback for the interpreting radiologists.

Box 12.2: Raw Data Needed for Medical Audit

Patient demographics
- Age
- Personal breast cancer history
- Hormone replacement therapy
- High-risk lesion on a previous biopsy (atypical ductal hyperplasia, lobular neoplasia)

Audit periods

Number of screening studies (asymptomatic women)

Number of diagnostic studies (abnormal screening mammogram and symptomatic women)

Number of first-time screens and number of repeat mammograms

Number of women recalled for additional studies (assessment category 0)

Number of women with biopsy recommendations (assessment categories 4 and 5)

Number of short interval follow-up recommendations (assessment category 3)

Number of benign and malignant biopsies tracking needle biopsy separate from fine-needle aspiration

Pathology tumor staging
- Tumor size, histologic type, and grade
- Nodal status

Table 12.1: Derived Data for Medical Audit

True positive (TP)	Breast cancer diagnosed within 1 year after a biopsy recommendation for an abnormal mammogram
True negative (TN)	No known breast cancer diagnosis within 1 year of a normal mammogram
False negative (FN)	Breast cancer diagnosed within 1 year of a normal mammogram
False positive (FP)	1. No breast cancer diagnosis within 1 year of an abnormal screening (categories 0, 4, and 5) 2. No breast cancer diagnosis within 1 year of an abnormal mammogram 3. Biopsy with benign findings within 1 year of a biopsy recommendation for an abnormal mammogram (categories 4 and 5)
Sensitivity	Probability of detecting cancer when cancer is present TP/(TP + FN)
Specificity	Probability of a normal mammogram when no cancer is present TN/(FP + TN); varies depending on FP definition used
Positive predictive value (PPV)	1. PPV of abnormal findings at screening: percentage of screening studies with abnormal findings that result in breast cancer diagnosis TP/(TP + FP1) 2. PPV of biopsy recommendations: percentage of patients with a biopsy recommendation with breast cancer diagnosis TP/(TP + FP2) 3. PPV of biopsies done: percentage of all known biopsies done that resulted in breast cancer diagnosis TP/(TP + FP3)
Cancer detection rate	Number of cancers detected per 1000 patients examined with mammography
Minimal breast cancers	Invasive tumor 1 cm or smaller or ductal carcinoma *in situ*
Interval breast cancers	Breast cancers that become clinically apparent after a negative mammogram but before next screening mammogram is due

Table 12.2: Desired Goals

Sensitivity	>85%
Specificity	>90%
Positive predictive value (PPV)	PPV1 = 5%–10%; PPV2 = 25%–40%
Tumor size	>50% stage 0 or 1 (screen detected) >30% are minimal (screen detected)
Node-positive breast cancers	<25% of screen detected cancers should be lymph node positive
Cancer detection rate	6–10/1000 among first screens (prevalent) 2–4/1000 among repeat screeners (incident)
Recall rate	<10%, ideally individual improves with experience

that there is more than one definition for several of the items evaluated, so be precise when discussing these issues. Desirable goals are detailed in Table 12.2 (10–13).

REFERENCES

1. American College of Radiology (ACR). *Breast imaging reporting and data system (BI-RADS(™)*, 3rd ed. Reston, VA: American College of Radiology; 1998.
2. D'Orsi CJ. Use of the American College of Radiology breast imaging and data system. *RSNA Categorical Course in Breast Imaging Syllabus.* RSNA, Chicago, 1995:77–80.

3. D'Orsi CJ, Kopans DB. Mammographic feature analysis. *Semin Roentgenol* 1993;28:204–230.

4. Sickles EA. Probably benign breast lesions: when should follow-up be recommended and what is the optimal follow-up protocol? *Radiology* 1999;213:11–14.

5. Sickles EA. Management of probably benign breast lesions. *Radiol Clin North Am* 1995;33: 1123–1130.

6. Sickles EA. Management of probably benign lesions. *RSNA Categorical Course in Breast Imaging Syllabus.* RSNA, Chicago, 1995:133–138.

7. Sickles EA. Nonpalpable, circumscribed, noncalcified solid breast masses: likelihood of malignancy based on lesion size and age of patient. *Radiology* 1994;192:439–442.

8. Sickles EA. Periodic mammographic follow-up of probably benign lesions: results in 3,184 consecutive cases. *Radiology* 1991;179:463–468.

9. Varas X, Leborgne F, Leborgne JH. Nonpalpable, probably benign lesions: role of follow-up mammography. *Radiology* 1992;184:409–414.

10. Sickles EA. Quality assurance: how to audit your own mammography practice. *Radiol Clin North Am* 1992;30:265–275.

11. Linver MN, Osuch JR, Brenner RJ, et al. The mammography audit: a primer for the Mammography Quality Standards Act (MQSA). *AJR Am J Roentgenol* 1995;165:19–25.

12. Linver MN. Plaudits for audits: the whys, wherefores and therefores. *Breast Imaging Categorical Course Syllabus.* New Orleans: American Roentgen Ray Society (99th annual meeting), May 9–14, 1999.

13. Sickles EA. Auditing your practice. *RSNA Syllabus Categorical Course in Breast Imaging.* RSNA, Chicago, 1995:81–91.

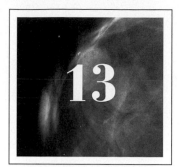

EMERGING TECHNOLOGIES

- Digital Mammography
- Computer-aided Detection
- Scintimammography
- Positron Emission Tomography
- Magnetic Resonance Imaging
- Ductal Lavage

This chapter is a brief introduction to some of the significant emerging technologies in breast imaging. Listed under each technology are some basic definitions, strengths and weaknesses, data, tips, and guidelines regarding their use.

DIGITAL MAMMOGRAPHY

- Image is acquired as an electronic signal that can be displayed on a monitor (soft copy display) or printed on film (hard copy display) (1–3).
- Different technologies are being evaluated for the acquisition of digital images, including scintillators with an array of charge-coupled devices (CCDs) and fiberoptic tapers, slot scanners with CCDs, photostimulable phosphor plates, and flat-panel amorphous silicone plates with scintillators (1–3).
- Status of workstation technology is not optimal; difficulties include resolution of monitors, how to compare current digital images to prior film-screen images, how to compare one side to the other and one projection to another, and length of time required to access studies (1–3).
- Most digital systems offer 5 line pairs per millimeter (lp/mm) of resolution (one digital system offers 12.5 lp/mm resolution) compared with 10 to 15 lp/mm that is typical with conventional mammography units. Significance of these resolution differences is not yet clear (1–3).
- Advantages of digital mammography include elimination of artifacts, noise, and variability related to film processing; postexposure processing of images that allows optimization of brightness and contrast; elimination of film and film storage costs; increased efficiency of technologist (no time spent developing films, reduced number of retakes); telemammography; easier application of computer-aided detection (CAD) and diagnosis; and application of new concepts such as tomosynthesis to eliminate superimposition of dense tissue (1–3).
- Disadvantages include availability of only one size of the image receptor, prohibitive costs of units given low reimbursement rates for mammography (mammography is already considered a "lost leader" in radiology); and suboptimal workstation technology. Although not yet clear, lower resolution of digital units may also be a disadvantage (1–3).

■ Because the mammographic images are large, image storage can be an issue, particularly if the facility is not working in a PACs environment.

COMPUTER-AIDED DETECTION

■ Computer is used to detect calcifications and masses. Computers are not subject to fatigue or distraction; however, the systems operate with high false-positive result rates as not to miss significant findings (2).
■ If using conventional film-screen mammography images, they need to be digitized.
■ Software programs have been developed that are good at detecting calcifications; detection of masses and distortion is more troublesome.

SCINTIMAMMOGRAPHY

■ Technetium-99m sestamibi (4)
Delivery depends on blood flow to tumor.
Tracer is taken up by mitochondria.
Many malignant lesions have increased blood flow and mitochondria.
For planar technique, positioning of patient is important. Early and delayed images are obtained to characterize lesions. Malignant lesions tend to have rapid uptake and washout, in contrast to benign lesions with delayed uptake and washout. There is a high degree of overlap in findings; however, a negative study is helpful.
   For single photon emission computed tomography (SPECT), lesion detectability is improved compared with planar images; acquisition and reconstruction parameters need to be monitored carefully.
   Not intended for use as a screening study.
   Size of lesions is important; study does not reliably identify lesions smaller than 1.2 cm.
   Study has limited use in small breasts and lesions that are close to the chest wall.
■ Thallium-201

POSITRON EMISSION TOMOGRAPHY

■ Study uses fluoro-2-deoxy-D-glucose; uptake of glucose level can be measured to quantitate metabolic activity of tumor.
■ Study is used for staging, restaging, and monitoring effect of chemotherapy on tumor; whole-body imaging enables assessment of axillary lymph nodes and presence of distant metastases.
■ Study has higher resolution and sensitivity than planar and SPECT scintimammography.

MAGNETIC RESONANCE IMAGING

■ Use of magnetic resonance imaging (MRI) in breast imaging continues to evolve.
■ There is no standardized protocol for breast MRI; in the United States, most breast MRI is being done with a high field strength, dedicated breast coil, high-resolution T2-weighted images, fast inversion recovery sequences with fat suppression, and dynamic, sequential imaging after contrast administration.
■ To decrease normal breast parenchymal enhancement secondary to estrogen effect, consider scanning premenopausal women in the second week of the menstrual cycle; in postmenopausal women, consider stopping hormone replacement therapy for 3 weeks

before scanning (unfortunately, neither of these is necessarily practical given tight MRI schedules). This decreases normal breast parenchymal enhancement that may obscure lesions. Ideally, both breasts should be imaged simultaneously—hormonal effects would be easier to establish.

■ Centers should have MRI biopsy capabilities available.

■ Rapid uptake and washout are seen with malignant lesions related to neovascularity and shunting occurring in tumors, compared with slow and continued uptake with no plateau or washout for breast parenchyma (5) (Figures 13.1 through 13.3).

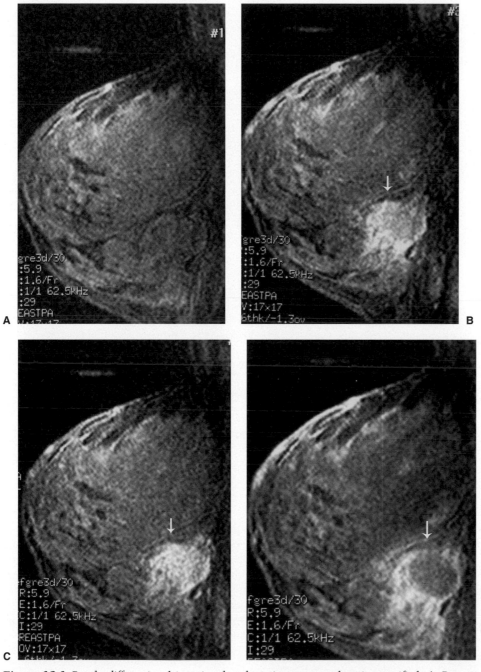

Figure 13.1 *Poorly differentiated invasive ductal carcinoma, not otherwise specified. A.* Precontrast image in a 42-year-old patient. *B.* Immediately after administration of contrast. *C.* Ninety seconds after contrast administration. *D.* Ten minutes after contrast administration. Lesion is seen with rapid uptake and washout of contrast and irregular margins. No additional lesions are detected.

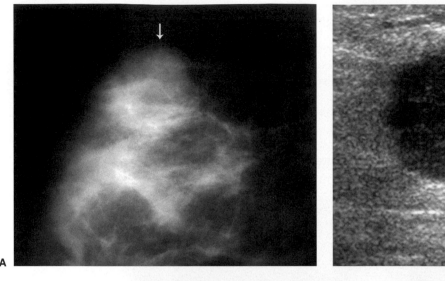

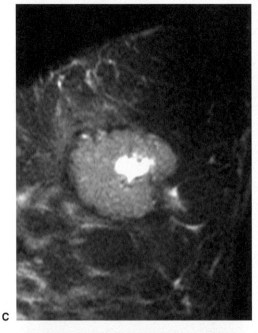

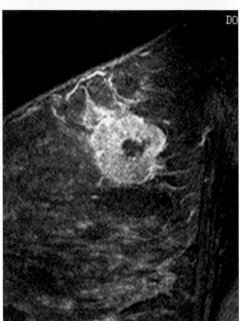

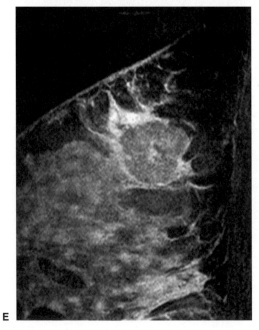

Figure **13.2** *Poorly differentiated invasive ductal carcinoma, not otherwise specified. A.* Round mass (*arrow*) in a 29-year-old patient. *B.* Round mass with irregular margins, heterogeneous echotexture (central area almost anechoic), and posterior acoustic enhancement. *C.* Precontrast magnetic resonance image shows lobular margin and high signal intensity corresponding to nearly anechoic area seen on ultrasound. *D.* Immediately after contrast administration, rapid enhancement of lesion is seen. *E.* Ten minutes after contrast administration, much of the contrast has washed out of the lesion; surrounding breast tissue is continuing to enhance. No additional lesions are detected. Neoadjuvant therapy is used.

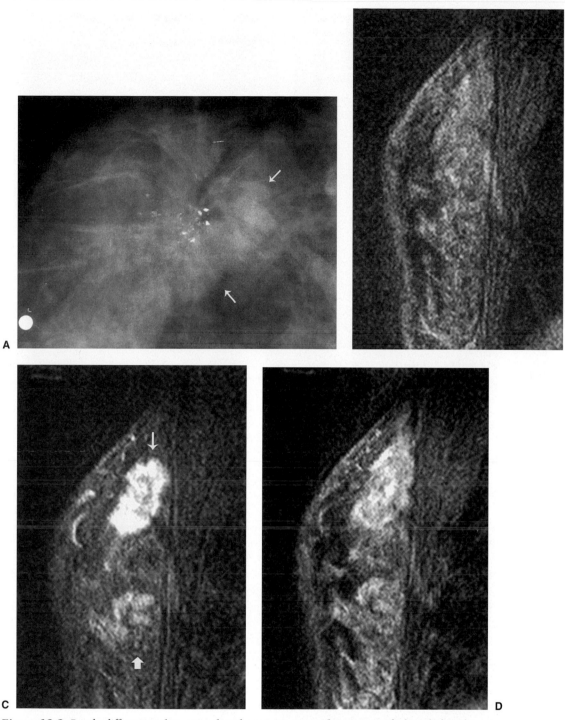

Figure 13.3 *Poorly differentiated invasive ductal carcinoma, not otherwise specified, with ductal carcinoma* in situ, *high nuclear grade.* A. Double spot compression magnification view demonstrates mass (*arrows*) with associated pleomorphic calcifications corresponding to palpable area in a 34-year-old patient. B. Precontrast image. C. Immediately after contrast administration, there is rapid enhancement of the mass corresponding to the area of clinical concern (*thin arrow*), and a second, unsuspected lesion (*thick arrow*) is detected. D. Ten minutes after contrast administration, contrast is washing out of lesions and accumulating in surrounding tissue.

(continued on next page)

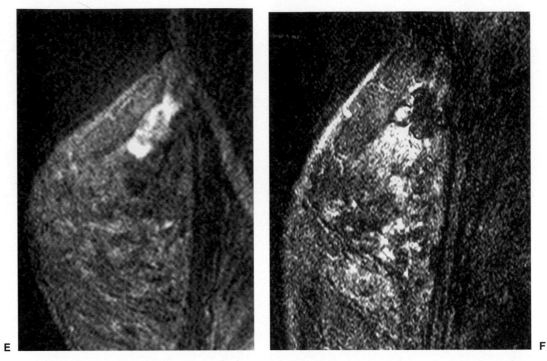

Figure 13.3 (continued) E. Follow-up study after two courses of neoadjuvant chemotherapy. Image is taken immediately after contrast administration. One lesion is now seen with rapid contrast uptake, and the mass has decreased in size. *F.* Follow-up study after four courses of neoadjuvant chemotherapy. Image taken immediately after contrast administration demonstrates nearly complete resolution of lesion. At the time of lumpectomy, residual tumor was identified at this site; however, no tumor was identified at second site seen on initial study.

- Potential false-positive results: cellular fibroadenomas and intramammary lymph nodes may overlap in contrast uptake with invasive lesions; hyalinized fibroadenomas have little or no enhancement.
- Potential false-negative results: invasive lobular carcinoma and ductal carcinoma *in situ* have unpredictable patterns of enhancement.
- MRI is used as an adjunctive test and is not intended to replace mammography and ultrasound. Indications include the following:

  Detection of breast primary in patients presenting with metastatic disease to the axilla and negative mammogram and ultrasound (6)

  Presurgical evaluation in women with breast cancer to define the extent of the disease, specifically to determine whether there is multifocal or multicentric disease (Figures 13.1 and 13.2)

  Assessment of response to neoadjuvant chemotherapy (Figure 13.3) (7)

  Evaluation of patients for local recurrence after conservative treatment

  Evaluation of implant integrity (does not require contrast administration)

  Emerging applications: screening of high-risk women with dense tissue mammographically and evaluation of women with nipple discharge (8).

DUCTAL LAVAGE

- Ductal lavage is a method of obtaining ductal cell samples for cytologic evaluation.
- Topical anesthesia is used on nipple surface.
- Discharge is either expressed or suctioned out to identify ductal openings with discharge.

- Thin catheters are used to cannulate the ducts with discharge; saline with lidocaine is injected into the cannulated ducts and then flushed out. The fluid obtained in this manner is evaluated cytologically.
- If atypical cells are identified, patient can consider increased number of evaluations (clinical, mammogram, and repeat lavage), use of tamoxifen as chemopreventive agent, or prophylactic mastectomy.
- No long-term data are available to evaluate effectiveness or significance of atypical cells obtained in this manner.
- Study may have associated false-negative and false-positive results, although there are no data addressing this possibility.
- Unfortunately, in some communities, this study is being marketed directly to patients, yet there is inadequate research to establish validity of procedure, findings, and proposed treatment approaches. Although it may prove to be beneficial, the appropriate role (if any) and application of this procedure have yet to be established.

REFERENCES

1. Feig SA, Yaffee MJ. Current status of digital mammography. *Semin Ultrasound CT MRI* 1996;17: 424–443.
2. Feig SA, Yaffee MJ. Digital mammography, computer aided diagnosis and telemammography. *Radiol Clin North Am* 1995;33:1205–1230.
3. Pisano ED, Yaffe MJ, Hemminger BGM, et al. Current status of full-field digital mammography. *Acad Radiol* 2000;7:266–280.
4. Khalkhali I, Mena I, Diggles L. Review of imaging techniques for a diagnosis of breast cancer: a new role of prone scintimammography using Tc-99m SestaMiBi for breast imaging. *Eur J Nucl Med* 1994;21:357–362.
5. Liberman L, Morris EA, Lee MJY, et al. Breast lesions detected on MR imaging: features and positive predictive value. *AJR Am J Roentgenol* 2002;179:171–178.
6. Orel SG, Weinstein SP, Schnall MD, et al. Breast MR imaging in patients with axillary node metastases and unknown primary malignancy. *Radiology* 1999;212:543–549.
7. Partridge SC, Gibbs JE, Lu Y, et al. Accuracy of MR imaging for revealing residual breast cancer in patients who have undergone neoadjuvant chemotherapy. *AJR Am J Roentgenol* 2002;179: 1193–1199.
8. Orel SG, Dougherty CS, Reynolds C, et al. MR imaging in patients with nipple discharge: initial experience. *Radiology* 2000;216:248–254.

Subject Index

Note: Numbers followed by *f* indicate figures; those followed by *t* indicate tables; and those by *b* for boxes.